Sustainable Development Goals Series

The **Sustainable Development Goals Series** is Springer Nature's inaugural cross-imprint book series that addresses and supports the United Nations' seventeen Sustainable Development Goals. The series fosters comprehensive research focused on these global targets and endeavours to address some of society's greatest grand challenges. The SDGs are inherently multidisciplinary, and they bring people working across different fields together and working towards a common goal. In this spirit, the Sustainable Development Goals series is the first at Springer Nature to publish books under both the Springer and Palgrave Macmillan imprints, bringing the strengths of our imprints together.

The Sustainable Development Goals Series is organized into eighteen subseries: one subseries based around each of the seventeen respective Sustainable Development Goals, and an eighteenth subseries, "Connecting the Goals," which serves as a home for volumes addressing multiple goals or studying the SDGs as a whole. Each subseries is guided by an expert Subseries Advisor with years or decades of experience studying and addressing core components of their respective Goal.

The SDG Series has a remit as broad as the SDGs themselves, and contributions are welcome from scientists, academics, policymakers, and researchers working in fields related to any of the seventeen goals. If you are interested in contributing a monograph or curated volume to the series, please contact the Publishers: Zachary Romano [Springer; zachary.romano@springer.com] and Rachael Ballard [Palgrave Macmillan; rachael.ballard@palgrave.com].

Aparajita Chattopadhyay ·
Akancha Singh · Samriddhi S. Gupte

Undernutrition in India

Causes, Consequences and Policy Measures

Springer

Aparajita Chattopadhyay
International Institute
for Population Sciences
Mumbai, Maharashtra, India

Akancha Singh
International Institute
for Population Sciences
Mumbai, Maharashtra, India

Samriddhi S. Gupte
International Institute
for Population Sciences
Mumbai, Maharashtra, India

ISSN 2523-3084 ISSN 2523-3092 (electronic)
Sustainable Development Goals Series
ISBN 978-981-19-8181-4 ISBN 978-981-19-8182-1 (eBook)
https://doi.org/10.1007/978-981-19-8182-1

This Springer imprint is published by the registered company Springer Nature Singapore Pte Ltd.
The registered company address is: 152 Beach Road, #21-01/04 Gateway East, Singapore 189721, Singapore

Foreword

Leading global experts have observed that a 1 cm increase in human height often led to a 4% increase in wages for men and a 6% for women. With 38.4% of children stunted and an estimated 447 million people suffering from anaemia, (which works out to India contributing almost one-quarter to the global burden of this disease) undernutrition is one of the major obstacles that prevent India from realizing its full economic potential.

Half a century back, a pediatrician practicing in one of the less affluent areas of a metropolitan area had informed me during an informal conversation that had the undergraduate curriculum of medicine includes a more in-depth coverage of nutrition, the state of health of the citizens of this country would have seen better days.

It took us a very long time to realize that nutrition plays a key role in the physical as well as economic well-being of a nation. Even now, globally, its importance is perhaps not as well appreciated, as it ought to have been. The fact that the key global health targets and systematic monitoring exclude diet, despite its health and environmental impacts, is a testament to this claim.

Nationwide surveys such as the National Family Health Survey and Comprehensive National Nutrition Survey do help us form an idea on the state of nutrition in the country, but they leave quite a few dots unconnected and many dimensions of undernutrition unexplained.

In *Undernutrition in India: Causes, Consequences, and Policy Measures*, Prof. Aparajita Chattopadhyay, Ms. Akancha Singh, and Ms. Samriddhi S. Gupte connect these dots admirably well. In this enlightening volume of moderate size, they bring together the many burdens of undernutrition in India. These include issues like the co-existence of India's around 62 million stunted children (2016 estimates) with adults and elderly who are suffering from both under and over-nutrition. There is a special focus on the status of undernutrition in the tribal population that throws light on a somewhat neglected issue. The authors also challenge the rather simplistic notion of linking undernutrition to poverty alone by highlighting the paradox of a state where there are high levels of children's undernutrition despite considerable economic development.

The authors address a whole range of questions that the researchers, policymakers, and lay readers have been asking for a long time; intriguing questions like—does economic growth translate into nutritional betterment? Do the states with higher GDP also do well in nutrition? What about the socio-economic inequality in nutrition? Do the tribes behave similarly in undernourishment? How far is undernutrition among women explained by diet and contraception? Why does Gujarat, a rich Indian state, have a high level of child undernutrition? Does women's empowerment lead to better nutrition? Does diet pattern, especially consumption of non-vegetarian food, help in addressing poor nutrition? What about elderly undernutrition? How far does food security play a role in addressing nutritional issues? Is there any comprehensive framework for addressing undernutrition?

The book explores the status of food and nutrition security in India based on several data and reports released at national and international levels along with visible gaps and suggests the kind of transformative action the country now needs to bridge these chasms.

The book could not have come at a more appropriate time. We are passing through a terribly challenging phase for the most vulnerable groups and people living in fragile states. There is a looming global nutrition crisis consequent upon the COVID-19 pandemic. We urgently need to address the underlying inequities and systems that lead to poor diet and malnutrition.

This book would be of immense help in understanding the many facets of undernutrition and in shaping up real clear policies and implementation practices that would, in the long run, help the nation realize all its potentials.

Dilip Ghosh IAS (Retd.)
Former Secretary
Department of Health
and Family Welfare
Government of West Bengal
Kolkata, India

Acknowledgments

The book deals with a multitude of questions pertaining to nutrition. The themes covered in the book are not only varied but also germane to the current development scenario in India. Through this book, we tried to address the issues surrounding nutrition with the aim of providing clues to handling nutritional challenges more effectively with the connotation of comprehensive development.

Having an idea and converting it into a book is as hard as it sounds. Our experience on formulating and completing this work is internally challenging, especially during the difficult time of COVID-19. We especially want to thank the individuals that helped make this happen.

We are grateful to Springer for extending us this wonderful opportunity for formulating a book on nutrition. It is our privilege to have this book as a part of their SDG series. We would like to thank the team of anonymous reviewers for their insightful comments. Further, we extend our gratitude to the wonderful team at Springer, including Ms. Satvinder Kaur, Senior Editor, and Mr. Gowrishankar Ayyasamy, Project Coordinator, for guiding us through the publication process. Special appreciation to Ms. Jayanthi Narayanaswamy of Springer Nature.

We extend our humble gratitude to Mr. Dilip Ghosh (IAS, Retd.) for his perfect Foreword message that enhanced the value of the work.

We are indebted to the International Institute for Population Sciences, Mumbai, for moulding us as researchers, instilling our interests in nutrition as an area of research, and providing access to large-scale datasets and academic references while writing the book chapters.

Last but not the least, we are eternally indebted to our families, and well-wishers for their constant support and encouragement in our academic endeavours.

Writing a book on nutrition, a topic that is already so much discussed in the Indian context is harder than we thought. However, this book perhaps could be more rewarding than we could have ever imagined, as the book is useful to a range of readers—starting from students, researchers to decision-makers as well.

Thank you, Readers. You are our greatest inspiration.

Book Summary

Undernutrition in India: Causes, Consequences, and Policy Measures

India is beset with multitudinous issues pertaining to undernutrition. These issues percolate through all sections of society. On one hand, India houses around 62 million stunted children (2016 estimates) which accounts for nearly 40% of the world's stunted children, while, on the other, both under and over-nutrition are serious issues among the adults and elderly in India. Nearly 31% of the elderly residing in rural areas are suffering from undernutrition a while higher prevalence of overnutrition is found among elderly residing in urban areas. Another subsection of the society that is often neglected in the discourse regarding undernutrition is the tribal population. While one may argue that poverty is the genesis of undernutrition, the paradox of the state of Gujarat proves otherwise. Gujarat, an Indian state displays a peculiar case of economic development with high levels of children's undernutrition. It accentuates the fact that while poverty alleviation is essential, it is not sufficient to solve the problem of undernutrition. Undernutrition has been a topic of concern since the advent of the Millennium Development Goals, which has further solidified with Sustainable Development Goals (SDGs). It becomes imperative to tackle the problem of undernutrition in order to achieve SGD 2 (Zero Hunger).

The book, *Undernutrition in India: Causes, Consequences, and Policy Measures*, encompasses all of these dimensions of undernutrition and tries to tie the loose ends. It covers multiple facets of undernutrition in India across various groups. The book further throws light on measures taken in order to curb the widespread problem of undernutrition in India and other countries. It not only speaks about the policies or state-specific interventions in India but also addresses the gaps in the existing policy framework and enlightens the way forward towards more comprehensive interventions. The authors use data from India's National Family Health Survey for analysis and estimation. In addition to it, data from Wave I of the Longitudinal Ageing Study in India has also been used to estimate elderly nutrition.

The book attempts to answer the following questions: How far has the economic advancement translated to nutritional betterment—Do the states with higher GDP also do well in nutrition? What about the socio-economic inequality in nutrition? Do the tribes behave similarly in undernourishment? How far is undernutrition among women explained by diet and contraception? Why is Gujarat, a rich state in India, criticized for its high level of child undernutrition? Does women's empowerment lead to better nutrition? Does diet pattern, especially consumption of non-vegetarian items, helps in addressing poor nutrition? What about elderly undernutrition? How far does food security play a role in addressing nutritional issues? Is there any comprehensive framework for addressing undernutrition? More questions are being dealt with in the chapters of the book that could be of good use for the researchers and policymakers.

Chapter 1 of the book positions India and its states on a global map concerning its nutritional outcome. The chapter talks about the global scenario pertaining to undernutrition and further throws light on where India stands along with its states. It is worth to note that the disparity within Indian states in terms of nutritional outcome is such that it would not be too farfetched to say that there exist nations within one nation. The chapter sets the pace for further discussion on the aforementioned dimensions while highlighting the compelling need for deliberation on these issues.

The book further attempts to uncover linkages, if any, of mother's economic independence in terms of asset ownership with her child's nutritional outcome. Existing literature does give a fair idea about women's diminished economic status to be a potential predictor of children's undernutrition. It becomes crucial to understand this dynamic relation in the Indian context given that India holds 104th rank out of 144 in global gender index. Chapter 2 of the book looks at this association and uncovers that, while mother's asset ownership does have a positive impact on child's nutritional outcome, it occurs at different parts of distribution, i.e. children who are already better-nourished benefit more from their mother's asset ownership.

To approach the topic of undernutrition from different directions, the book goes further to understand the nutritional status of the elderly in India. With the global elderly population gradually moving to cross the 10% mark and expected to escalate to 16% by 2050, it becomes imperative to understand those policy interventions should not only be focused on maternal and child nutrition but also accommodate the needs of the growing population of elderly and the hurdles faced by them. The problem of nutrition takes a new shape with the simultaneous existence of both over and undernutrition among the elderly. Hence, it becomes crucial to start early interventions and not let the problem aggravate. Chapter 3 in the book provides information with an overview of essential nutritional facets associated with the changes that occur with aging.

While one may point towards concerns around elderly nutrition being relatively new and, hence, lesser talked about, it is important to note that poor rural sections such as tribes are also often neglected on nutrition. Anaemia, which is an important indicator of nutrition among women, is not well explored using large-scale data. Hence, the next two chapters of the book (Chaps. 4 and 5) delve into the realms of tribal nutrition, specifically, anaemia among women and children. Tribes, despite efforts by the government, remain geographically isolated, economically marginalized, and far from the mainstream. It becomes important to understand the prevalence and predictors of anaemia among tribes. Association of use of modern contraceptives with anaemia among women is also brought out quite evidently here.

One of the predictors of anaemia that does come up often is wealth index. Existing literature talks about poverty alleviation being a key factor to eradicate undernutrition. However, the paradoxical relationship that economic development has with children's nutritional indicators in the state of Gujarat proves that economic growth is essential but not always sufficient for improved nutritional outcomes. Chapter 6 of the book brings this paradox under the lens. One of the crucial findings of the chapter suggests that, despite years of rapid advancements made in all sectors, it is still the poor section of the society that shoulders the disproportionate burden of undernutrition in Gujarat. Socio-economic inequality remains an important contributor to determining the nutritional status of children.

The final two chapters of the book (Chaps. 7 and 8) bind the book and tie all the loose ends together. They talk about the book's SDG relevance, particularly in the context of Sustainable Development Goal 2, Zero Hunger. The chapters try to understand the status of food and nutrition security in India based on data and reports released at national and international levels along with visible gaps, and the need of the hour to engage in transformative action to overcome these chasms. More, it outlines areas that are lacking policy attention and thereby, inhibiting India's journey towards achieving the SDG targets. The chapter, Policy Perspectives, also highlights the actionable interventions and a simplified framework to handle undernutrition.

The book would be useful to those dealing with nutrition and health. As it has multidisciplinary approach, a number of professionals working as economists, sociologists, geographers, anthropologists, demographers, nutritionist, medical professionals, social workers, healthcare providers, public health and policy analysts, decision-makers, and program managers may find the book interesting.

Contents

About the Authors

Aparajita Chattopadhyay is currently associated with the International Institute for Population Sciences (IIPS) as a professor, Department of Population and Development where she has invested significant time in academic research and postgraduate teaching for two decades. An area expert in geography and demography, Chattopadhyay has also served at the Banaras Hindu University as a faculty with the Department of Geography for a brief period. Her teaching and research career include a portfolio of wide-ranging research projects and peer-reviewed academic publications. She has been a recipient of awards and grants for academic achievements/research from reputed universities and organizations including the likes of the Presidency College Calcutta, University of Calcutta, International Institute for Population Sciences, Indian Association for the Study of Population, University of Karachi, RAND corporation, Columbia University, USA, to highlight a few. She handled different research projects funded by the Government of India, UNICEF, etc., like Longitudinal Aging Study in India (LASI), Comprehensive Nutrition Survey in Maharashtra and Gujarat, SWABHIMAAN base line study, and Population, Environment and Settlement Project (Pop-Envis). Springer Nature published two of her books in 2020. Her area of research interests includes environment, development, gender issues, aging, nutrition, and health.

Akancha Singh is a Ph.D. scholar at the International Institute for Population Sciences (IIPS). Having done her graduation in economics from the Banaras Hindu University, she has good understanding in economic theories and statistical analyses. She has received awards and medals for her academic performance from esteemed institutions like the Banaras Hindu University and the International Institute for Population Sciences. Her area of interest is adolescent and child nutrition, gender studies, aging, and public health. She is currently working on nutritional issues among the elderly in India. She strongly believes in the power of one-to-conversations and aspires to bridge the nutrition-knowledge gap for young women, children and elderly. She is an ardent believer in the efficacy of grass-root level interventions in eradicating inequality and aspires to build efficient community-based network to deal with social and economic challenges.

Samriddhi S. Gupte is an M.Phil. graduate from the International Institute for Population Sciences, Mumbai. She has done her Master's in Economics from the Banaras Hindu University and has a Masters' degree in Population Studies from the International Institute for Population Sciences. She has won accolades for her academic performances. Her areas of interest are gender and development studies, nutrition, and public health. She thoroughly believes that any change starts with self, and she aims to touch the lives of as many people as she can, in a positive manner, through her words and works. She is currently working as a research analyst at Max Institute of Healthcare Management, Indian School of Business (ISB).

List of Figures

List of Tables

1 The Problem of Undernutrition: Positioning India and Its States

Akancha Singh, Samriddhi S. Gupte, and Aparajita Chattopadhyay

Abstract

The nutritional scenario of India is often criticized due to its heavy burden of undernutrition of mothers and children. As per the recently published Global Nutrition Report 2020, India along with 87 other countries would fail to achieve the Global Nutrition Targets, 2025. Besides the burden of undernutrition, India has one of the highest rates of domestic inequalities in malnutrition. Owing to the diversity within states in India, each state is equivalent to a country with its distinct socio-economic and cultural level, food habits, health infrastructures, lifestyle, and state economic level and communication facilities. Thus, this chapter highlights the position of India in world context followed by the position of states in terms of nutritional status, especially in the context of states' economic development.

Keywords

Nutrition · SDGs · South Asia · Food security · Nutrition policy · India

1.1 The Global Picture

A prerequisite for pinpointing and identifying the drivers of unjust and inequitable nutrition outcomes and enables swift and correct action for impact is shared responsibility on global nutritional scenario. Estimates suggest that 1 in 9 people, amounting to a global number of 820 million people, suffer from hunger or some form of nutritional deprivation. It is also astonishing that despite sustained efforts, a consistent increase in these numbers is being observed continually, especially in Latin America, West Asia, and Africa (FAO, 2019). Sheltering more than 50% of stunted children globally, Asia presents an acute global nutrition challenge (Global Nutrition Report, 2020). Some of the major factors causing nearly 113 million people across 53 countries around the world falling prey to acute hunger are economic disturbances, armed conflicts, food insecurity, and climate shocks (Food Security Information Network, 2019). Another interesting trend that has risen in the past decade is the simultaneous rise in the prevalence of overweight and obesity, with more

A. Chattopadhyay et al., *Undernutrition in India*, Sustainable Development Goals Series,
https://doi.org/10.1007/978-981-19-8182-1_1

than 33% of the global population reporting this condition (Ng et al., 2014). Undernutrition is perseverating at alarmingly high levels, with stark intra-country, inter-country, and within population differentials.

The Global Nutrition Report (2020) states that the world is not on course as far as attaining the Global Nutrition Targets by 2025 is concerned. The problem becomes increasingly complex because of countries' experience of dual malnutrition burden and the resultant co-existence of diet and lifestyle-related non-communicable diseases, overweight, and obesity. The report also states that, while the progress made by only 8 out of 194 countries is sufficient to meet four targets, no country in the world is expected to meet all the set targets by 2025 (Table 1.1). Additionally, while nearly one fourth of children aged five years and below are stunted globally, almost every country in the world is experiencing a massive rise in the proportion of the overweight and obese population, with no signs of a fall in the pace of its increase. Advancements made on achieving nutrition targets so far have not just been painfully slow; they have also been inequitable and unjust. Latest research shows that observing global and national trends and patterns camouflages the widespread inequalities persistent within countries and sub-groups of populations, with the worst impact being borne by the marginally neglected and susceptible groups. It is also important to note that there are substantial variations in nutritional outcomes between countries. While underweight is a persistent problem in economically laggard countries, with the prevalence in such countries being ten times higher than that in the richer countries, the richer countries are dealing with an exceptionally high prevalence of overweight/obesity, these rates being up to five-fold as compared to their poorer counterparts.

Further, it is hard to achieve the set reduction in anaemia, when almost 613.2 million (32.8%) women of reproductive age and adolescent girls report being anaemic. It is also worth noting that a higher proportion of pregnant women and adolescent girls are found to be anaemic (40.1%) than their non-pregnant counterparts (32.5%). However, impressive strides have been made towards increasing the prevalence of exclusive

Table 1.1 Progress of South Asian countries in attaining global targets 2025

Countries	Stunting	Wasting	Anaemia (15-49)
Afghanistan	Some Progress	Some Progress	No progress or worsening
Bangladesh	On Course	Some Progress	Some Progress
Bhutan	No data	No data	Some Progress
India	On Course	No progress or worsening	No progress or worsening
Iran	No data	No data	No progress or worsening
Maldives	No data	No data	No progress or worsening
Nepal	Some Progress	Some Progress	Some Progress
Pakistan	Some Progress	Some Progress	No progress or worsening
Sri Lanka	Some Progress	No progress or worsening	No progress or worsening

On Course Some Progress No progress or worsening No data

Source Based on Global Nutrition Report, 2020

breastfeeding, with nearly 42% of infants aged 6 months and below being breastfed exclusively. It is, thus, crucial that expedited enhancements are made to meet the target by 2025 in this context. With nearly 149 million (21.9%) and 49.5 million (7.3%) children aged 5 years and below being affected by stunting and wasting, respectively, the progress made by the global community is hardly sufficient to achieve any of those targets (Global Nutrition Report, 2020).

Lack of proper diets and poor nutrition are among the prominent current societal problems, causing massive challenges from the health, economic, and environmental perspectives. In order to arrive at an equitable solution to the global nutrition crisis, it is imperative to transform our approach tremendously in a couple of ways: focusing on the different facets of food and health. First, it is necessary to eliminate the widespread inequalities that are present in food systems, affecting both primary producers and end-product consumers. Concurrent food systems lack the ability to empower people to make healthy and sustainable choices from the various food options that are available. A balanced and healthy diet is beyond the access and affordability of a vast majority of people. The reasons behind the above dilemma are complicated and multifarious.

The focus of the existent agriculture systems is primarily on a profusion of staple food grains like maize, wheat, and rice, instead of targeting the production of an extensive range of diversified and robust foods, like fruits, nuts, and vegetables. In the meantime, there is an elaborate network of processed foods that are affordable and aggressively marketed; with their sales being historically high in upper income quintile countries and soaring rapidly in upper middle- and lower middle-income countries. Second, it is also equally imperative to tackle the widespread nutrition-based inequalities in health system as well. Nutritional deprivation, in all its forms, is one of the prime causes of morbidity and mortality, and the massive escalation of non-communicable diseases related to diet and unhealthy lifestyles is putting the health systems at an intolerable strain. Additionally, quality nutrition preventive and curative care is still beyond the affordability of the masses. Globally, only about a quarter of the 16.6 million children aged 5 years and below with severe acute undernutrition were included in interventions in 2017, putting forth the dire need to combat this inadmissible burden (Global Nutrition Report, 2020). Although targeted nutrition interventions constitute a small fragment of national health budgets globally, they can go a long way in curtailing healthcare expenditures and offering cost-effective and sustainable solutions.

1.2 The Indian Scenario: Development Versus Welfare

With a Global Hunger Index score of 27.5, India is placed at 101st rank among 116 countries in the recently released Global Hunger Report, 2021 (von Grebmer et al., 2021). While India's overall rating has certainly risen as compared to 2019, India has fared the worst in child wasting rates. Though India's current rank is an improvement over past years, but her performance is still worse than Pakistan (88th rank) and Bangladesh (75th rank). In the recent past, the high prevalence of child undernutrition in South Asia was puzzling for researchers (Ramalingaswami, 1996). This, however, is not the case any more. India's neighbouring countries like Nepal and Bangladesh have registered an impressive decline in the prevalence of child undernutrition in recent years (Cunningham et al., 2017; Nisbett et al., 2017). The impressive performance of Sri Lanka, however, makes it an exception. Cues can also be taken from Bangladesh. This country has made a commendable breakthrough in initiating nutrition-sensitive interventions. In addition, it has interventions targeted towards improving access to clean water, sanitation, immunization coverage, and school enrolment rates and reducing infant and child mortality (Naher et al., 2014). This has led to massive enhancements in child nutrition scenario in Bangladesh. The steep downturn in the under-five mortality rate in Bangladesh from 1990 to 2011 has been accompanied by a staggering decline in infant mortality and neonatal

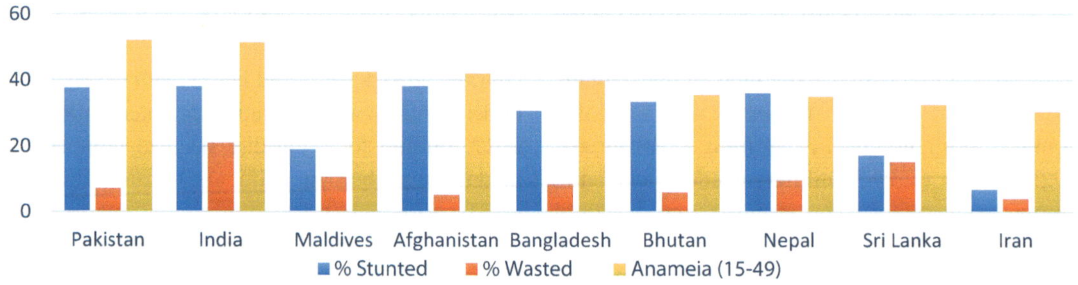

Fig. 1.1 Positioning India, along with other South Asian nations, in key nutrition indicators. *Source* Based on Global Nutrition Report, 2020

mortality rate. Along similar lines, under-five mortality rate has reduced from 151 to 53 in the two decades following the 1990s. The infant mortality rate (IMR) and neonatal mortality rate stand at 43 and 32 per 1000 live births, respectively. The decline in under-five mortality is suggestive of improvements in the immunization scenario to 84% in 2014 (Suri, 2019). The few countries of South Asia that are still laggards include India as well (Fig. 1.1).

Developments in child health are one of the important indicators of advances towards attaining Goal Three of the United Nations' Sustainable Development Goals, that advocates a ubiquitous assurance of a "healthy life and well-being at all ages". Undernutrition places an elevated risk of disease susceptibility on children while also having detrimental impacts on their physical, cognitive, and mental well-being (Black, 1995; Sánchez, 2017). This has severe ramifications on their economic productivity in later life (Strauss & Thomas, 1995) and it increases economic inequality (Pickett & Wilkinson, 2015). Globally, India's performance across standard child nutritional measures has been rather unsatisfactory (Haddad et al., 2015). As far as child nutritional indicators are concerned, recent estimates place India at 114th place among 132 countries, only marginally ahead of Pakistan and Afghanistan (IFPRI, 2016). Data from Indian Demographic and Health Survey (DHS) also second these statistics, registering only marginal improvements in child nutrition indicators from 1992 to 2016. Despite a massive reduction in stunting and underweight prevalence among children aged 5 years and below from 52 to 38% and 53 to 36%, respectively, between 1992 and 2016, the prevalence is still disquietingly high (Khan & Mohanty, 2018). In 2016, there were about 62 million stunted children in India, which accounted for 40% of the global stunting burden (Khan & Mohanty, 2018).

1.2.1 Regional Divergences in Child Nutrition in India: Nations Within a Nation?

About 38% of world's stunted children were housed by India alone in 2011 (UNICEF, 2013), and the number of nutritionally deprived children in India were more than that in all of Africa (Headey, 2013). Current estimates suggest that 149 million children aged 5 years and below are stunted globally, with India making up the lion's share of the above. This makes it an anomaly even among the developing countries (UNICEF, 2013; UNICEF et al., 2018). It is surprising to note that certain regions within India have a higher prevalence of childhood stunting than some of the most socio-economically laggard regions of sub-Saharan Africa (Spears, 2013). While the aggregate level of undernutrition in the country is declining slowly, the economic and social inequities, i.e. income divide, rural–urban inequality, and gender disparity, further compound the magnitude of this problem. An increasing number of researchers and policymakers have recently shown increasing interest in examining socio-economic inequalities in health outcomes (Mohanty and Pathak, 2008; Poel et al., 2008; Wagstaff and Watanbe, 2000; Zere and McIntyre, 2003). Data points towards the presence of extant socio-economic inequalities in health both within countries and between countries, regardless of their position in the development process. Massive regional disparities persist between Indian states, with the proportion of stunted children under 5 in two of the populous states of India, Uttar Pradesh and Bihar, being over 46 and 48%, respectively (Sunny et al., 2018). An inverse relationship has been found between socio-economic status, illness, and death, with the economically deprived population at the highest risk of mortality and morbidity. This highlights the crucial role played by social and economic disparities, more so in a country like India that is grappling with the issue of food and nutrition security since decades.

Table 1.2 sheds light on the following aspects of nutrition scenario in India:

- While states like Mizoram and Kerala are front-runners in child nutrition, the status of under-five nutrition is exceptive in the States/UTs of Bihar, Jharkhand, Uttar Pradesh, and Dadra and Nagar Haveli.
- States that have a high proportion of adults with low BMI are Uttar Pradesh, Madhya Pradesh, Bihar, and Jharkhand; Sikkim is one of the states that are performing better in this arena.
- The proportion of overweight/obese adults is the highest in the UTs of Delhi, Lakshadweep, Andaman and Nicobar Islands, and Puducherry; the states that fare better here are Bihar, Jharkhand, Rajasthan, and Meghalaya.
- The states/UTs that have the highest prevalence of anaemia are Ladakh, Tripura, Jammu and Kashmir, and Jharkhand; Goa, Kerala, Lakshadweep, Manipur, and Mizoram are the states that are performing well in this area.

From the above points, it is evident that there are wide disparities and differences as far as the nutrition profile of Indian States/UTs is concerned. These disparities are also manifested at the micro level, with more and more literature and data suggesting that the situation of poor and deprived population, as far as the consumption of micronutrients, proteins and calories is concerned, is in a worrisome situation in rural areas and slums in cities in the poorer states. Contrarily, an increase is being registered in the prevalence of lifestyle-related non-communicable diseases and excessive eating among the elite population groups in cities as a consequence of the massive escalation in the availability of processed and refined foods and drinks (Allison, 2011).

There are a myriad of reasons that could possibly explain the high prevalence of undernutrition in India (Mishra et al., 1999). The term, "South Asian Enigma", coined by Ramalingaswamy et al. (1997) and accorded the poor nutritional situation in India to low birth weight of babies, lack of women empowerment, and poor water, sanitation, and hygiene practices. The poor and deprived state of females can be traced back to the patriarchal norms in Indian society, which manifests itself in gender-biased distribution of food and healthcare choices in the household (Gragnolati et al., 2005; Smith et al., 2003; World Bank, 1998). In addition to the above, undernutrition is also pervaded by the existing socio-cultural norms of child-feeding practices in India. Informational hurdles result in a lack of awareness and education among women and have affected breastfeeding and other child-care practices, causing undernutrition among children. There is a plethora of evidence to suggest that the disproportionate burden of undernutrition falls on the economically deprived and marginalized sections of the society (Mishra & Retherford, 2000; World Bank, 1998). However, the factors affecting nutritional status and their share in the persistent inequality in undernutrition and the role played by economic status in determining the same have not been fully explored by studies as yet (World Bank, 1998). It is certainly possible that the factors affecting nutritional status may not play an equally important role when dealing with socio-economic inequality in nutritional outcomes

Table 1.2 Statewise nutritional profile of children and adults, India (2019–21)

States/UTs	Children (under 5 years)				Adults (15–49 years)					
					BMI below normal		Overweight/Obesity		Anaemia	
	Stunting (%)	Wasting (%)	Underweight (%)	Anaemia (6–59 months) (%)	Females (%)	Males (%)	Females (%)	Males (%)	Females (%)	Males (%)
Andaman and Nicobar Islands	22.5	16.0	23.7	40.0	9.4	4.0	38.1	45.3	57.5	16.1
Andhra Pradesh	31.2	16.1	29.6	63.2	14.8	16.5	36.3	31.1	58.8	16.2
Arunachal Pradesh	28.0	13.1	15.4	56.6	5.7	4.9	23.9	27.6	40.3	21.4
Assam	35.3	21.7	32.8	68.4	17.6	13.4	15.2	16.2	65.9	36.0
Bihar	42.9	22.9	41.0	69.4	25.6	21.5	15.9	14.7	63.5	29.5
Chandigarh	25.3	8.4	20.6	54.6	13.0	15.1	44.0	34.4	60.3	8.1
Chattisgarh	34.6	18.9	31.3	67.2	23.1	17.4	14.1	14.9	60.8	27.0
Dadra and Nagar Haveli + Daman and Diu	39.4	21.6	38.7	75.8	25.1	18.3	26.8	21.4	62.5	24.6
Goa	25.8	19.1	24.0	53.2	15.1	12.5	36.1	32.6	39.0	12.0
Gujarat	39.0	25.1	39.7	79.7	13.9	20.9	22.6	19.9	65.0	26.6
Haryana	27.5	11.5	21.5	70.4	5.2	14.5	33.1	28.3	60.4	18.9
Himachal Pradesh	30.8	17.4	25.5	55.4	26.2	11.8	30.4	30.6	53.0	18.6
Jammu and Kashmir	26.9	19.0	21.0	72.7	17.2	4.3	29.3	31.6	65.9	36.7
Jharkhand	39.6	22.4	39.4	67.5	10.1	17.1	11.9	15.1	65.3	29.6
Karnataka	35.4	19.5	32.9	65.5	4.4	14.3	30.1	30.9	47.8	19.6
Kerala	23.4	15.8	19.7	39.4	8.0	10.0	38.1	36.4	36.3	17.8
Ladakh	30.5	17.5	20.4	92.5	23.0	2.1	28.3	37.8	92.8	75.6
Lakshadweep	32	17.4	25.8	43.1	20.8	5.5	33.5	41.3	25.8	5.6
Madhya Pradesh	35.7	19.0	33.0	72.7	7.2	20.8	16.6	15.6	54.7	22.4
Maharashtra	35.2	25.6	36.1	68.9	10.8	16.2	23.4	24.7	54.2	21.9
Manipur	23.4	9.9	13.3	42.8	5.3	8.0	34.1	30.3	29.4	6.0

(continued)

Table 1.2 (continued)

States/UTs	Children (under 5 years)				Adults (15–49 years)					
					BMI below normal		Overweight/Obesity		Anaemia	
	Stunting (%)	Wasting (%)	Underweight (%)	Anaemia (6–59 months) (%)	Females (%)	Males (%)	Females (%)	Males (%)	Females (%)	Males (%)
Meghalaya	46.5	12.1	26.6	45.1	11.1	9.0	11.5	13.9	53.8	25.5
Mizoram	28.9	9.8	12.7	46.4	10.0	5.1	24.2	31.9	34.8	15.6
Nagaland	32.7	7.9	26.9	42.7	20.8	7.5	14.4	23.9	28.9	10.0
Delhi	30.9	11.2	21.8	69.2	9.0	9.1	41.3	38.0	49.9	12.6
Odisha	31.0	18.1	34.4	64.2	12.7	15.3	23.0	22.2	64.3	28.5
Puducherry	20.0	12.4	29.7	64.0	19.6	11.1	46.2	43.3	55.1	19.5
Punjab	24	10.6	15.3	71.1	5.8	12.5	40.8	32.2	58.7	22.6
Rajasthan	31.8	16.8	27.6	71.5	12.6	14.0	12.9	15.0	54.4	23.2
Sikkim	22.3	13.7	13.1	56.4	18.8	4.9	34.7	36.3	42.1	18.7
Tamil Nadu	25.0	14.6	22.0	57.4	16.2	12.1	40.4	37.0	53.4	15.2
Telangana	33.1	21.7	31.8	70.0	19.0	16.2	30.1	32.3	57.6	15.3
Tripura	32.3	18.2	25.6	64.3	13.9	12.4	21.5	23.4	67.2	36.9
Uttar Pradesh	39.7	17.3	32.1	66.4	14.8	17.9	21.3	18.5	50.4	21.5
Uttarakhand	27.0	13.2	21.0	58.8	9.4	16.2	29.7	27.1	42.6	15.1
West Bengal	33.8	20.3	32.2	69.0	14.8	15.1	22.7	16.2	71.4	38.9
India	**35.5**	**19.3**	**32.1**	**67.1**	**18.7**	**16.2**	**24.0**	**22.9**	**57.0**	**25.0**

Source NFHS-5 (2019–21)

(Van de Poel et al., 2007; Zere & McIntyre, 2003). It is crucial that evidence base be derived from an in-depth understanding of such factors causing undernutrition that play a role in the affecting the prevalence of undernutrition across the population and this evidence base should be put to use for targeting program interventions at the severely marginalized and susceptible groups.

A pertinent question, then, that keeps sprawling up in the undernutrition debate is the role of economic growth and its efficacy in curtailing the prevalence of undernutrition. However, there have been numerous studies addressing this question; the results have been inconclusive. A cross-country analysis suggests that a one percentage point reduction in stunting can be attained by a 5.5% increase in per capita economic growth (Headey, 2013). Other sets of studies report contradicting findings, stating that the role played by economic growth in averting child undernutrition in India is only minimal (Joe et al., 2016; Subraam et al., 2011). This set of mixed findings necessitates that the role played by economic growth in alleviating child undernutrition can neither be overestimated nor be underestimated. Besides economic growth, other important determinants of child nutrition have been identified by previous studies such as educational and nutritional enhancement among mothers, economic profile of households, better child-feeding practices, dietary diversity, and better sanitation for improvement in child nutrition (Aguayo & Menon, 2016; Corsi et al., 2016).

India creates the perfect setting for understanding the nexus between impoverishment and undernutrition. India has made impressive improvements on population health front, as evident from falling fertility rates, maternal, child and infant mortality rates, increase in immunization coverage, improvements in life expectancy, and reduced prevalence of communicable diseases (Peters et al., 2002), and concomitant carving out of a quicker orbit of economic development. Despite these advancements, India has not been successful in achieving the aspirational outcomes as far as health parameters are concerned. The ensuing waves of the National Family Health Survey have facilitated the comparison in child undernutrition indicators over decades. Despite there being substantial reduction in child undernutrition in almost three decades, it is undeniable that the prevalence is still quite high and needs intervention.

1.2.2 Quadrant Analysis: Nutrition Vis-a-Vis Development

In order to understand the correlation between undernutrition and economic development, it will be insightful to paint a picture of levels of undernutrition in the Indian states and compare them with the prevalence of poverty and the levels of economic development. To facilitate this, a scatter plot has been created, wherein the y-axis consists of proportion of undernourished children aged 5 years and below and the x-axis consists of poverty prevalence as defined by the state-specific poverty lines and the natural logarithm of per capita net states domestic product at current prices. In order to develop a better understanding of the above, a quadrant analysis has been adopted and the overall averages have been used as quadrant demarcations (Mazumdar, 2010). Four regions have been identified using quadrant demarcations based on national averages. The first region (Region I) is the pitfall region. The characteristics of this region include high rates of undernutrition along with high inequality in their prevalence. The second region (Region II) is the intensity region. The characteristics of this region include high rates of undernutrition along with low inequality in their prevalence. Region III represents the do-gooders. These are the states that are characterized by both low prevalence of undernutrition and low inequality in the prevalence. Region IV is called the disparity region. It consists of the states that have lower prevalence of undernutrition, but the levels of inequality in the prevalence are high.

Figure 1.2a, b show the unidirectional nature of the relationship between nutritional status and the levels of economic development and deprivation at the macro level. The R2 values of 0.40

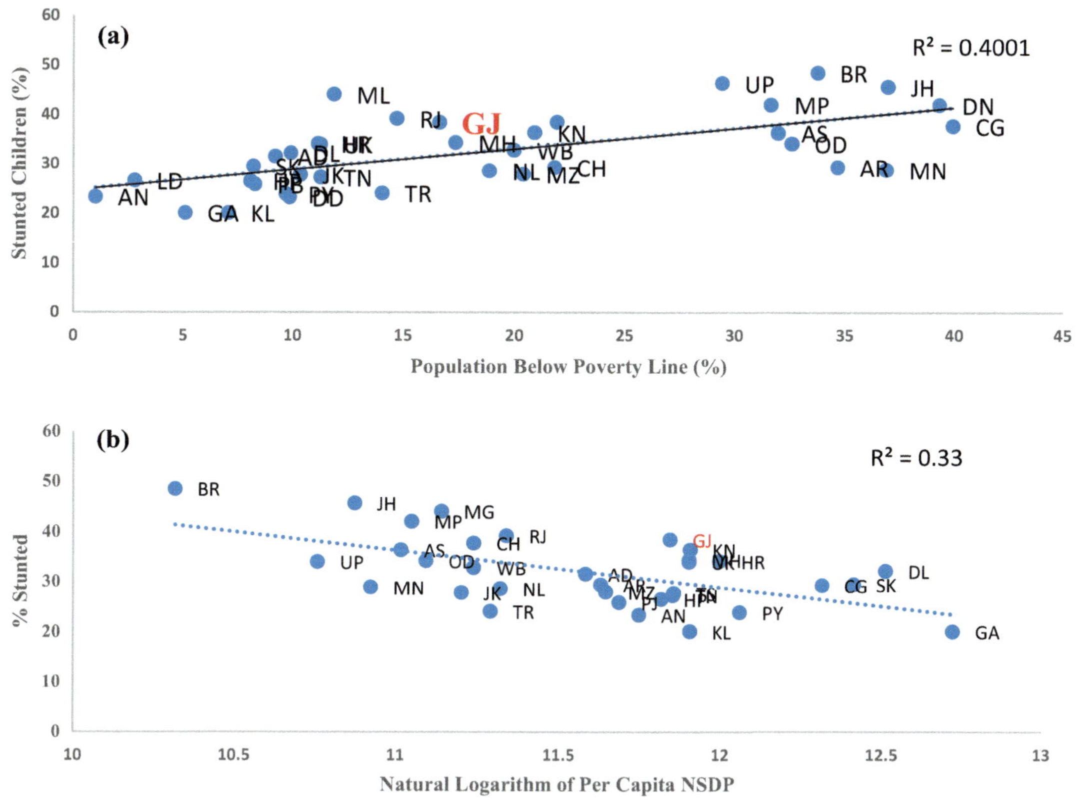

Fig. 1.2 **a** Child undernutrition and proportion of population below poverty line, India (2015–2016). *Source* Authors. **b** Child undernutrition and per capita gross state domestic product (GSDP), India (2015–2016). *Source* Authors

and 0.33 depict that the strength of the relationship between populations below poverty line and child stunting is 40%, while that of per capita NSDP and child stunting is 33%. In Fig. 1.2a, the states towards the northeast quadrant, i.e. Chhattisgarh, Madhya Pradesh, Jharkhand, Bihar, and Uttar Pradesh are those with concomitantly high levels of undernutrition and proportions of the population living below the poverty line. Along similar lines, states towards the south-west quadrant, i.e. Punjab, Himachal Pradesh, and a few northeastern states, have both lower levels of undernutrition, and a lower proportion of population staying below the poverty line, when compared to the national average value. The outliers, Kerala and Goa, for instance, also present pertinent policy implications. Despite having identical levels of proportion of population below poverty line, these states differ considerably in nutritional outcomes, with the prevalence of undernutrition in Kerala being far lower than that in Gujarat. One of the most plausible explanations behind this is that the role played by improved access to health care in Kerala is quite important in improving nutritional outcomes for children in the state and making its prevalence rates one of the lowest in the country (Ramachandran, 1997). This proves that social and economic development and human capital formation are prerequisites if undernutrition levels are to be curtailed.

The plausible relationship between child undernutrition and the overall economic development of the states is explained in Fig. 1.2b. The results are consistent with predictions. Once more, it is discovered that states with a high prevalence of undernutrition tend to cluster in the northwest quadrant, with the concentration dispersing as one travels south-east along the regression line. This shows that the rates of undernourishment are still extremely high, even with adequate rates of economic growth. This reaffirms the necessity of other proximate factors, which must cooperate with economic development in order to reduce undernourishment in the Indian setting.

The quadrant analysis is displayed in Fig. 1.3. The first area, known as the "pitfall region," is made up of states like Gujarat, Odisha, and Assam for both stunting and underweight cases. This area is characterized by significant undernutrition rates as well as considerable inequality in these rates. The second region, known as the intensity region, is made up of states like Jharkhand, Bihar, Uttar Pradesh, and Madhya Pradesh for underweight, and Rajasthan, Chhattisgarh, and Meghalaya in addition for cases of stunting. This region is characterized by a high prevalence of undernutrition and relatively low inequality in this prevalence. The do-gooder states that makeup Region III have lower average undernutrition levels and less evident inequality in these levels; for stunting, Region III contains Tamil Nadu, Pondicherry, Lakshadweep, and Uttarakhand, and Sikkim and Tripura are also included. Region IV, which encompasses Goa, Kerala, the Andaman and Nicobar Islands, Himachal Pradesh, Telangana, Nagaland, and

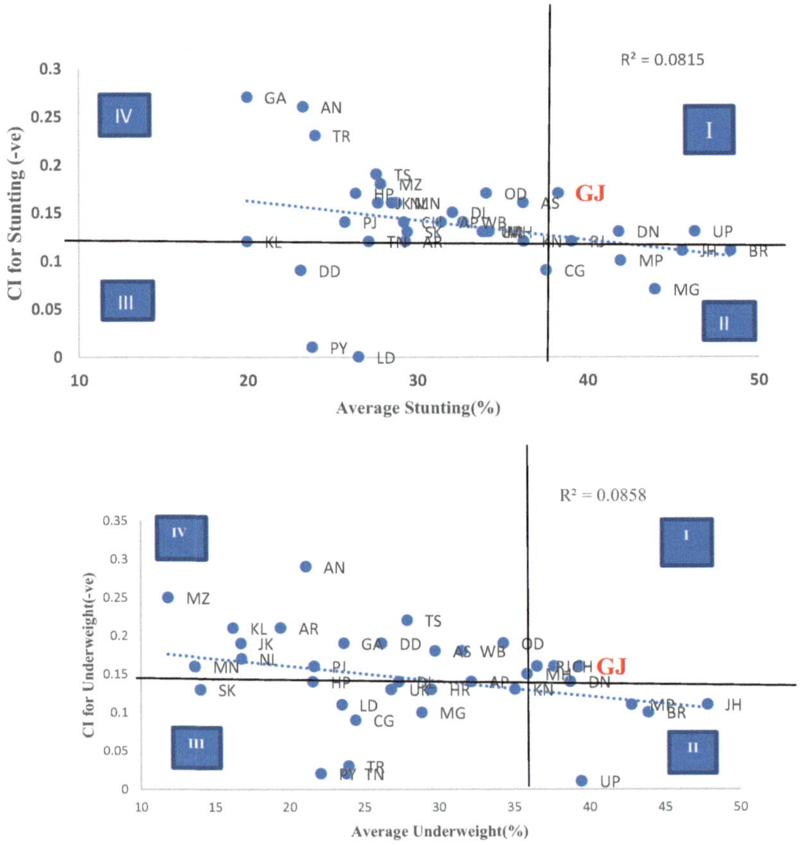

Fig. 1.3 Child undernutrition versus socio-economic inequality in the prevalence of undernutrition in children under the age of five in India. *Source* Authors. *Notes* Legend for the states: AP*Andhra Pradesh; CG*Chhattisgarh; GA*Goa; TR*Tripura; HR*Haryana; MZ*Mizoram; NL*Nagaland; HP*Himachal Pradesh; PB*Punjab; KL*Kerala; UT*Uttaranchal; BR*Bihar; JH*Jharkhand; MH*Maharashtra; GJ*Gujarat; MN*Manipur; AS*Assam; DL*Delhi; OR*Orissa; SK*Sikkim; J and K*Jammu and Kashmir; MP*Madhya Pradesh; UP*Uttar Pradesh; TN*Tamil Nadu; RJ*Rajasthan; KA*Karnataka; ARN*Arunachal Pradesh; ML*Meghalaya; WB*West Bengal

Jammu and Kashmir, represents the discrepancy of having considerable inequality in the distribution of undernutrition even at lower levels of this phenomena.

Gujarat is the only state that stands out in the previous research. It is located in the danger zone and, compared to the other states, not only has a higher prevalence of child undernourishment, but also a higher inequality in that prevalence. Gujarat, one of the nation's wealthier states economically, is a fascinating example since it shows that economic growth and development alone are insufficient to guarantee equitable and better nutritional results for children.

There is a distinct association between poverty and undernutrition at an aggregate level, with states having higher levels of average poverty, suffering from higher levels of undernutrition among children. A similar pattern is being followed in better-developed states, i.e. the level of economic development in the states resonates with lower levels of undernutrition. Nevertheless, Gujarat, a developed state, highlights the point that economic development per se would not ensure better nutritional outcomes unless it is effectively backed by improvements in social and human development, as well as institutional coverage. The states of Kerala and Tamil Nadu reestablish the hypothesis that the quintessential approach to assure reduction in undernutrition levels involves a coordination of collective action at all the levels—individual, household, and community. It is very evident from the results that India faces the twin challenges of reducing widespread undernutrition levels, in of the larger states, and of reducing inequality in the extent of undernutrition.

Hence, what India is witnessing today is the domino effect of socio-economic inequality, which morphs into an endless loop of undernutrition. The following chapters attempt to understand and shed light on this multi-pronged issue. It tries to bring together aspects and linkages of undernutrition, build a bridge towards understanding the multifaceted problem that undernutrition is, and thus, help the policymakers to reach a cohesive approach in order to fulfill the Sustainable Development Goal.

Another important aspect that acts as a barrier to India's nutrition goal is the prevalence of anaemia among women. In 2011, the estimated global prevalence of anaemia was nearly 29% (469 million) among non-pregnant women belonging to the reproductive age group (Stevens et al., 2013). In India, nearly 57% of women fall under the category of suffering from anaemia (NFHS-5). Anaemia, defined as the insufficiency of haemoglobin in blood, has detrimental physical, social, and economic effects (Bharati et al., 2008). Although anaemia has been identified as an area that requires urgent attention, there is little to no concrete evidence established at a national level. Smaller and more focused studies do highlight contributors to anaemia. It is crucial to note that determinants of anaemia are manifold; the primary cause in developing countries is the lack of bioavailable dietary iron (Scrimshaw, 1991). Consequences of anaemia range from reduced cognitive ability hindered capacity to work to aggravated risk of disease and infection and, in some cases, maternal and child mortality (Schloz et al., 1997). The concept and perspective of undernutrition have been changed from protein-energy undernutrition to hidden hunger in 1991, at the UNICEF/WHO international conference on "Ending Hidden Hunger" in Montreal. Micronutrient undernutrition is a significant public health issue for low- and middle-income countries, essential for the human body's proper growth and development. Micronutrient deficiency or "Hidden Hunger", affects health, learning ability, and productivity due to high rates of illness and disability. These contribute to a vicious cycle of undernutrition, underdevelopment, and poverty. Children born to anaemic mothers are more susceptible to being born prematurely and with low birth weight (Hirve et al., 1994; Klebanoff et al., 1991). Hence, the cycle of intergenerational undernutrition continues. As per the World Bank (1994), India loses 5% of the gross domestic product (GDP) due to the burden of iron deficiency anaemia (IDA) in low- and middle-income countries. It is observed that the same population often shoulders the disproportionate burden of multiple micronutrient deficiencies, which is concurrent to 7% of annual

GBD and 9% of childhood Disability-Adjusted Life Years (DALYs).

While India has various policies that aim to tackle nutritional challenges, a sub-section of the population that still is disproportionately worse off are the tribes. India is home to al half the tribal population of the world. Over 10 crore individuals belonging to 689 tribes are identified as Scheduled Tribe by the Constitution of India (Indian Ministry of Tribal Affairs). Every tribe is different from the other. Yet, there is a dearth of an inclusive pan-India study when it comes to tribes. Various pocket studies do point us towards a plethora of determinants that can be associated with anaemia. Some socio-economic determinants of tribal anaemia are household wealth, place, and region of residence (i.e. belonging to eastern, western, northern, southern, or north-eastern India) (Unisa et al., 2011). Lack of diverse diet, consumption of only vegetarian diet is also suggested as determinants of anaemia among tribes (Abriha et al., 2014; Jemal, 1999). A handful of studies also point towards the use of modern contraceptives to be associated with lower anaemia levels (Haile et al., 2016).

On the one hand, as India grapples with undernutrition among the children, nutritional status of the elderly is also steady becoming a cause of worry. As a result of a considerable global increase in the average human life expectancy, a detailed understanding of the nutritional state of the elderly has been the subject of extensive investigation in recent years. According to a fact sheet released by the World Health Organization (WHO), forecasts show that, while over 12% of the world's population—or roughly 900 million individuals—were 60 years of age or older in 2015, this number will more than double to 22% (or about 2 billion people) by 2050 (WHO, 2018). Similar predictions have been made in other studies, with some estimating that by 2050, roughly a quarter of the world's population will be at least 60 years old (Zhao et al., 2018). According to a different UN estimate, 962 million people over the age of 60 lived in nations in Asia in 2017, making up the majority of the world's old population (549.2 million). In India, the elderly make up roughly 9.4% of the population, and by 2050, that percentage is expected to soar to 19.1% (UNDESA, 2017). Keeping one's health and reducing the risk of chronic disease are made possible by nutrition, which is a major factor in the ageing process (Agarwal et al., 2013; Ahmed & Haboubi, 2010; Cederholm et al., 2017; Zhao et al., 2018). An aged person's poor nutritional quality increases their chance of developing chronic diseases like cardiovascular disease and sarcopenia as well as overall ill health (Agarwal et al., 2013; Cederholm et al., 2017; Zhao et al., 2018). A generalized state of low nutrition, including a lack of macro- and/or micronutrients, is referred to as undernutrition. Negative health conditions, frequent hospital visits, and mortality are all effects of poor nutrition in the elderly. This has consequences for not only the out-of-pocket costs but also causes a significant increase in the economic load (Robinson, 2018). According to studies, the prevalence of undernutrition among elderly Indians varies significantly by location, with Central India having the greatest prevalence and Northern India coming in second (Kushwaha et al., 2020).

1.2.3 Programs and Policy Interventions

There have been numerous policy interventions to tackle all the above-mentioned problems. The Indian Constitution (Article 47) makes it compulsory for the state to bolster the nutritional status and the standard of living of its citizens and buttress public health infrastructure. Adherence to this clause is shown in the form of nutrition missions spearheaded by certain state governments. For instance, the nutrition mission of Maharashtra (2005) seeks to end all types of undernutrition. Delivering evidence-based interventions, focusing on adolescent girls' nutrition, education, and empowerment, combining facility, outreach, and community-based interventions to make services and support accessible and affordable for the public, especially for those belonging to the marginalized sections, and auditing pregnancy weight gain at every antenatal visit are some of the elements included in the mission strategy. A multi-sectoral plan has been implemented with this objective in mind. The mission is now regarded as a role model because it has succeeded in improving people's nutritional status. Following the mission's allocation of $500 million to Madhya Pradesh in 2010, the following actions were taken: creating district-level action plans; starting pilot projects; keeping track of and evaluating progress indicators; and providing nourishing meals to expectant mothers at Anganwadi centres. Similar initiatives were also carried out in states like Uttar Pradesh in 2014 and Gujarat in 2012, as well as Karnataka in 2010. In 2015, a similar project was also initiated with technical support from UNICEF in Jharkhand, where the situation regarding maternal and child undernutrition is serious.

- National Nutrition Policy

On the basis of a thorough understanding of the causes of undernutrition, India's Nutrition Policy of 1993 was developed (Ministry of Human Resource and Development, 1993). To accomplish the objective of balanced nutrition for everyone, the policy called for the adoption of a multi-sectoral strategy and the implementation of a wide variety of initiatives. As a result, numerous ideas, projects, and missions were occasionally launched (Table 1.4). The health sector's policy and program initiatives, which were planned to address many aspects of nutrition, have been crucial in reducing the current problem. The trends of decline in some of the crucial health indicators for the nation are as follows: (i) a decrease in the infant mortality rate from 80 per 1,000 live births to 41 per 1,000 live births between 1990 and 2015–16 (NIMS et al., 2016); (ii) a decrease in maternal mortality ratio from 398 per 100,000 live births to 167 per 100,000 live births in 1997–98 and 2011–13 respectively; (iii) a decrease in the proportion of undernourished people in the overall population from 24 to 15% between 1990–92 and 2014–16 (FAO et al., 2015); and (iv) reduction in under-five mortality rate from 115 per 1,000 live births in 1991 to 50 per 1,000 live births in 2015–16; (v) (iii) decrease in the percentage of underweight, stunted, and anaemic children from 115 per 1,000 live births in 1991 to 50 per 1,000 live births in 2015–16 (IIPS & ICF, 2017). The Sustainable Development Goals are a series of global progression objectives established by the UN to track the development of social, economic, and environmental injustices.

- MDGs to SDGs

The United Nations noted that India was still falling behind (slow or off-track) the 2015 target of halving the percentage of people who experience hunger between 1990 and 2015 with regard to the first Millennium Development Goal (i.e. eradicate extreme poverty and hunger), and the government must take immediate measures to ensure India expedites advancements on reducing hunger (UN, 2015). Nearly 54% of all Indian children were underweight in 1990, when the objective was established. By 2015, only 40% of people were undernourished. Particularly noticeable was this shift in the percentage of underweight children under three years old. Therefore, the goal of lowering the proportion of malnourished children by half, to 26% (which is the proportion recorded in 1990), was not met (MoSPI, 2016; UNDP, 2015). The UN announced 17 Sustainable Development Goals (SDG) in 2016 for the time period ending in 2030 after the Millennium Development Goals' era ended in 2015. Ending hunger, achieving food security and improved nutrition, and promoting sustainable agriculture are the objectives of the second Sustainable Development Goal (UNDP, 2015).

- National Food Security Act

The National Food Security Act's implementation is one effort to address the problem of hunger (and nutritional deficiencies). The law, which has been in place since 2013, intends to provide increased access to an adequate supply of wholesome food at affordable rates. Under the Targeted Public Distribution System (PDS), which was introduced in June 1997, up to three-fourths of eligible rural and half of eligible urban population, as determined by States/UTs, are entitled to receive food grains (5 kg of rice, wheat, and coarse grains per person per month at subsidized prices of INR 3/2/1 per kg, respectively). The Act includes provisions for monetary maternity benefits as well as the development of a grievance retribution process to guarantee compliance by the state/district government employees, in addition to guaranteeing access to food grains. Inadequate progress has been made in the implementation of the Act, according to data gathered from a survey by the political organization Swaraj Abhiyan (Drèze, 2015). Less than half of the poor families had eaten any pulses in the month preceding the poll, according to the same statistics for Uttar Pradesh's drought-like regions. According to Drèze, these issues will persist until coordinated efforts are undertaken to support the existing programs (such as the Public Distribution System, Mid-day Meal Scheme, Integrated Child Development Services Scheme, Village and Child Development Centers) (Drèze, 2015).

- Integrated Child Development Scheme

Inadequate access is also caused by the food grains that are wasted in Food Corporation of India's warehouses (due to rotting and theft). Additionally, the Integrated Child Development Services (ICDS) Scheme, which benefits over 100 million Indians, including kids, pregnant women, and nursing moms, has been a success. However, there are issues with supplying high-quality food and distributing it fairly. Anganwadi centres were established under ICDS to offer services and education in primary health care to the entire nation. Because of poor pay and inadequate training, workers are unable to effectively address the issue of undernourishment. Thus, if there was a mechanism for regular orientation programs, regarding exposing workers to new techniques available for tracking the growth of every child, organized and workers are supported in the implementation of schemes, it would be helpful in improving the country's nutrition situation.

There are many instances to illustrate the poor quality of service delivery. For instance, the Village Child Development Centres (VCDC) were set up in 36 districts of Maharashtra in 2016 with assistance from the central government to offer undernourished children medical care and nourishing meals for a month. However, it has been shown that the majority of these centres are ineffective because of a lack of funding. The state government is under pressure from non-governmental organizations and local self-governments to step in and take the necessary steps for the revival of these centres and continuation of their funding because, without them, the state's nearly 80,000 severely malnourished children are at serious risk. The domination of social and cultural issues that frequently work against the very purpose of a nutrition intervention is another significant barrier to the previously existing economic and political reasons that support undernutrition. Over 200 million people (16.6%) in the diverse community groups that make up India's population are classified as "scheduled castes." Because some alleged beneficiaries refused to eat the food prepared by Anganwadi workers from the scheduled caste community, who have historically been labelled as untouchables by the upper castes, Hausla Poshan Yojana, an effort to provide nutritious food to pregnant women and undernourished children in Uttar Pradesh, failed to even start off (Aijaz, 2017).

In addition to the foregoing, Census data from 2011 reveals that child marriage is extremely common in India (30% of all marriages). A recent study in the British Medical Journal found that infants in India born to underage brides (married before the age of 18) have a higher risk of malnutrition (Raj et al., 2010). These infants are simply born into the cycle of undernourishment because their moms are themselves young, defenceless, and frequently malnourished. Steps are being taken toward widespread food fortification to improve the nutritional value of food products (Ministry of Women and Child Development, 2016). A suggested strategy would deal with adding essential vitamins and minerals (iron, folic acid, vitamin, iodine) to foods sold in markets, such as rice, wheat flour, salt, edible oil, and milk. Nutritional standards have been developed by the Food Safety and Standards Authority of India (FSSAI) to ensure that food manufacturers who are in charge of fortifying food supply the necessary levels of micronutrients to the food items. Insightful lessons in this regard can be drawn from procedures used in the Gajapati district of Odisha, where school personnel tasked with preparing midday meals for students are given training and assistance so they can fortify the rice with iron to increase its nutritious content. While the central government has expressed interest in extending the scope of this effort to other regions of the country, only about 1,449 schools in the district are currently covered by it.

Continued nursing for the first year after delivery, according to the Department of Biotechnology (DBT), Ministry of Science and Technology, GOI, raises iron levels and lowers the prevalence of anaemia in school-age children (PIB, 2017). There is evidence to show that an increase in iron levels may be a risk factor for diabetes; thus, it is crucial to keep iron consumption below recommended limits. It follows that a significant fiscal allocation is necessary for any nutrition-related program to succeed. According to data from India, monetary provisions have decreased over time for centrally backed programs like the Integrated Child Development Scheme. The amount of money allocated was exactly cut in half between 2014–15 and 2015–16, from 166 to 83 billion. However, it is crucial to note that even while the allocations have increased in absolute terms, the annual rate of change has decreased to 12.76% (Table 1.3). The central government's position on this is that the state governments must take a more proactive role in combating undernourishment and raise money for this purpose.

In addition to the already discussed programs and interventions, the judiciary and advocacy groups have started playing an instrumental role in curtailing the prevalence of undernutrition in India. An interesting example in this context is the Right to Food Campaign. Officially launched in March 2014, it is an unofficial group of organizations and individuals that came together because of PILs. This platform is used to persuade state governments to take cognizance of matters related to public interest, one of the core areas of this being nutrition (Table 1.4).

1.2.4 What Can Be Done?

Despite a plethora of nutrition-centric interventions in India, India is still far behind her South Asian counterparts. There have, undoubtedly, been commendable strides in fields like exclusive breastfeeding. However, whether the programs address the inherent inequalities based on gender and socio-economic differentials is a policy concern that needs to be taken into consideration as well. Launching of the National Nutrition Mission was an achievement in the sense that it conveyed an acknowledgement of a convergence between individual-level and community-level factors and underlying determinants of

Table 1.3 Central budgetary allocations for integrated child development services scheme

Financial year	Budgetary allocations (in INR billions)	Annual change (%)
2013–14	163.12	–
2014–15	165.61	1.53
2015–16	83.36	−49.66
2016–17	148.50	78.14
2017–18	167.45	12.76

Source Ministry of Women and Child Development

Table 1.4 Nutrition-centric government interventions

Direct policy measures	Program interventions
• Making programs inclusive by enlarging the safety nets to include the more nutritionally vulnerable population, such as expecting mothers, adolescents, and infants • Food fortification with essential nutrients such as iron and iodine • Increase the production and popularity of affordable and nutritionally dense food • Curtail micronutrient deficiencies among susceptible sections	• Mid-day Meal Programme, 1962–63 • Goitre Control Programme, 1962 (now known as National Iodine Deficiency Disorders Control Programme) • Special Nutrition Programme, 1970–71 • Balwadi Nutrition Programme, 1970–71 • Nutritional Anaemia Prophylaxis Programme, 1970 • Prophylaxis Programme against Blindness due to Vitamin A Deficiency, 1970 • Integrated Child Development Services (ICDS), 1975
Indirect policy measures • Improving food production to ensure bolstered food security • Enhancing per capita availability of nutritionally dense food items and improving diet structure by stimulating production • Improving the purchasing power of the poor and deprived sections of the population by making the public distribution system more inclusive • Implementation of land reform laws to downsize susceptibility of the impoverished, improve education and accessibility at all levels and of all programs related to health, nutrition, immunization, and encourage community participation to ensure maximum benefits	• Bi-annual Vitamin-A Supplementation • Establishment of: Nutritional Rehabilitation Centres; Village Health Sanitation & Nutrition Committee • Village Health & Nutrition Days (at Anganwadi centres) • Promotion of Infant & Young Child Feeding Practices Guidelines, 2013 • National Diarrhoeal Diseases Control Programme, 1981 • Weekly Iron & Folic Acid Supplementation, 2015 • Wheat-based Supplementary Nutrition Programme, 1986 • National Plan of Action on Nutrition, 1995 • Public Distribution System, 1997 • National Nutrition Mission, 2003 • National Health Mission, 2013 (subsumes former Rural & Urban Health Missions) • National Iron+ Initiative, 2013 • National Deworming Day, 2015

Source National Nutrition Policy, 1993; Ministry of Health and Family Welfare. Annual Report 2015–16
Note Years after program names denote the year of launch of the program in India

undernutrition, with a special focus on the marginalized sub-sections of the population. While such an acknowledgement is an impressive first step, there is an ardent need to take into cognizance, other factors that contribute to the persistent problem of undernutrition like women's empowerment, nutrition-related awareness, the need for behavioural change, and the importance of ensuring that households have access to a variety of foods throughout the year, which is also easily affordable. The UN Decade for Action on Nutrition (2016–25) emphasizes on the 'leave no one behind' approach (Global Nutrition Report, 2017). This reiterates the importance of the idea of inclusivity, which refers to a universal approach that ensures that all people have the capability and affordability to avail such resources as may be needed by them to be able to attain a healthy and safe living. This is the idea that needs to be incorporated into the policymaking of all the countries globally.

Combatting undernutrition requires harmonized planning and engagement both within sectors and across sectors, which entails a juxtaposition of horizontal and vertical coordination at all levels of governance. This is hindered by the complexity in the governance and institutional structure, lack of responsibility and accountability pertaining to nutrition, and structural setbacks (Balarajan, 2014; Balarajan & Reich, 2016; Benson, 2007; Gillespie et al., 2015; Hoey & Pelletier, 2011; Kennedy et al., 2015; Mejia-Costa, 2011; Meija-Costa & Fanzo, 2012; Natalicchio et al., 2009; Nisbett et al., 2015; Pelletier et al., 2012). The formulation of legitimized integrating departments and structural frameworks with carefully laid out strategies to tackle undernutrition is crucial in swamping these threats through such structural reforms by involving all the stakeholders, including policymakers, NGOs, and audit teams. This will also facilitate simultaneous policy development at all levels and help in monitoring and evaluation activities by marshalling resources at all levels, including financial and technical resources and human capital (Balarajan, 2014; Balarajan & Reich, 2016; Benson, 2007; Haddad et al., 2014; Hawkes et al., 2016; Lapping et al., 2012; Levitt et al., 2011; Meija-Costa & Fanzo, 2012; Pelletier & Pelto, 2013). This often fundamentally involves the systemic coordination between the two most obvious sectors, which are the agriculture and health departments. This coordination, however, needs to be expanded to include partnerships between several different ministries such as economic development, finance, gender, education, water and sanitation, social justice, industry, and trade (Benson, 2007; Clayton et al., 2015; Gillespie et al., 2015; Hawkes et al., 2016; Hoey & Pelletier, 2011; Kennedy et al., 2015; Levitt et al., 2009, 2011; Meija-Costa & Fanzo, 2012; Taylor et al., 2015; Thow et al., 2010; van den Bold et al., 2015; Walls et al., 2016).

Irrespective of the problem being dealt with or the country being discussed, it is crucial to have smart indicators and data systems in place to enable informed policy choices through: (i) identification of the problem (i.e. showcasing the change in prevalence of undernutrition and the persistent inequality in them), (ii) designing new policies and improving existing policies, (iii) monitoring and evaluation activities, (iv) the development of a framework for auditing of policies and programs, and (v) as a groundwork for competent financing and accountability systems (Baker et al., 2017; Balarajan, 2014; Balarajan & Reich, 2016; Chung et al., 2012; Craig et al., 2010; Haddad et al., 2014; Hawkes et al., 2016; Huicho et al., 2016; Kugelberg et al., 2012; Lapping et al., 2012; Levisnon et al., 2013; Levitt et al., 2011; Meija-Costa & Fanzo, 2012; Mejia & Haddad, 2014; Mohmand, 2012; Nathan et al., 2005; Nisbett et al., 2015; Pelletier et al., 2011, 2012; Reich & Balarajan, 2012; Thow et al., 2010; Yeatman, 2003). Data-driven and "policy success" enabled interventions will, thus, go a long way in aiding India's combat against maternal and child undernutrition (Balarajan, 2014; Hajeebhoy et al., 2013; Hoey & Pelletier, 2011; Levitt et al., 2011; Yeatman, 2003).

It is crucial to understand that nutrition is both the start as well as end-product of the Sustainable Development Goals. Nutritional deprivation is not just a result of dietary insufficiency, but a web of factors such as women's education and empowerment, access to and quality of healthcare, economic well-being both at the macro and micro levels, water, sanitation and hygiene practices, and other related facets. Nutritional outcomes are affected by several factors such as food choices made by individuals and their production and marketing, the food that is consumed by them and their families, and the quality of care provided to those members who are nutritionally at risk (children and their mothers, in particular). Improved nutritional status results in improved cognitive abilities, further leading to improved earnings and better income. This, further, is translated to economic growth at the macro level and societal upliftment. Dismal nutritional status (reflecting itself in nutritional deprivation, or dual burden of malnutrition) hinders productive capacity of individuals, which further leads to staggered growth of national income. Without suitable investments, poor nutrition remains persistent, making significant contributions to the global burden of disease and debilitated quality of life. In this sense, undernutrition acts as a nefarious, oftentimes unnoticed, hurdle in achieving all the SDG targets.

This book makes an attempt to establish the central role played by social and economic development in affecting undernutrition rates and the persistent inequality in such rates in India. The widely varying rates of undernutrition in India can be singlehandedly accorded to the prevalence of social and economic inequalities in India. This means that even after controlling for other confounders, the economically laggard sections of the society bear the brunt of higher rates of child undernutrition in India. This analogy can also be extended to poorer states and regions of the country, in the sense that these regions report the highest prevalence of undernutrition rates in the country. The situation is further aggravated by this as poorer states are also the ones with a huge proportion of infant and child population, given their high fertility rates and dismal quality of health services. Therefore, it is important to understand the connection between socio-economic development, poverty, and nutritional status to devise effective policies to curtail the same. It is also important to realize that social and economic equality is a pre-condition to ensuring egalitarian nutritional outcomes and reduces the persistent inequality in their prevalence.

There are not only a plethora of reasons available for the occurrence of undernutrition but also an expansive range of ideas to solve this issue. It is, however, crucial to pay attention to develop an in-depth understanding of the factors that hinder the attainment of nutrition-related goals. It goes beyond doubt that the policymakers and stakeholders have to move forward with a multi-pronged and all-inclusive approach that is devised after having taken into consideration the variable nature of local-level challenges. It is equally imperative to demonstrate better governance. In addition to the above, it is also beneficial to develop collaborative initiatives with the civil society. In particular, there is an ardent need to pay attention to building and strengthening the health and nutrition profiles of the immediate neighborhood and devising policies and interventions based on a need-based approach.

The book tries to answer the following research questions pertaining to the Sustainable Development Goals:

- What is the extent of progress made by India and the states in covering SDG-2 of Zero Hunger?
- How is food security instrumental in buttressing nutritional outcomes for women and children in India?
- What are the ramifications of socio-economic inequality for nutritional situation among women and children in India?
- Does contraceptive usage help in averting the risk of anaemia among women?
- How is the nutritional status of children benefitted by the economic empowerment among women?

The book deals with numerous issues related to undernutrition and anaemia in India and tries to establish its inextricability with poverty, empowerment, tribal living conditions, usage of contraception, dietary diversity, and socio-economic inequality. The book also attempts to put forth the linkages between mother's economic empowerment and children's nutritional status, anaemia of women with special reference to tribal women and children and the issues associated with anaemia in India. Another compelling yet relatively less explored aspect that this book delves into is the relationship between contraceptive usage and anaemia level. The book tries to measure the progress made by India and its states in achieving the targets laid down by the SDGs. In addition to the above, it deals with socio-economic inequalities and the ramifications it can have on women and children, especially those belonging to the marginalized communities. The high and worrying prevalence of anaemia is widely criticized and, thus, dissecting this issue may play an important role in aiding India in realizing the target of reduced anaemia among women of reproductive age and improving maternal and child health.

What makes the book stand out is, however, the fact that it tries to explore the immediate and distal factors affecting undernutrition at the state level in India. It also tries to understand the linkages between women's asset ownership and the nutritional status of their children by using large-scale data on asset ownership of women to comprehend how the children's health and nutrition are affected directly by the economic of their mothers. In addition to the above, the book not only attempts to dig into the determinants of anaemia among tribal women but also understands the geographical variation in dietary diversity and its role in determining the anaemia prevalence among tribal women who are rarely highlighted in nutrition research using nationally representative data. The book also deals with multiple facets of SDG5 of Gender Equality, more particularly Targets 5.1 and 5.C talk about doing away with every kind of favoritism against women and girls everywhere and adoption of policies for enforceable legislation of gender equality, respectively. The book also encapsulates the first and tenth SDGs of No Poverty and Reduced Inequalities and touches upon environmental health aspects as well. The book is, thus, an attempt to understand the determinants of undernutrition in the context of the SDGs and suggest policy measures to further bolster the improvements made thus far.

2 Women's Asset Ownership and Its Linkages with Child Undernutrition in India

Akancha Singh and Aparajita Chattopadhyay

Abstract

This chapter tries to analyse different aspects of women's ownership of assets and its linkages with child nutritional outcomes. Studies suggest that women's authority in household decision-making is greatly linked to the value of their assets compared to those of their husbands. Moreover, ownership of property not only gives women the option of falling back but also proves to be a powerful leverage in negotiations in household-related issues. The study found that women's ownership of assets has positive ramifications for the nutritional status of their children. However, the beneficial impact on children's nutritional status due to mother's asset ownership happens at different parts of the distribution, with children who are already better nourished benefitting more from their mothers' asset ownership.

Keywords

Assets · Stunting · Children · India · Quantile regression

2.1 Introduction

2.1.1 Indicators of Women's Empowerment

Achieving gender equality and women's empowerment are prime elements that facilitate the improvement of the well-being of all people (United Nations, 2015). Sustainable Development Goal five (SDG 5) talks about achieving gender equality and empowering all women and girls (Goal 5: Achieve gender equality and empower all women and girls). The primary aims of this goal are to end all forms of inequity against women and girls, to eliminate violent/harmful practices that affect women and girls, to identify the unpaid caregiving/domestic jobs performed by women, to assure equal opportunities for women's participation and leadership, and to capture universal access to sexual and reproductive health and rights (SRHR) for all women and girls (United Nations, 2015).

Empowerment is defined as the change in a person's ability to exercise choice (Kabeer, 1990). Existing literature focuses on the impact of gender equality and women's empowerment (GEWE) on maternal and child health and family planning (FP), and sexual and reproductive health rights. Women's empowerment is a social determinative of maternal and child health (Pratley, 2016). It is conversely linked with

A. Chattopadhyay et al., *Undernutrition in India*, Sustainable Development Goals Series,
https://doi.org/10.1007/978-981-19-8182-1_2

increased contraceptive usage among women in LMICs (James-Hawkins et al., 2018) and attrition in under-five mortality rates (Doku et al., 2020). Conceptual frameworks for quantifying women's empowerment exist. The prominent aspects of women empowerment mentioned in the literature are resources, agency, and achievements (Kabeer, 1990). Resources ameliorate a woman's capacity to exercise choice, while agency provides her with the capacity to act according to those choices. Another conceptual model of empowerment perceived by Van Eerdewijk et al. includes agency and resources, but goes on to add institutional structures to the realm (van Eerdewijk et al., 2017). In this framework, however, agency is further extended to include collective agency, decision-making, and leadership; resources pertaining to the bodily integrity of women and girls, analytical consciousness, asset ownership, and organizational structures dealing with the formulation of laws and policies concerning women and traditions that affect the capability of women and girls to command resources (Van Eerdewijk et al., 2017).

Although definitions of women's empowerment have been put forth, there is, at present not one homogenized, conceivable way to define women's empowerment. However, those definitions can be encapsulated as the process through which a woman attains agency. Agency is defined as "what a person is free to do and achieve in the quest of whatever goals or values he or she believes to be crucial" (Sen, 1985). This decision-making, more often than not happens through manoeuvering related and social dynamics through negotiation and manipulation (Cornwall & Edwards, 2010; Kabeer, 1990). The second concept that is pertinent in these definitions is processed, which places emphasis on a change from one state (gender inequality) to another (gender equality) over time (Malhotra & Schuler, 2005). Myriad works on women's empowerment state that its importance lies on women's active involvement in this process and the accompanying psychological change (e.g. gain in self-efficacy) that occurs along with it (Alsop et al., 2006; Cornwall & Anyidoho, 2010; Ibrahim & Alkire, 2007; Kabeer, 1990; Malhotra & Schuler, 2005).

The definition that has been used throughout this study is: "Women's status is women's power in comparison to men's in the households, communities, and countries in which they live" (Smith et al., 2003a). Three facets of the above definition are crucial to understand. First, women's status is not usually considered to be absolute or relative to that of other women but relative to men's. The definition, therefore, inherently assimilates the notion of gender disparity as proposed by Ramalingaswami et al. (1996) to be so deleterious to nutritional status of children. Second, it is established on the concept of power. To simplify it further, power entails the capability to make choices and exert them. It is a person or a group's capability to identify goals and seek after them, even amidst hostility and resistance from others.

Power, exerted through decision-making, takes the form of real decisions made on one's own or collectively through bargaining and negotiation. It can also take the form of deceit and duplicity, destruction and defiance, brutality, intimidation, threat, or even "non-decision making", in which a person or group accepts the state of affairs as given without contemplation or has others take a decision for them (Kabeer, 1999; Riley, 1997; Safilios-Rothschild, 1982; Sen, 1990). A person's control over different resources such as economic, human, and social, augments their capacity to choose. Economic resources include food availability, time, monetary resource, productive inputs, and financial assets. Human resources include education, skills, and knowledge. Membership in groups and approachability to kith and kin and other social networks constitute social resources (or "social capital") (Kabeer, 1999; Quisumbing & Maluccio, 2003; Sen & Batliwala, 2000). The definition of women's status, therefore, takes into account inequities in the competence of both women and men to choose, which may be a reflection of the discrepancy in authority over resources.

Third, the definition has both the elements—intra- and inter-household. Women experience disparities in their power when compared to their male counterparts both within households and in the communities and countries where they reside.

Traditions and customs entrenched in deeply rooted archaic beliefs, values, and attitudes often mandate differentiated roles, respectable behaviours, rights, privileges, and life options for both men and women (Agarwal, 1997; England, 2000; Kevane, 2000; Kishor, 1999; Safilios Rothschild, 1982; Sen & Batliwala, 2000; World Bank, 2000). For instance, women and men may face discrepancies in incentives or disincentives while engaging in any employment at all or in a certain type of employment, as well as different accolades and remunerations for similar terms of service. Women may amass less respect than their male counterparts may and face elevated risks of assault or be seen as inferior (intellectually) to men when they encounter people, groups, and organizations outside of their household. They may discover that female-specific health services, such as gynaecological or maternity needs, are not readily available, or not easily accessible. More integrally, traditions and customs administering social behaviour mean that some substitutes are not even considered as viable choices for women. They are not assumed to be within the sphere of possibility. These social group (men and women) differences have their roots in inequitable power dynamics between them (Barosso & Jacobson, 2000; Kabeer, 1999; Riley, 1997; Sen & Batliwala, 2000). Owing to the extra-household differences in the power dynamics between the two sexes, irrespective of their power relative to their husbands, women may come across more hurdles in achieving their goals and aspirations than men. One may omit crucial pathways through which women's status influences outcomes by ignoring the broader institutional context in which men and women conduct themselves (Mason, 1986, 1993; Safilios-Rothschild, 1982; Sen & Batliwala, 2000).

While the disparate power of women and men out of their household sphere is not compulsorily correlated with their distinctive power within the household sphere, the former influences the latter. As mentioned above, traditions and norms play a significant role in determining who has more clout in decision-making, meaning, who engages in and, thus, affects them all (Agarwal, 1997; Katz, 1997). Incidents under which negotiations can be engaged in, for example, norms may call for complacent concurrence of women when men display rage, are limited due to set customs and norms (Kevane, 2000). They also set the terms of the "outside options" of both the sexes and, therefore, their competence in negotiating with their husbands. For instance, if a woman has no better alternative than to reside with her husband in order to safeguard her livelihood because of inequitable labour policies and/or the absence of enforceable laws against domestic violence, she might refrain from disagreeing with him in the case of a strife (England, 2000; Haddad et al., 1997; Hoddinott & Adam, 1998; Katz, 1997; McElroy & Horney, 1981).

2.1.2 Why Is Tracking Child Undernutrition Important?

Developments in child health are crucial indicators of stride towards achieving the goal three of the United Nations' Sustainable Development Goals: A comprehensive assurance of a healthy life and well-being at all ages. Undernutrition not only makes children more susceptible to disease vulnerability but also hinders their holistic development (physical, cognitive, and mental) (Sánchez, 2017) which may affect productivity in later life (Strauss & Thomas, 1995) and increase economic inequality (Pickett & Wilkinson, 2015). Apart from the lack of adequate and nutritious food, there are factors that cause undernutrition, including, but not limited to recurring illnesses, poor childcare practices, and lack of access to health and other social services. These multifactorial determinants of health and nutrition have been classified into immediate, intermediate, and underlying factors (UNICEF, 1990). Undernutrition is particularly precarious because it has implications not only at the individual level but also at macro-level outcomes (WFP & MOSPI, 2019).

While the prevalence of stunting and underweight has declined to 35.5 and 32.1%, respectively, in 2015–16, the prevalence of wasting and severe wasting has slightly increased, which is a cause of serious concern for the authorities (NFHS-5, 2019–21. Globally, India fares poorly as far as standard child nutritional measures are concerned (Haddad et al., 2015). India ranked 114 out of 132 countries for child undernutrition indicators, just ahead of Afghanistan and Pakistan (IFPRI, 2016). In addition to the above, India had 62 million stunted children, which accounted for nearly 40% of the global share of stunting in 2016 (Khan & Mohanty, 2018). The condition is particularly dubious in India because there are large regional differences among different states, with stunting over 46 and 48%, respectively, in the states of Uttar Pradesh (India's populous state) and Bihar (Sunny et al., 2018). The cycle of intergenerational undernutrition stems at an early stage of life for an individual. From an undernourished mother to baby with low birth weight, undernutrition perpetuates through childhood and adolescence and is exacerbated by inadequate feeding, constrained access to healthcare facilities, early marriages, and early and intermittent pregnancies (WFP & MOSPI, 2019). The reason behind the global impetus on nutrition is that it is pertinent in achieving the national and global targets of SDGs and is, thus, more of a determinant than an aftermath of a country's future and a measure of its development. An increased understanding of this over the recent years has guided policy decisions and provides for a compelling case for higher attention and investments in nutrition.

2.1.3 Women's Asset Ownership and Child Nutrition

Over the past decades, there have been substantial improvements in the nutritional status of children in developing countries. However, South Asian countries lag behind in achieving advancements in child's nutritional status. Concurrent estimates suggest that, while 37% of South Asian under-5 children are stunted, nearly 46% are underweight (Gulati, 2010; Stevens et al., 2012). Attempts to resolve the Asian Enigma, in which economic advancements have not led to a concomitant decrease in child undernutrition, have shed light on a plethora of factors contributing to incessant child Undernutrition including, but not limited to poor water, sanitation, and hygiene practices (including open defecation), which contribute significantly to elevated concerns, particularly, gastrointestinal diseases and environmental enteropathy (Bhutta, 2006; Checkley et al., 2008; Dangour et al., 2012). Women's diminished social status has been identified as one of the crucial factors that acts as a potential contributor to child Undernutrition in the region (Ramalingaswami et al. 1996). Regional statistics based on national data buttress the claims that women's status is relatively lower than that of men's in South Asia as compared to sub-Saharan Africa. When economic indicators are compared in Table 2.1, it is indisputable that gender-based inequalities act in favour of males across the regions. One indicator providing evidence of the lower value placed on women's health and well-being as compared to their male counterparts is the ratio of female-to-male life expectancy and literacy, the values of which are much lower in South Asia when compared to Sub-Saharan Africa. In addition to the above, women's labour force participation and their share of earned income are lower for South Asian women as compared to their sub-Saharan African counterparts, pointing towards the gender disparities in ownership and access to economic resources in South Asia. Finally, at the national level, disparities in political power dynamics between the two sexes are far higher in South Asia than in sub-Saharan Africa.

Regional statistics further buttress the claims that women's and child nutritional status are the worst in regions that have the largest disparities between women and men. While the maternal mortality rate in South Asia is marginally higher than that in sub-Saharan Africa, the proportion of underweight women in South Asia quadruples when compared to sub-Saharan Africa. It is worth noting that, although studies and their descriptive statistics using national-level data back the Asian Enigma hypothesis (Smith & Haddad, 2000), ramifications on women's status

Table 2.1 Comparison of progress made by South Asia and Sub-Saharan Africa in some determinants of child nutritional status

Determinants	South Asia	Sub-Saharan Africa
GDP per capita (USD)	1804.9	1483.8
Poverty headcount ratio (%)	15.2	40.4
Democracy index (0–10; 0 = lowest)	5.6	4.2
Per capita dietary energy supply (Kcal/day)	2700	2360
Access to safe water (%)	93	61
Health expenditure as a % of GDP	3.5	5.1
Gross school enrolment ratio (%)	99.3	98.9

Source United Nations, World Bank, Economist Intelligence Unit, Food and Agricultural Organization, 2020

and child's nutrition actually take place at a household level. Micro-level data analysis on individual women, their husbands or partners, and their children is ardently needed for an exhaustive understanding of the pathways through which women's status affects the nutritional status of children. There is a dearth of empirical research that establishes linkages women's status and child's nutritional status on a cross-regional basis using household-level data to spell out the impact of women's status on the nutritional status of their children and the particular pathway through which it does so…

Economic and political structures and socio-cultural traditions create possibilities of inequalities that often result in women's inaccessibility to (or control over) resources, ineptitude in making household decisions, and restricted social support. This, in turn, may have ramifications in the form of household decisions that do not provide the required resource to buttress child nutrition and growth. For instance, without access to required monetary resources, mothers may be incapable in purchasing relevant food to meet the special needs of their young children or engage in beneficial health-seeking behaviour (Bhagowalia et al., 2012; Bhutta et al., 2004; Smith et al., 2003a, 2003b). Maternal care resource constitutes characteristics that may have an impact on how mothers are able to meet the requirements for the care of their children and include education and knowledge; physiological health; mental wellness and three areas pertaining women's empowerment; autonomy and control of household resources; workload and availability of time; and social support networks. There is abundant evidence to suggest that women's diminished status and lack of empowerment in South Asia may be a significant contributor to the recurrent problem of poor child nutrition in the region (Haddad, 1999; Ramalingaswami et al., 1996; Smith et al., 2003a, 2003b). However, the specific dimensions of women's empowerment that are crucial for childcare practices and nutritional status still remain inadequately understood and there is still a dearth of a holistic evidence base for the same.

Additionally, a significant number of studies have linked increased maternal autonomy to better nutrition of children, girl children in particular (Brennan et al., 2004; Glewwe, 1999). An amelioration in maternal autonomy is expected to bring about improvements in a mother's ability to decide about her children's health and nutrition, and a more autonomous mother is expected to have increased access to resources, which may lead to the acceptance of healthy and varied diets, boost the nutritional content of diets, contribute to better food hygiene and sanitation, and thereby reduce the risk of infection and disease. Since undernutrition is the outcome of insufficient food intake and repeated infectious diseases (UNDP, 2006), it is imperative to understand the links between household-level socio-economic factors (the role of maternal autonomy and asset ownership, in particular) and the extent to which it has manifestations for poor nutritional outcomes for children.

Figure 2.1 outlines the prime pathways through which children and their nutritional status

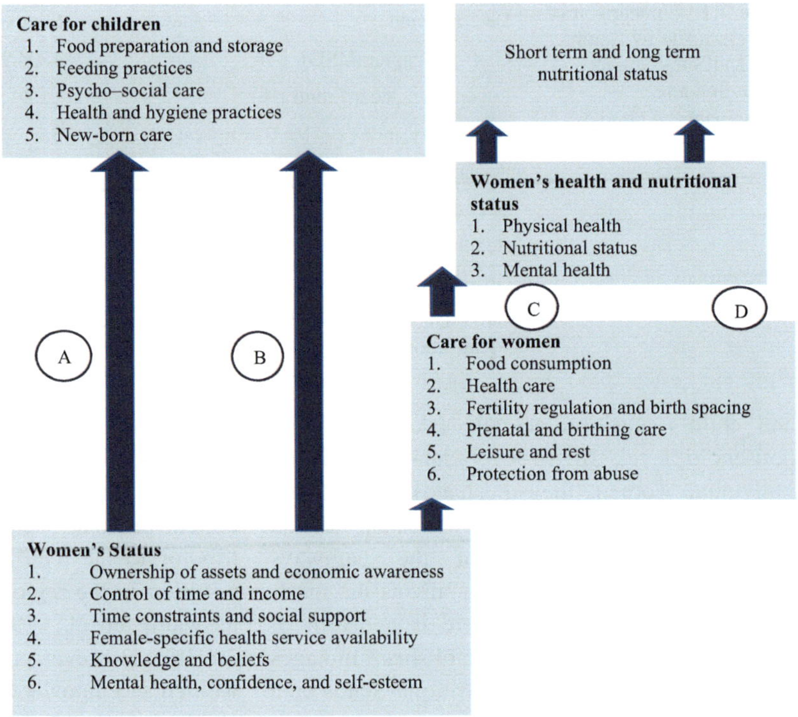

Fig. 2.1 Relationship between women's status and childcare practices and nutritional status. *Source* Adapted from Engle et al. (1999)

are influenced by women's status. The five pertinent caring practices that are imperative for children and their nutritional well-being are ways of food preparation and storage, feeding practices, psychosocial care, hygiene and home health practices (Engle et al., 1999), and post-natal care. Foods purchased by the household must be stored properly in a hygienic manner and prepared keeping the nutritional value of foods intact so that it is beneficial for children. It is crucial to take care of the timing and frequency of the foods given to children. In addition to the above, it is important for the child to get sufficient psychosocial care, including affection and warmth, receptivity, and the encouragement of self-determination and expedition. The child's environment needs to be sanitized sufficiently to protect him or her from diseases. Finally, the child must receive efficient care in the first 28 days of life which are extremely critical, including support during child-birth and throughout the neo-natal period by healthcare workers trained in antenatal and post-natal care. The pertinent areas of care for women include satisfactory quality and quantity of food, knowledge about fertility regulation and birth spacing, care during pregnancy and breastfeeding, safe prenatal and natal care, abundant time for rest and recreation (crucial for stress management), and safeguard from physical and emotional abuse (Engle, 1999). As laid out in Fig. 2.1, women's status impacts the quality of care for children not only directly (arrow A) but also indirectly through the quality of the care that the women themselves get (arrow B). Thus, the care received by women influences both the quality of care for children via the medium of women's own health and nutritional status, (arrow C) and children's nutritional status (arrow D).

In a majority of societies, women are the primary caregivers for young children, bearing the fundamental responsibility of health, well-being, and survival. Additionally, women are also the primary caregivers for themselves. Yet women with relatively low status to men usually have very little or no control over household and resources, face time constraints, and have negligible social support to deal with such constraints.

They have been found to have insufficient knowledge or inappropriate beliefs, along with poor mental health, low self-confidence, and self-esteem. In addition to the above limitations, women residing in communities with limited value placed on women's well-being than their male counterparts find accessing reproductive health services for themselves challenging and debilitating. These circumstances make it challenging for women to undertake the caring practices that are in the best interest of their children. They also tamper with a woman's ability to provide enough care for herself, further constraining her ability to give the care required by her children.

Extant literature shows that any additional income that is controlled by mothers leads to a higher household expenditure, with a major chunk being allocated towards child well-being including their food, education, and health services (Doss, 2006; Kumar & Quisumbing, 2012; McElroy, 1990; Quisumbing & Maluccio, 2003; Thomas, 1997). However, studies that trace this direct effect of women's asset ownership on child's health are scarce; the important reason being that there is hardly enough sex-disaggregated data on asset ownership. This study helps to bridge the gap that exists in knowledge by examining the linkage between women's asset ownership and children's nutritional status in India, a country with some significantly high rates of child stunting and wasting in the world and is a glaring example of *Asian Enigma* (Fig. 2.2). India proves to be a perfect case study for such research given the blatant gender discrimination and poor children's nutrition. The country ranks 104 out of 144 countries in the global gender index (WEF, 2017). Furthermore, the widely prevalent socio-economic inequalities and the challenges it poses (Mohanty and Pathak, 2008; Poel et al., 2008; Wagstaff et al., 2003; Zere and McIntyre, 2003) also make India eligible for this study.

2.1.4 How Are Asset-Based Interventions Important?

During the past decade, awareness and policy scrutiny on women's property rights had been increasing but the progress made so far has been majorly on ease of access, not ownership rights

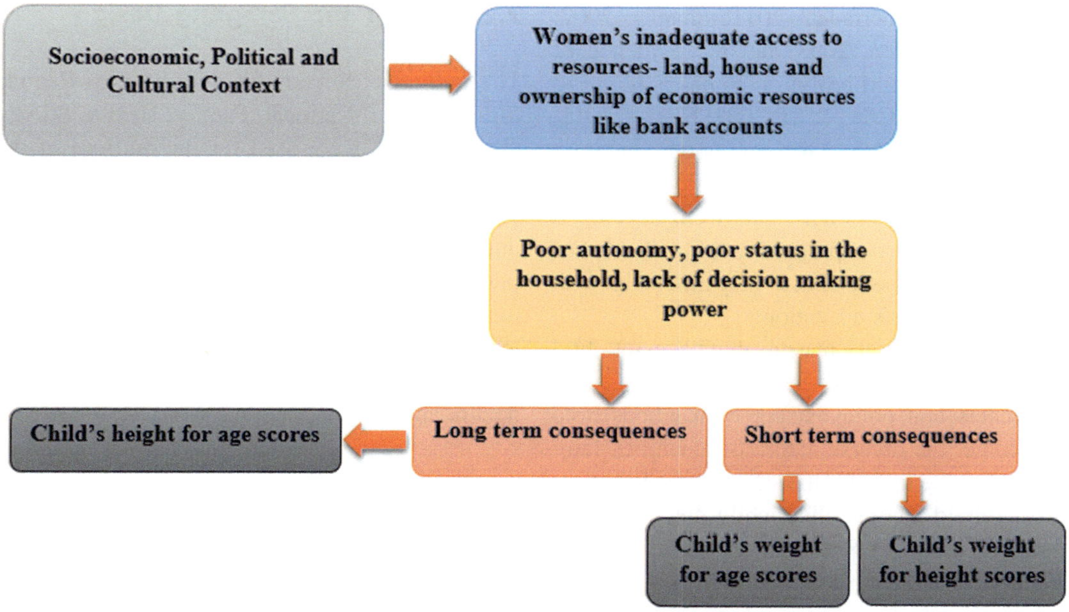

Fig. 2.2 Conceptual framework linking mother's asset ownership to child nutritional indicators. *Source* Authors

(International Center for Research on Women, 2005). An emerging arena of research is to understand the impact of women's asset ownership on various household-level determinants. A number of initial findings focus on the impact of assets, including improved usage of modern reproductive health services, better empowerment and social status, and ameliorated general household well-being. The impact on children's educational success and health due to asset holding has also been explored but the evidence has been rather limited. In recent years, policymakers have shown keen interest in implementing child development programs through asset-based interventions rather than traditional income support models (Loke, 2013).

Assets are looked upon as critical elements for poverty mitigation as they can have multifarious effects not only at the individual and household levels but also at the community levels. In the last decade, there has been an abundance of empirical studies on the role of assets family's welfare including child well-being. Various studies have singled out that household assets (net worth) positively affect children's educational outcomes (Conley, 2001; Chowa et al., 2013; Deng et al., 2014; Elliott & Sherraden, 2013; Filmer & Pritchett, 2001; Huang, 2011, 2013; Kim & Sherraden, 2011; Shanks, 2007; Zhan & Sherraden, 2003) but the evidence of asset effect on child health outcomes is found to be insubstantial (Chen & Li, 2008; Huang, 2011; Shariff & Ahn, 1995). Of the previous literature on the impact of asset accumulation on child education has always used data from developed countries, a massive proportion of such studies have estimated asset effects in partnership with effects of mother's education.

One of the primary reasons that the asset-child well-being linkage has been a topic of interest to researchers and policymakers is that household wealth, i.e. the diverse nature of amenities families can make use of rather than a small figment of household income affect child outcomes. For instance, assets (household or financial) may decrease economic stress, act as an alternative source of income, and empower people to flatten their consumption. Along similar lines, public assets such as provision of health services, water, hygiene and sanitation, schools, and transportation facilities can have a direct bearing on individual's well-being in myriad ways.

There are four prime hypotheses by which the assets-child development linkages are established. First, assets are pictured as household wealth that administers economic cohesion through a substitute source of income as well as easier trans-generational transfers of parental property as inheritance and gifts. Second, asset ownership reduces economic and psychological stress which may ultimately lead to better parenting and improved health condition. Third, parental behaviour that leads to asset aggregation may also lead to high demand for child quality and vice versa. The fourth hypothesis that networks public assets to individual welfare states that asset-rich households tend to live in localities where goods and services are located nearby providing their children with better opportunities. Based on the above-mentioned four hypotheses, this chapter tries to assess the effect of maternal asset holding on child health outcomes.

2.2 Data and Methods

2.2.1 Data and Sampling Design

The Individual Recode file and the Kids Recode file from the National Family Health Survey (2015–16) IV were used for the purpose of the analysis. With the first round beginning in 1993–93, three rounds of the survey have been conducted. The survey provides state and national information for India on fertility, infant and child mortality, the practice of family planning, maternal and child health, reproductive health, nutrition, anaemia, utilization and quality of health, and family planning services.

2.2.2 Study Population and Sample Size

The National Family Health Survey IV collected data from all 29 States and 7 Union Territories.

Sample size for males and females and children under 5 years of age were 112,122, 699,686, and 259,627, respectively.

2.2.3 Outcome Variable

A combined variable for asset holding was created by using four separate variables, namely, ownership of land, house, mobile phone, and having a bank account. The variable ranked from 0 to 1, with 0 indicating that a woman has none of the assets and 1 indicating that she owns at least one of the assets.

The data are used to examine the height-for-age (HAZ scores), weight-for-age (WAZ scores), and weight-for-height (WHZ scores) which are the determinants of children's nutritional status. At the lower tail of the distribution, this measure is an indicator of nutritional deprivation: children whose HAZ, WAZ, and WHZ scores are more than two standard deviations below the median of the international reference population for children of the same gender are considered stunted, underweight, and wasted, respectively. Only children in the age group of 6 months–2 years have been considered in the analysis to eliminate the effect of breastfeeding on child nutritional indicators. The HAZ scores are also used to create a Stunting Variable wherein 0 means the child is not stunted and 1 means the child is stunted. The Wasting and Underweight variables have been created in a similar way.

2.3 Statistical Analyses

2.3.1 Distribution of Asset Ownership of Women: Descriptive Statistics

Bivariate analysis along with descriptive statistics have been used to show the levels of asset ownership by females across different states in India. An asset index, called the basic asset index, simply adds the dummy variables for individual asset ownership together. The range for this index is from 0 (when a woman owns none of the asset types) to 4 (when a woman owns all four of the asset types).

2.3.2 Association of Women's Ownership of Assets with Child Stunting: Binary Logistic Regression

Z scores of height-for-age (stunting) were used to measure the nutritional status. The z-score measures based on children from a diverse set of countries such as Brazil, Ghana, India, Norway, Oman, and the USA (WHO, 2006, p. 1) put forward by WHO (2006) were used. Following WHO (1997), we define z-score as

$$\text{z score} = (x_i - x_{median})/\sigma_x$$

where x_i is the height of the ith child, x_{median} is the median height of the same age and gender from the reference population, and σ_x is the standard deviation from the mean of the reference population. The reference population's z-score has a standard normal distribution in the limit. Binary logistic regression has been used to establish the relationship between child stunting and background characteristics of both the parents. The binary category (1 = Child is Stunted, 0 = Child is not Stunted) for each respondent is related to a set of categorical predictors, X, by a logit function:

$$\text{logit}\ [P(Y = 1)] = \beta_0 + \beta_1 X + \varepsilon$$

In the above equation, β_0 estimates the log odds of the child being stunted for the reference group, while β_1 estimates the maximum likelihood, the differential log odds of the child being stunted associated with a set of predictors X as compared to the reference group and ε represents the residuals in the model.

2.3.3 Impact Estimation of Mother's Asset Ownership on Child Stunting: Quantile Regression

Quantile regression helps to analyse the impact of independent variables on different sections of the dependent variable distribution. Compared to the OLS comparison at the mean, it offers a more whole picture of the effects of female asset ownership. The parameter of quantile regression explains the marginal effect of an independent variable on a specified quantile of the dependent variable. And, thus estimated coefficients from various quantiles are comparable to each other. Given the structure of the anthropometrics, children at the left tail (poor health) of the distribution may have a disparate marginal response to a given independent variable than healthier children at the median or right tail of the distribution. The quantile regression equation is given below:

$$(Y_i) = \alpha(\tau)_0 + \alpha(\tau)_1 A_i + \alpha(\tau)_2 X_i + \varepsilon(\tau)_i$$

Here, τ indicates the specified quantile. We estimate the model at $\tau = 0.10, 0.25, 0.50, 0.75,$ and 0.90. The endogeneity of the assets may cause serious bias of causal effect of asset ownership on child outcomes. This endogeneity of assets may come from simultaneity, i.e. reverse causality or both. Simultaneity may occur when assets and the outcomes of interest cause each other. Similarly, reverse causality occurs when the asset growth is caused by the outcome of interest. In addition to this, the systematic differences among people may lead to some people to accumulate more assets than others. We rule out the endogeneity resulting from simultaneity and reverse causality because child health outcomes may not directly lead to asset accumulation.

Research has explained that estimating the impact of socio-economic variables (land ownership, etc.) on children's nutritional score can be deceptive given their differing impact along the conditional nutritional distribution (Aturupane et al., 2011). It is probable that some variables may have a significant impact at the lower end of the distribution even though they might not be as significant for a child's z-score on average. Thus, quantile regression model has been applied to enhance the understanding of the relationship between the variables of interest.

2.4 Results

2.4.1 Women's Ownership of Assets Across India

About 37, 28, 46, and 53% of females own a house, land, mobile phone, and bank account, respectively, in India. It is quite evident that the ownership of mobile phones and bank accounts is higher than that of house and land. States like Odisha (62.8%) and Bihar (57.8%) in the East and Manipur (66.8%), Arunachal Pradesh (58.6%), and Meghalaya (56.8%) in the Northeast have high ownership of house. States like Karnataka (50.6%) and Telangana (46.7%) in the South also have a comparatively higher proportion of 30 women who own a house. Coming to land ownership, the pattern is nearly the same as that of house ownership. States like Bihar (49.6%) and Odisha (46.5%) in the East have quite a high proportion of women who own a land either alone or jointly or both alone and jointly. Other states, which closely follow these states, are Arunachal Pradesh (49.8%), Assam (45.3%), and Meghalaya (42.5%) in the Northeast. It is surprising that, in a developed state like Kerala, a comparatively lower number of women own land and house but the ownership of mobile phones and bank accounts is quite high in Kerala (nearly 81% women own a mobile phone that they themselves use and 71% women have a bank account that they themselves use). When observing the pattern of ownership of mobiles, it is observed that states in the North like Chandigarh (74.2%), Delhi (66.6%), and Himachal Pradesh (73.9%) have a considerably higher proportion of women who own a mobile phone that they themselves use. States in the Northeast like Mizoram (77.0%), Nagaland (70.4%), and Sikkim (79.8%) also have a quite high proportion of women who have a mobile phone that they themselves use. In totality, the ownership of land and house is higher in some Eastern states like Odisha and North-eastern states like Assam and Manipur and the ownership of mobile phones and bank accounts is higher in some selected Northern states like Chandigarh and Southern states which are more developed like Kerala (Table 2.2).

Table 2.2 Women's ownership of assets in India

State/union territory	Own a house alone or jointly	Own a land alone or jointly	Have a mobile phone that they themselves use	Have a bank or savings account that they themselves use
India	37.2	28.3	45.9	53.0
North				
Chandigarh	20.7	14.9	74.2	79.6
Delhi	34.1	23.9	66.6	64.5
Haryana	35.1	27.2	50.5	45.6
Himachal Pradesh	9.8	8.9	73.9	68.8
Jammu and Kashmir	32.8	26.9	54.2	60.3
Punjab	31.7	22.2	57.2	58.8
Rajasthan	23.3	19.0	41.4	58.2
Uttarakhand	28.7	21.8	55.4	58.5
Central				
Chattisgarh	25.6	19.5	31.0	51.3
Madhya Pradesh	42.7	33.2	28.7	37.3
Uttar Pradesh	33.4	25.5	37.1	54.6
East				
Bihar	57.8	49.6	40.9	26.4
Jharkhand	48.9	40.8	35.2	45.1
Odisha	62.8	46.5	39.2	56.2
West Bengal	22.6	17.3	41.8	43.5
North-east				
Arunachal Pradesh	58.6	49.8	59.8	56.6
Assam	51.6	45.3	46.0	45.4
Manipur	66.8	37.0	63.1	34.8
Meghalaya	56.8	42.5	64.3	54.4
Mizoram	17.8	14.8	77.0	57.1
Nagaland	33.5	25.3	70.4	38.8
Sikkim	24.1	20.6	79.8	63.5
Tripura	56.2	33.8	43.9	59.2

(continued)

Table 2.2 (continued)

State/union territory	Own a house alone or jointly	Own a land alone or jointly	Have a mobile phone that they themselves use	Have a bank or savings account that they themselves use
West				
Dadra & Nagar Haveli	21.1	18.6	36.9	36.9
Daman & Diu	25.4	16.6	60.6	61.9
Goa	33.4	14.0	80.9	82.8
Gujarat	26.8	18.8	47.9	48.6
Maharashtra	33.2	23.0	45.6	45.3
South				
Andaman & Nicobar Islands	28.1	17.5	66.9	81.8
Andhra Pradesh	42.7	26.4	36.2	66.3
Karnataka	50.6	40.1	47.1	59.4
Kerala	29.2	23.4	81.2	70.6
Lakshadweep	38.0	30.4	64.9	74.4
Puducherry	39.3	24.6	67.3	68.2
Tamil Nadu	34.7	26.6	62.0	77.0
Telangana	46.7	30.3	47.4	59.5

Source NFHS-4, 2015–16

2.4.2 Nutritional Status of Children by Selected Characteristics and Across India

While nearly 38% of female children have height-for-age scores below −2SD, the percentage is 39% for male children. The gap increases when only children −3SD are considered. The case for wasting and underweight is identical. The percentage of children stunted, wasted, and underweight increases with the increase in the birth order of children. The figures are even higher when we consider height-for-age scores below −2SD. While only 12 and 31% children, respectively, have height-for-age scores below −3SD and −2SD in urban areas, the figures increase to 18 and 41%, respectively, for rural areas. Similar trend is observed for wasting and underweight as well. While 27 and 53% of babies whose birth size is very small have height-for-age scores below −2SD and −3SD, respectively, the percentage is comparatively lesser for those babies whose birth size is average or bigger. As the educational level of mothers increases, the percentage of children who have height-for-age scores below −2SD and −3SD decreases. With the increase in mother's BMI, the percentage of children stunted, wasted and underweight decreases. Also, with the increase in wealth quintile, the percentage of children who have height-for-age scores, weight-for-age scores, and weight-for-height scores below −2SD and −3SD decreases.

Percentage of under-5 children categorized as malnourished according to three anthropometric indices of nutritional status: height-for-age, weight-for-height, and weight-for-age, by background characteristics, India, 2015–16.

Nearly 38, 21, and 36% of children in India are stunted, wasted, and underweight, respectively. Bihar (48%), Uttar Pradesh (46%),

Jharkhand (45%), Meghalaya (44%), and Madhya Pradesh (42%) are the states in which the prevalence of stunting is among the highest. Similar observations can be made for wasting and underweight as well (Table 2.3 and Fig. 2.3).

2.4.3 Women's Ownership of Assets and Its Linkages with Child Undernutrition in India

2.4.3.1 Mother's Characteristics

This table shows the odds of a child being stunted, wasted, and underweight given the background characteristics of the mother and father. Since asset ownership is our main variable, we analyse the impact of asset ownership on child stunting first. The children of those females who are in the highest category of asset ownership are least likely to be stunted, that is, the odds of children being stunted decrease as mothers move higher in the category of asset ownership. Thus, the children whose mother owns all the four assets are nearly 0.8 times less likely to be stunted, wasted, and underweight as compared to children of those mothers who do not own any asset at all. The children whose mothers having the highest level of education are 0.4, 0.7, and 0.3 times less likely to be stunted, wasted, and underweight than those with mothers having no education.

Table 2.3 Nutritional status of children by background characteristics

	Height-for-age		Weight-for-height		Weight-for-age	
Background characteristics	Percentage below −3SD	Percentage below −2SD	Percentage below −3SD	Percentage below −2SD	Percentage below −3SD	Percentage below −2SD
Age in months						
<6	9.3	19.9	14.9	31.9	9.3	26.4
6–23	16.3	36.1	8.5	23.9	10.5	33
24 and above	17.1	42	5.9	18.2	11.4	38.3
Sex						
Male	16.9	38.9	7.9	21.9	11.1	36.1
Female	15.6	37.9	6.9	20.1	10.9	35.3
Birth interval (months)						
First birth	13.0	33.4	7.2	20.5	9	31.6
<24	21.7	46.9	7.4	21.1	14.5	42.5
24–25	19.4	43.4	7.9	22.2	12.8	40.5
36+	15.5	36.9	7.5	20.9	10.4	34.1
Birth order						
1	13.0	33.4	7.2	20.5	9	31.6
2–3	16.4	39.0	7.4	21.1	10.9	36.1
4 and above	24.7	50.4	8.2	22.4	16.8	46
Residence						
Urban	12.0	31.0	7.5	20	8.2	29.1
Rural	17.9	41.2	7.4	21.4	12.1	38.3

(continued)

Table 2.3 (continued)

	Height-for-age		Weight-for-height		Weight-for-age	
Background characteristics	Percentage below −3SD	Percentage below −2SD	Percentage below −3SD	Percentage below −2SD	Percentage below −3SD	Percentage below −2SD
Size at birth						
Very small	26.9	52.8	10	28.1	23.3	53.5
Small	20.0	45.1	8.4	24.5	15.9	44.6
Average or larger	15.5	37.1	7.3	20.5	10	34.2
Mother's schooling						
No schooling	24.8	50.7	8.1	22.7	16.7	46.8
<5 years complete	18.5	45.3	7.6	22.2	12.6	41.9
5–7 years complete	16.0	39.8	7.5	21.6	11	37.6
8 and above	10.7	29.3	7	19.7	7.3	27.5
Religion						
Hindu	16.4	38.3	7.6	21.5	11.3	36.3
Muslim	17.1	39.8	6.9	19.4	10.6	34.9
Christian	12.4	29.9	6.4	18.5	7	27.2
Others	12.6	33.0	7.8	20.5	9.4	31.3
Caste						
Scheduled Caste	19.0	42.8	7.5	21.2	12.6	39.1
Scheduled Tribe	19.7	43.8	10.3	27.4	16.1	45.3
OBC	16.4	38.7	7.2	20.5	10.7	35.5
Others	11.9	31.2	6.5	19	7.8	28.8
Mother's BMI						
Underweight	20.5	45.8	8.9	26.7	16.3	47.8
Normal	16.2	38.2	7.5	20.4	10.3	34.3
Overweight	9.4	27.1	4.8	14.2	5	21.7
Wealth index						
Poorest	25.7	51.4	8.7	24.2	17.8	48.6
Poorer	18.3	43.5	7.5	21.7	12.5	40.4
Rich	13.5	36.5	7	20.2	8.9	33.2
Richer	10.6	29.2	6.8	19.3	6.8	27.4
Richest	7.9	22.2	6.6	17.9	5.1	20.1

Footnote −2 standard deviations (SD) includes children who are below −3 standard deviations (SD) from the international reference population median
Source Based on NFHS-4, 2015–16

Stunting

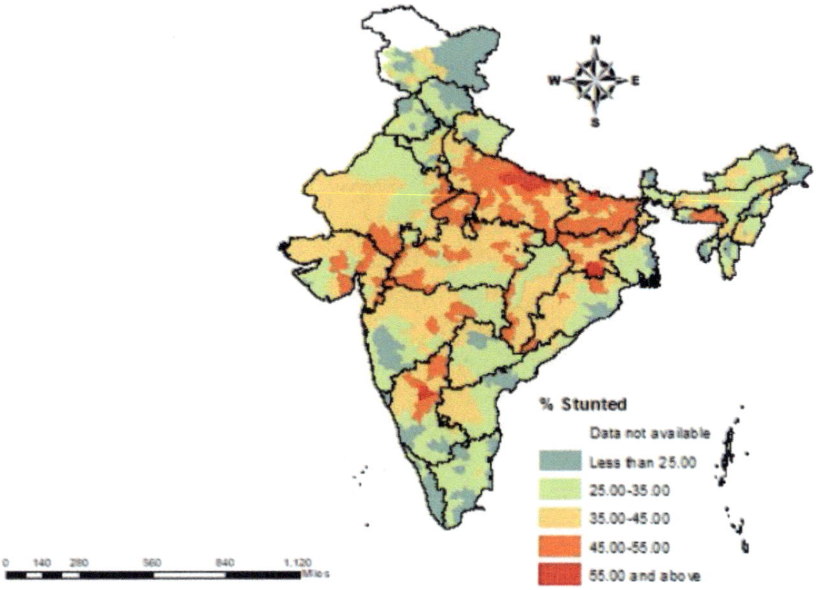

Source: *Made by authors based on estimates from NFHS-4, 2015-16*

Wasting

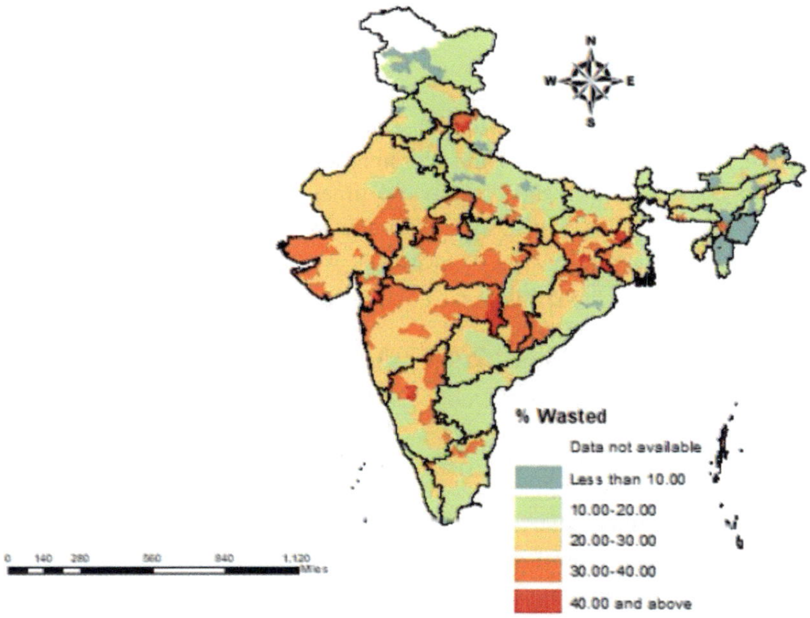

Source: *Made by authors based on estimates from NFHS-4, 2015-16*

Fig. 2.3 Nutritional status of children by Indian districts: 2015–16

Underweight

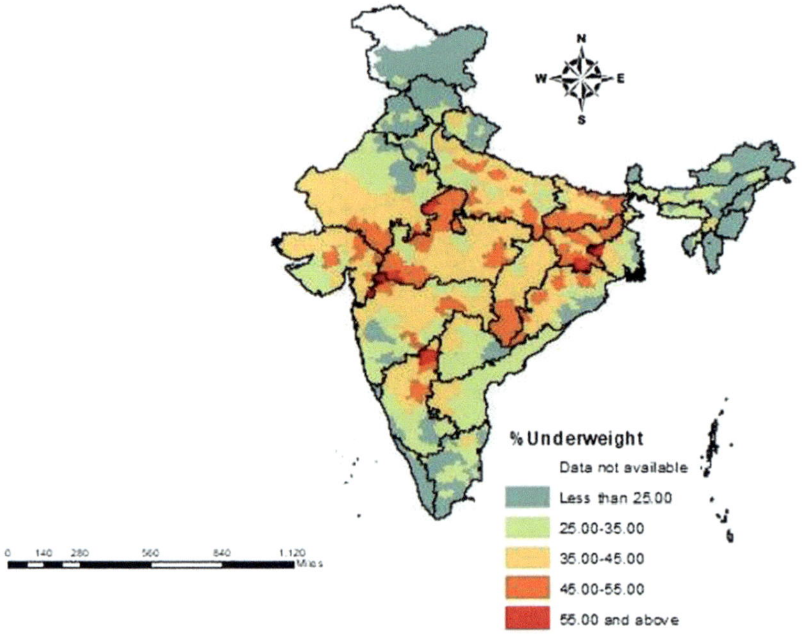

Source: *Made by authors based on estimates from NFHS-4, 2015-16*

Fig. 2.3 (continued)

2.4.3.2 Father's Characteristics

Just like mothers' education, the odds of children being stunted are indirectly associated with the educational qualification of fathers. Thus, children whose fathers are in the higher category of education are 0.5, 0.9, and 0.6 times less likely to be stunted, wasted, and underweight, respectively, than those whose fathers have no education at all. Talking about the geographical regions, children belonging to the Central, Eastern, and Western states are 1.6, 1.4, and 1.3 times, respectively, more likely to be stunted that those children who belong to the Northern states (which is the reference category). Similar observations are recorded for wasting and underweight as well (Table 2.4).

2.4.3.3 Child's Characteristics

A female child is nearly 0.9 times less likely to be stunted, wasted, and underweight as compared to a male child. The odds of children being stunted, wasted, and underweight increase with the increase in the birth order of children. Thus, the children who are of order 4 and above are nearly 1.3 times more likely to be stunted, wasted, and underweight than those children who are of second or lesser order.

2.4.4 Analysis of Effects of Mother's Asset Ownership on Different Parts of Distribution of Child Height-for-Age Scores

Quantile regression permits an analysis of the impact on different sections of the dependent variable distribution of the independent variables. Compared to the OLS comparison at the mean, it can offer a more comprehensive picture of the effects of female asset ownership. The quantile regression parameter explains the marginal effect on a specified quantile of the dependent variable of an independent variable.

Table 2.4 Odds ratio of child undernutrition indicators based on mothers' background characteristics

Socio-demographic variables	Stunting	Wasting	Underweight
Mother's characteristics			
Asset ownership (ref. none)			
1	0.90*	0.91**	0.95**
2	0.87*	0.88*	0.89*
3	0.89	0.82*	0.88
4	0.81*	0.84	0.81*
Level of education (ref. no education)			
Primary	0.87**	0.90*	0.85*
Secondary	0.66*	0.82*	0.64*
Higher	0.40**	0.65*	0.37*
Mother's BMI (ref. Low)			
Normal	0.85**	0.91*	0.79**
High	0.72*	0.82*	0.65*
Father's characteristics			
Father's education (ref. no education)			
Primary	0.94*	1.10	0.98**
Secondary	0.76**	0.93**	0.76*
Higher	0.58**	0.89**	0.60**
Geographic regions (ref. north)			
Central	1.61*	1.17*	1.84*
East	1.41*	1.23	1.78*
Northeast	1.00	0.67*	0.71*
West	1.38**	1.56*	1.84*
South	1.03	1.22*	1.25*
Child's characteristics			
Sex of the child (ref. male)			
Female	0.93*	0.88**	0.95**
Birth order (ref. less than 2)			
2–3	1.11**	1.01	1.11*
4 and above	1.24**	1.02	1.18**

The notation ** is $p < 0.05$, * is $p < 0.01$
Sample is children of married mothers (n = 40,729)
Regression is controlled for mass media exposure variables
Note It excludes children less than 6 months to eliminate the impact of breastfeeding
Source Authors' calculation from NFHS-4, 2015–16

These estimated coefficients from various quantiles are comparable. Given the structure of the anthropometrics, the response to a given independent variable maybe disparately mariginal at the left tail (poor health) of the distribution than the healthier children at the median or right tail of the distribution. These differences are not visible with the OLS estimated coefficients. Quantile regression analysis may be used to study specific portions of the child nutrition z-score distributions. Studies have used this method to detect crucial asymmetrical effects of various treatments on child health in developing countries. This table presents quantile-regression estimated

Table 2.5 Summary of quantile regression estimates for mother's asset ownership indices

	Quantiles				
Asset index coefficients for HAZ scores	0.10	0.25	0.5	0.75	0.90
Asset ownership	3.84*	4.14*	4.27**	4.89*	5.45*
Asset index coefficients for WHZ scores	**0.10**	**0.25**	**0.5**	**0.75**	**0.90**
Asset ownership	4.22**	4.69*	4.99*	6.02*	6.77*
Asset index coefficients for WAZ scores	**0.10**	**0.25**	**0.5**	**0.75**	**0.90**
Asset ownership	3.64*	3.81*	4.09*	4.46*	6.33**

The notation ** is $p < 0.05$, * is $p < 0.01$
Sample is children of married mothers (n = 40,729)
Source Authors' calculation from NFHS-4, 2015–16

coefficients for the asset ownership of mothers. It is evident that HAZ scores are greater for children of mothers with asset ownership. The table indicates that the basic additive index has a positive impact on the HAZ scores, which are an indicator of long-term nutritional status. Focusing on the asset ownership, at the median, a one-unit increase in this asset index increases the HAZ score by 4.3 points compared to 4.9 and 5.5 points at the 75th and 90th quantiles, respectively. Similarly, a one-unit increase in this asset index increases the WHZ score by 5.0 points compared to 6.0 and 6.8 points at the 75th and 90th quantiles, respectively. Results obtained for WAZ scores are along similar lines. The findings suggest that women's asset ownership influences the nutritional status of those who are already relatively healthy (Table 2.5).

2.5 Discussion

In recent years, the allocation of land rights and ownership of other assets has become a pertinent issue in India because of their established role in ameliorating the welfare of both the household and the community. There is significant evidence in developing countries that women's asset ownership increases women's autonomy and positively impacts children's health outcomes. There has been, however, a dearth of literature in India on women's asset ownership and its impact on child health outcomes. This study is not only limited to filling this decisive gap in the literature but also aims to shape collective understanding of the association between mothers' asset ownership and its impact on the health of her children's nutritional security. By using nationally representative data from India, this study provides empirical estimates of the relationship between women's asset ownership and children's nutritional status. Additionally, the study tries to understand the differential impact of mothers' asset ownership on different sections of distribution of child HAZ, WHZ, and WAZ scores. The results indicate that women's asset ownership helps reduce childhood stunting, wasting, and underweight in India. It was also found that the beneficial impact of mother's asset ownership on children's nutritional status occurs at different parts of the distribution, with children who are already better nourished benefitting more from their mothers' asset ownership.

The important finding of this study is that women's asset ownership helps to reduce child stunting, wasting, and underweight. This result is consistent with previous studies (Menon et al., 2014; Quisumbing & Maluccio, 2003; Rehman et al., 2019; Smith et al., 2003; World Bank, 2010), which stated that not only women's own welfare but also intra-household food security and nutritional status of children improve with women's access to and control of assets. Previous research has also suggested that it is not just the ownership of assets that influences development outcomes but also who has control over it.

Furthermore, the study confirms the hypotheses that women's status has a considerable impact on child nutrition given their higher household status translating to better nutritional status themselves, better cared for, and provide higher quality care to their children. However, the strength of the impact of women's status and the linkages through which it affects child nutrition differ substantially across regions. The implication of this study's results is lucid: in the interest of sustainably buttressing the nutritional status of children, it is imperative that necessary steps be taken towards improving women's status across all regions. It is extremely pertinent to do so for South Asia, especially India. Accomplishing this mammoth task reckons policy measures that eradicates gender discrimination and policies that limit power inequities between women and men by actively promoting women. Examples of the above include enabling women to gain access to new resources, contriving cash transfer programs that encourage girls' education and health care, advancing technologies that save household labour, funding childcare for working parents, and instituting programs to ameliorate the nutritional status of adolescent girls and young women.

Studies differentiate between individual and joint ownership of assets for women and look at their impacts on children's welfare separately (Rehman et al., 2019). However, given the limitation of the small sample size in the dataset that has been used in the study, the two categories have been clubbed together to form a single category. It is worthwhile to mention that there is certainly a difference in the impact of individual and joint ownership of assets on child nutritional outcomes. There are reasons that are put forth for this. Studies state that one of the probable reasons for the differing impact of individual and joint asset ownership on children's nutritional outcomes could be due to the benefits of individual or joint ownership not being straightforward (Razavi, 2003). For instance, if a land is shared, a woman may not enjoy equal authority and flexibility to manage her plot from production, to claiming land after divorce. Conversely, if the land is owned by a woman alone, although she might have all the rights, there could be resource constraints, especially if the land that she owns is small. Another possible reason could be that the variables used in the current study define ownership, but do not provide ample information about who actually controls the assets in joint ownership. This is especially pertinent in developing countries like India where joint ownership of assets may be biased towards men. This entails that policies aimed at encouraging joint ownership of assets should be designed and implemented in a prudent way, only after ensuring that women have equal access to and control over assets. In addition to the above, there is also a need to design future research endeavours to use more detailed survey data to understand both the ownership and control of assets.

The role played by a woman as the food producer, and nutritional and household food security caretaker is extensively commended in the development literature. A household's decision to spend a considerable amount of monetary resource on food consumption and human resource formation is governed by the gender pattern in the control over economic resources, especially monetary (Tangka et al., 2000; Thomas, 1997). With women committing more to the household income via agriculture, animal husbandry, and caregiving they are expected to have a more important role in household decision-making, especially those pertaining to food and nutrition. Rogers (1996) has reported that, with an increased control over household resources, the consumption inclinations of women customarily places the welfare of children prior to anything else and favour their basic needs. The literature on intra-household kinetics also shows that developmental outcomes of the child are limited to not only the household assets but also who asserts controls ove those assets. It has been proven that women's access to and control over assets lead to an amelioration not only in their own welfare but also plays an instrumental role in augmenting household food security and child nutrition and education (Quisumbing & Maluccio, 2003; Smith et al., 2003a; World Bank, 2010).

In communities that confront alterations in the power balance between genders, policies can help alleviate the unintended impacts of this imbalance, rather than targeting it directly. Directing the focus of health services towards communities where women's status is low is one of the prominent examples of this indirect approach to address the gender imbalance issue. This study produces results that state unequivocally that making policy decisions aimed at improving women's status produces considerable benefits. Its impact would not be limited to improvement in a woman's own nutritional status but also the nutritional status of her children. Ameliorating women's status today is a powerful force for buttressing the physical, mental capacity, and productivity of the coming generation of young adults.

2.6 Implications for Policy and Program Development

In this chapter, we have presented the findings of our research on the affect that assets have on women and children in India. A comprehensive asset-building policy manifestation that targets women and children and pursues to ameliorate their well-being would act as a colossal step in the correct direction. The findings of the chapter make it clear that there is an ardent need of more focused research to investigate the effects of asset ownership on women and children. As per the above discussion, it is recommended that women's rights to land and other productive assets should be reinforced more effectively through the adoption of an integrated framework approach, whilst also manoeuvring efforts towards changing traditional attitudes and institutional arrangements. For instance, there should be concerted efforts to promote the mobility of women to boost their participation in financial activities and encourage the usage of these incomes to ensure the well-being of themselves and their children. Additionally, there is also a need for architecture financial institutions so as to provide women easy access to credit (Ahmad, 2011) and provide them with necessary skills needed to manage their assets. It is noteworthy that India already has a set of lucid formal laws pertaining to asset ownership and control for both men and women. However, the predominance of customary laws and traditional notions leaves little scope for these laws to actually empower women. Thus, besides enacting stricter laws and policies, there is also an ardent need to create mass awareness about women's rights in the society. This can be done using influential people such as clerics and priests. This will not only help in bringing about systemic changes in the social fabric of our country but also help women and others in society to understand their rights and the benefits accruing from the same to their children.

The ideal situation would be to have more longitudinal studies that could give a glimpse of the causal relationships with changes in asset accumulation pathways. These avenues might also include savings programs for over a period of time targeted towards women and children with alteration of whether government and/or other donors are providing stimuli, whether the children are committing towards the accounts, and grades of community association. Better and more convincing insights on the relevance of targeted programs and policies for women and children might be extracted from these findings.

However, it would need a multipronged approach. Other policy initiatives that tackle the legal concerns to safeguard the assets of women and children would need to coordinate and complement these policies. The outcome of such a policy is, thus, best placed in the mainstream economy with financial establishments that are overseen by the law. This ensures that savings would be safeguarded and recipients would have easy ingress to their savings. Similarly, legal systems should also frequent asset ownership protection that would otherwise not place women's ownership under the ambit of their protection. Research on asset effects for women and children will help in knowledge and consensus building for reformist asset-building initiatives that will prove to be catalytic for policies that augment household well-being. The key players building this knowledge on the impact of asset ownership on women and children and their well-being could be large-scale longitudinal and random assignment of women and children to asset-building programs and controls.

2.7 Conclusion

This study is especially germane when considered within the current context of India being committed to achieving the *Zero Hunger goal* of Sustainable Development Goal by 2030, and with food security and nutrition being made a public health priority. Additionally, there has been an increased recognition of women's property rights and empowerment in recent times. This study expects to aid policymakers dealing with food security and nutrition by providing empirical evidence that improving women's lives, their right to assets, and financial independence will also lead to better nutritional outcomes for their children. The results of our study largely support all initiatives or programs designated to promote women's land rights. This study is one of the first of its kind to directly measure the impact of women's asset ownership on the nutritional status of their children, to the best of our knowledge. This study concludes that women's ownership of assets positively impacts children's nutritional status in both the short term and long term. However, to reap potential benefits from women's ownership of assets, concerted efforts on various fronts would be required, including changes in cultural attitudes, perceptions, and institutional frameworks in the country. In totality, the results suggest that assets are a pertinent component of social policies that cast focus on both individual and public welfare programs. As the impact of assets on child outcomes is based on the class of assets owned, policy initiatives that encourage and support build-up asset endowment should be implemented, however, with a note of caution. Policies that amalgamate asset transfers with the traditional income support module may be more efficient than the income support module alone.

Key Findings
About 43.3%, 54% and 78.6% females own a house/land, mobile phones and bank account respectively in India (2019-21).
Nearly 35.5% 19.3% and 32.1% of children in India are stunted, wasted and underweight respectively (2019-21).
Bihar and Kerala, with 48% and 20% of stunted children, has the highest and lowest prevalence respectively of child stunting in India. Similar observations can be made for wasting and underweight as well.
Male children are more likely to be stunted, wasted and underweight than female children are.
Both mothers' and fathers' education have positive impacts on the nutritional status of their children.
Women's asset ownership impacts the nutritional status of those who are already relatively healthy

Nutrition Scenario Among Elderly in India

3

Abstract

This chapter is an attempt to delve into the current scenario of elderly nutrition in India. With the global elderly population crossing the 10% mark in 2020 and expected to escalate to 16% by 2050, it becomes crucial to understand that the elderly is a vulnerable and heterogeneous group that reckons attention and concerted policy interventions. With all the policy focus on maternal and child nutrition, the nutritional requirements of the elderly population are often neglected and not catered to. Through this chapter, we argue that there is a considerable proportion of elderly in India who suffer from undernutrition and should, therefore, be a focus of policymaking initiatives. The ageing process manifests itself through changes in physical, and psycho-social conditions of a person. Being an important part of health of elderly, nutrition has a massive impact on the entire process of ageing. The proportion of elderly suffering from both undernutrition and overnutrition is increasing rapidly, both globally and in India and this leads to functional limitations, anaemia, hindered muscle function, reduced bone density, decreased cognitive function, issues with the immune system, dismal wound healing capacity, delayed recovery process, higher hospitalization rates, and death. Recent changes in family and kinship structure have resulted in elderly staying alone and taking care of themselves. This may prove to be detrimental for their nutritional status. Routine prognosis of the nutritional status among elderly necessitates the need for increased awareness about their nutrition and health, and, thus, this chapter aims to provide information with an educational overview of different facets related to nutrition and associated changes that occur with ageing.

Keywords

SDGs · India · BMI · Elderly · Life-course approach

3.1 Introduction

3.1.1 Global Population Ageing: A Victory and a Challenge

As stated by Gro Harlem Brundtland, Director-General, World Health Organization, 1999, "*Population ageing is first and fore a success story for public health policies as well as social and economic development. ...*". There is a continuous change in the age structure of the population globally, primarily heralded by an increase in life expectancy along with a concomitant reduction in fertility and mortality rates. People all over the world are living longer and, consequently, both the share and absolute number of

A. Chattopadhyay et al., *Undernutrition in India*, Sustainable Development Goals Series,
https://doi.org/10.1007/978-981-19-8182-1_3

elderly in the total population are rapidly escalating. The number of elderly aged 65 and above was 727 million globally in 2020. Projections place this estimate at 1.5 billion in 2050, over the next three decades. It is estimated that all regions will witness rapid advances in the share of their elderly population in the next three decades. Unsurprisingly, the global share of elderly aged 65 years or above is estimated to rise to 16.0% by 2050 from the current level of 9.3% (United Nations, 2019a). About 67% of the estimated increase in the share of elderly population is expected to happen in Asia, where studies project a threefold increase in their numbers from 330 million in 2015 to 956 million in 2050 (UNDESA, 2017). Similarly, the older population of Latin America and the Caribbean is projected to grow nearly three times, while that of Africa is expected to increase 3.5-fold. Relatively meagre changes are expected in Oceania, where the increase is expected to be a little over two times, and in Europe and Northern America, where the corresponding share is expected to increase by 44 and 50%, respectively. While Europe will observe an increase in the proportion of population aged 65 and above, this will be accompanied by a decrease in the proportion of the younger age groups by 2050 (UNDESA, 2017) (Fig. 3.1).

Age composition, defined by the proportion of people in all age groups, i.e. children, adolescents, middle-aged adults, and elderly in any given country, is a crucial aspect for policymakers to consider. Ageing of population is said to occur when there is a marked rise in the proportion of people aged 60 years and above with a decline in the proportion of children and people in the younger age groups. With this change in population age, the triangular shape of the population pyramid of 2000 will be replaced with a more cylindrical structure in 2050, with the area of the bottom of the pyramid becoming smaller and the top becoming broader (Fig. 3.2).

Until recently, the developed regions of the world have been associated with population ageing. For instance, Europe houses nine out of ten countries with the largest proportion of elderly population and more than ten million inhabitants. It is expected that the ranking will remain more or less unchanged by 2025 elderly aged 60 years and above will constitute about 33% of the population in countries like Germany, Italy, and Japan, followed closely by other European countries (WHO, 2002).

3.1.2 Global and Regional Trends in Population Ageing

Recent trends point towards the faster rate of growth of elderly population in the developing countries as compared to their developed counterparts (UNDESA, 2019). As a consequence of the above, the developing regions house a rapidly increasing share of the global elderly population (Fig. 1.3). While the developing regions housed about 56% of elderly aged 60 years and above in 1980, this share grew to two-thirds of the total population in 2017. The number of elderly residing in developing regions are projected to more than double between 2017 and 2050,

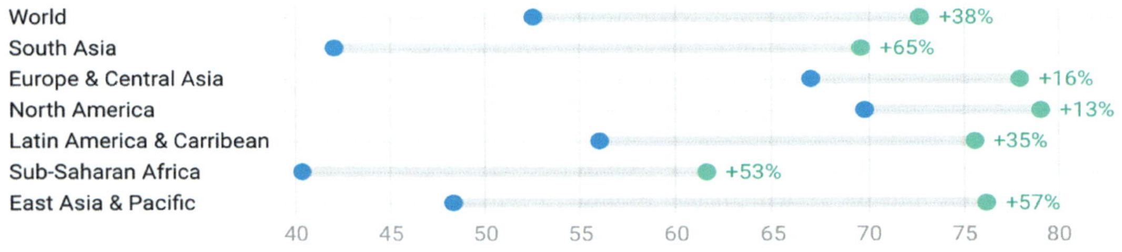

Fig. 3.1 Percentage change in global life expectancy at birth, 1960–2019. *Source* Created by authors using World Bank Data

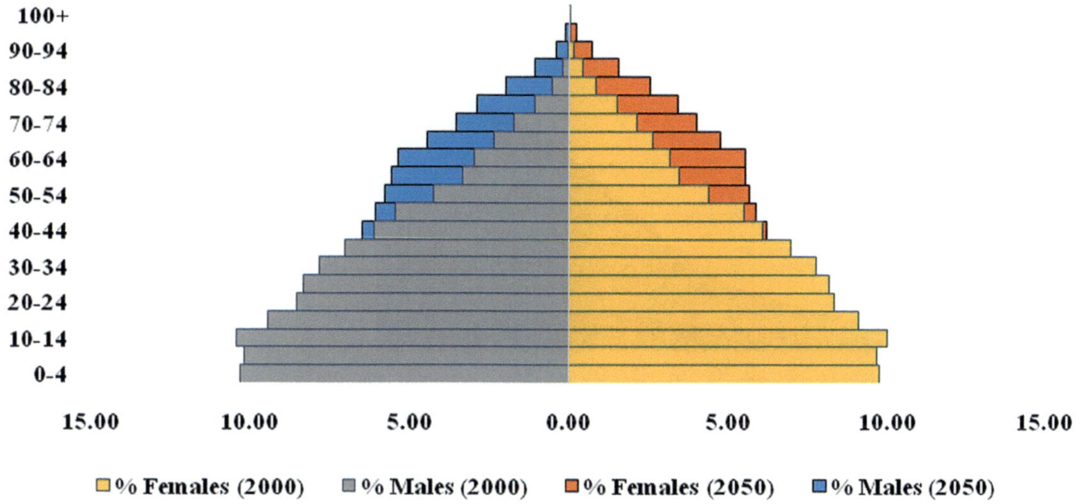

Fig. 3.2 Global population pyramid in 2000 and 2050. *Source* Created by authors using World Population Prospects: the 2019 Revision data

jumping to 1.7 billion from 652 million. The developed regions, on the contrary, are expected to see an increase of 38% in the proportion of elderly during the same period. The figures are expected to rise from 310 million elderly in 2017 to 427 million in 2050. Estimates suggest that the developing regions will be home to nearly 79% of the global elderly population in 2050 (UNDESA, 2019).

Increase in the proportion of elderly is happening globally: estimates suggest that al all the countries will witness a considerable rise in the size of population aged 60 years and above between 2017 and 2050 (UNDESA, 2019). It is, however, worth noting that there are widespread differentials in the growth rates of the elderly population not only between regions but also within regions and income groups. Globally, the rate of increase in the number of elderly is expected to surpass the population in the younger age groups. In 1980, children aged 10 years and below surpassed the elderly population by a substantial amount (1.1 billion children versus 0.4 billion elderly). However, estimates suggest that the global elderly population will have surpassed the population of children aged 10 years and below by 2030 (1.41 billion elderly versus 1.35 billion children) (Fig. 3.3). Estimates also suggest that there will be a greater proportion of elderly as compared to the younger age groups in 2050 (2.1 billion versus 2.0 billion). It is also noteworthy that the number of oldest-old people is also increasing rapidly: the global population of elderly aged 80 years and above is projected to increase three folds between 2017 and 2050, increasing from 137 to 425 million (UNDESA, 2019).

In most of the countries, a decline in fertility leads to an increase in the proportion of elderly population. Globally, one in eight people was aged 60 years and above in 2017. This figure is expected to increase to one in five in 2050 (UNDESA, 2019). Although the developed regions of Europe and North America are in much advanced stages of population ageing, where more than one in five persons was an elderly in 2017, a rapid increase in the proportion of elderly is being observed in other regions as well. The elderly population is projected to account for nearly 9% in Africa, 23% in Oceania, 24% in Asia, 25% in Latin America and the Caribbean, 25% in Latin America and the Caribbean, 28% in Northern America, and 35% of the population in Europe, by 2050 (Fig. 3.4).

In 1980, the top ten countries with world's highest proportion of elderly population were

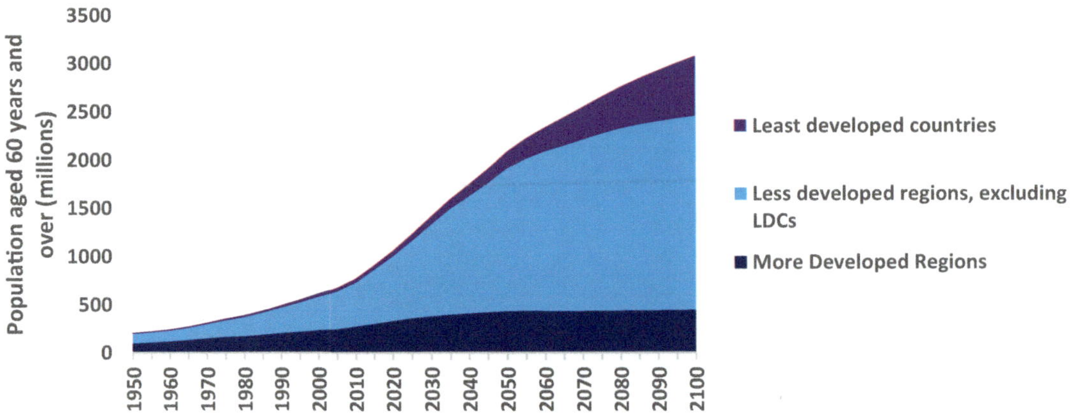

Fig. 3.3 Region-wise number of persons aged 60 years or above, 1950–2100. *Source* Created by authors using World Population Prospects: the 2019 Revision data

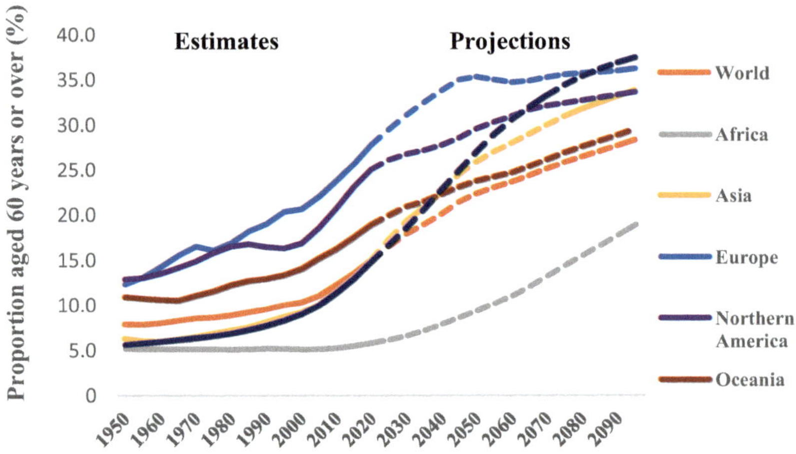

Fig. 3.4 Proportion of elderly population by region, from 1950 to 2100. *Source* Created by authors using World Population Prospects: the 2019 Revision

situated in Europe and the proportion of elderly population globally had not breached the 25% mark in any region or country (UNDESA, 2019). However, in 2017, this proportion surpassed the 25% mark in those top ten aged countries and it is estimated that the elderly population will constitute more than 39% of the population of each of the ten aged countries in the world by 2050. In 2017, Japan was home to world's aged population (33% elderly aged 60 and above) and it is projected that the status quo will be maintained till 2050 (42% elderly aged 60 and above). Along similar lines, Europe is projected to house five of the ten aged countries or regions in 2050 (UNDESA, 2019).

3.1.3 Elderly in India: An Expanding Age Group

Comprising 17% of the global population, India's population of 1.31 billion is the second largest population globally after China, and India is expected to overtake China by 2028 (United Nations, 2015) (Table 3.1). The proportion of elderly population in India is becoming increasingly noticeable with India's growing population. The rate of growth of elderly population in India at present is thrice that of the total population as a whole (Giridhar et al., 2014). The prominent increase in the proportion of elderly population is being driven by three important demographic

Table 3.1 Countries with the greatest absolute number of elderly, 2015 and 2050

2015		2050	
Country	Number of elderly (thousands)	Country	Number of elderly (thousands)
China	209,240	China	491,533
India	116,553	India	330,043
USA	66,545	USA	108,326
Japan	41,873	Japan	69,882
Russia	28,730	Russia	61,896

Source United Nations (2015)

processes, first, a decline in fertility owing to the ready availability and increased usage of contraceptive methods, an increase in the mean age at marriage (especially among females) and a reduction in the infant mortality rate, second, advancements in life expectancy due to progress on different fronts such as health, nutrition, medicine, water, and sanitation facilities and, third, progression of large cohorts to older ages (Bloom et al., 2014b). There have been tremendous improvements in life expectancy at birth (LEB), with LEB increasing from 41.4 years in 1960 to 69.7 years in 2018 and expected to increase to 75.9 years by 2050 (World Bank, 2019) (Fig. 3.5). Another factor playing an instrumental role in increasing the proportion of elderly in certain communities is the high rate of international out-migration, especially among middle-aged working individuals. In 2013 itself, India was the highest sender of international migrants, with more than 14 million people of Indian origin living outside India (Pew Research Center, 2013).

According to the Technical Group on Population Projections for India and States 2011–2036 report, the number of senior people increased by over 34 million over the population census of 2011 in 2021, and this number is predicted to increase by another 56 million elderly people in 2031. It is interesting to notice that, up until 1991, older women outweighed older men. Since then, however, the pattern has reversed, with older men now outnumbering older women (Fig. 3.6). In addition, it is predicted that by 2031, there will be more old men than women. A rise in life expectancy, which is a result of better healthcare and medical facilities, a decline in childbearing rates, and economic prosperity, may be the cause of this rise in the share of the old population. Another intriguing finding is that, whereas the general population increased at a rate of 12.4% from 2011 to 2021 and at an 18% rate from the previous decade, the old population increased at a rate of 36% from 2001 to 2011 and 36% from 2021 to 2023, respectively (NSO, 2021).

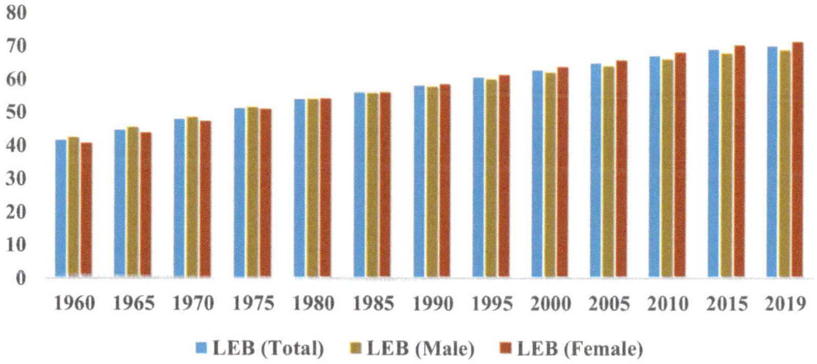

Fig. 3.5 Life expectancy at birth in India, 1960–2019. *Source* Created by authors using World Bank data

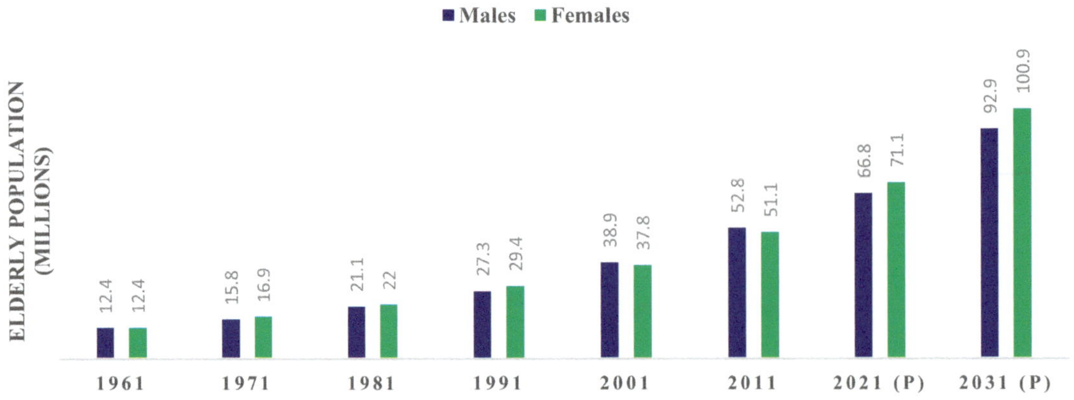

Fig. 3.6 Distribution of Elderly Population (60 Years & Above), India. *Source* NSO, 2021. *Note* P- Projections

When compared to the overall population, the senior population saw a similar high growth rate between 1961 and 1981. Since 1961, there has been a rising tendency in India's senior population as a percentage of the country's overall population. About 5.6% of Indians were 60 and older in 2016, but that number increased to 10.1% in 2021 and is projected to reach 13.1% in 2031. (NSO, 2021). Similar patterns have been seen in both urban and rural settings. While in rural areas, the proportion of elderly has risen from 5.8% to 8.8% between 1961 and 2011, the corresponding proportion in the urban areas has increased from 4.7% to 8.1% between 1961 and 2011 (Fig. 3.7).

3.1.4 Elderly Nutrition in India: The Uncharted Territory

Ageing has been found to be linked with nutritional inadequacies, which is a public health challenge and is characterized by a state of multifactorial physiology (Van der Pols-Vijlbrief et al., 2014; Streicher et al., 2018). Undernutrition for aged people is defined as the lack of nutritious food intake or absorption of food, which causes a reduction in both fat and muscle mass of an individual (Hickson, 2006; Corish & Bardon, 2018). The European Society for Clinical Nutrition and Metabolism (ESPEN) defines undernutrition as being judged primarily by a body mass index (BMI) of less than18.5 kg/m^2 or by meeting two of the below-mentioned three criteria: unintentional weight loss (greater than10% in an indefinite time period or greater than 5% over the last 3 months) in combination with either a low BMI (BMI of less than 20 kg/m^2 if age is less than 70 years, or less than 22 kg/m^2 if age is greater than 70 years), or a low fat-free mass index (FFMI) score (FFMI of less than 15 and less than 17 kg/m^2 in women and men, respectively) (Cederholm et al., 2015).

BMI levels are categorized as underweight (BMI less than 18.4), normal (BMI 18.5–24.9),

Fig. 3.7 Distribution of Elderly population (60 years & above) by residence, India. *Source* Based on NSO, 2021

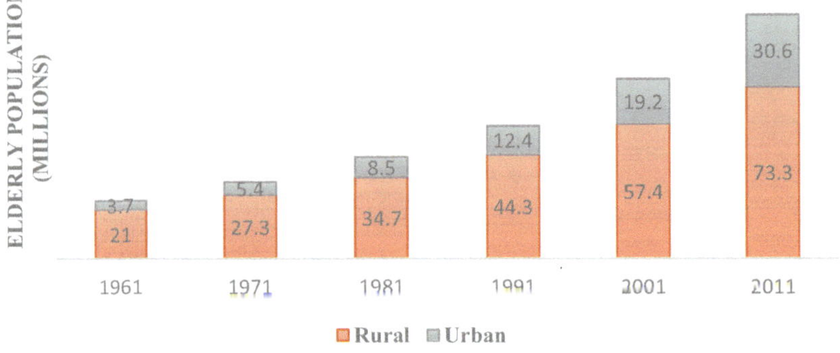

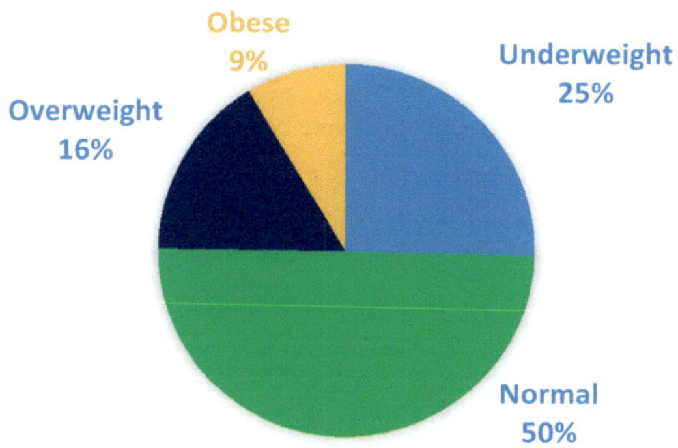

Fig. 3.8 Prevalence of undernutrition and over-nutrition among elderly aged 60 and above* in India, 2017–18. *Source* Longitudinal Ageing Study in India, 2017–18. * Includes spouse irrespective of age

overweight (BMI 25–29.9), and obese (BMI greater than 30) based on the WHO definition. The prevalence of underweight, overweight, and obesity in India is covered in the section that follows. According to Fig. 3.8, 51% of Indian seniors aged 60 and older have a BMI that is within the normal range, whereas 25% are underweight, 16% are overweight, and 9% are obese.

Elderly adults who live in rural areas are more likely to be underweight (30.9%) than those who live in urban areas (11.6%). Contrarily, senior people in urban regions are more likely to be overweight or obese (26.6% vs. 14.7%, respectively) than those in rural areas (12% vs. 6.2%, respectively) (Fig. 3.9).

Nearly 44% individuals fell in the age group 60 and above in the 2017–18 LASI data collected. Table 3.2 presents a rough sketch of indicators related to nutrition among the elderly. While nearly 61% of undernourished elderly have a PDS card, nearly 62% were still facing food insecurity constraints. It is rather intriguing to see that only 24% and 23% of elderly belonging to poor and poorer categories were underweight and overweight respectively, indicating that malnourishment cuts across wealth. The prevalence of both underweight and overweight was more among females, with nearly 83 and 50 males per 100 females being underweight and overweight, respectively. The prevalence of chronic diseases was more among those elderly who were overweight, with the prevalence of at least one chronic disease being 31% and 57% among underweight and overweight elderly, respectively.

3.1.5 Nutritional Screening Tools For the Elderly

Reduced anthropometric and biochemical values are the first step in the development of nutritional deficiencies, which is characterized as a continuous process (Jeejeebhoy et al., 1990; Vellas et al., 1999). Because of the aforementioned, serum proteins and anthropometric measurements are frequently employed to assess the nutritional

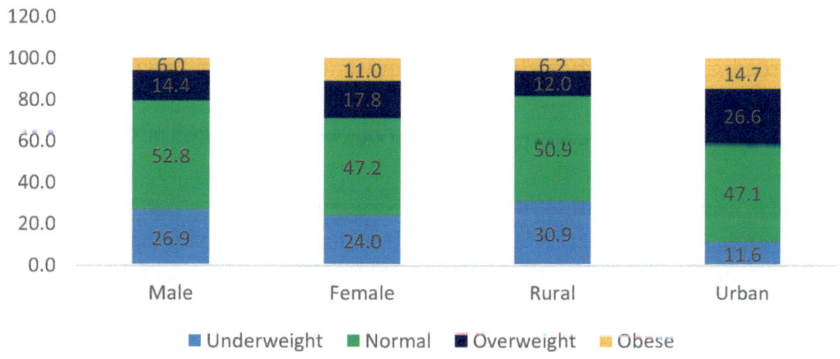

Fig. 3.9 Sex and residence-wise proportion of elderly* according to their nutritional status, India, 2017–18. *Source* Longitudinal Ageing Study in India, 2017–18. * Includes spouse irrespective of age

Table 3.2 A snapshot of elderly nutrition indicators in India, 2017–18

Indicators	
Among undernourished having PDS card %	61.11
Among undernourished, having food insecurity (low or severe constraint) %	62.25
Among undernourished, engaged in work (currently) %	60.95
Among undernourished, with at least 1 chronic disease %	31.03
Among poor and poorer-percent undernourished %	23.53
Among undernourished, educated above 10 %	18.36
Among undernourished, having edentulism %	73.49
Among underweight, male to female ratio per 100 (M/F)	82.96
Among overweight, having at least 1 chronic disease %	57.09
Among overweight, heavy alcoholic behaviour %	2.1
Among overweight, male–female ratio per 100 (M/F)	49.91
Among poor and poorer, percent overweight %	22.7

Source Authors' calculation based on LASI data, 2017–18

condition of aged people. However, the assessment of anthropometric and biochemical values has limits of its own (Charney, 1995), and in some circumstances, the presence of just one parameter has low specificity (Jeejeebhoy et al., 1990). Anthropometry, the primary assessment (Lansey et al., 1993; de Onis & Habicht, 1996), is impacted by a variety of factors, including serum protein levels, fluid retention, liver function (Thuluvath & Triger, 1995), inflammation (Rosenthal et al., 1998), and long-term stress (Fleck, 1988; Boosalis et al., 1989). Studies demonstrate that utilizing a combination of at least one anthropometrical and one biochemical indicator to determine the nutrition status improves the assessment's sensitivity (Symreng et al., 1983; Lansey et al., 1993). Determining whether to utilize the 5th or 10th percentile as the cut-off point for the amount of subnormal anthropometrical readings is another difficulty that comes up in the computation (Joosten et al., 1999).

However, it is essential to employ proven techniques to assess the risk of undernutrition before determining the need for an aged patient's nutritional status (Cederholm, 2015; Corish & Bardon, 2018). The Mini Nutritional Assessment (MNA), which is made up of four areas including anthropometry, clinical status (illness, medications, psychological stress, and neuropsychological problems), dietary assessment, and self-perception about health and nutrition, is the most efficient tool, according to the ESPEN, for identifying and assessing the risk of undernutrition in the elderly (Kondrup et al., 2003; Donnini et al., 2016; Corish & Bardon, 2018). (Donnini et al., 2016). The Malnutrition Screening Tool (MUST) and the Nutrition Risk Screening (NRS) are two additional frequently used instruments for evaluating the risk of undernutrition; however, they lack the criteria to measure crucial undernutrition risk variables like functional, psychological, and cognitive parameters (Donnini et al., 2016).

3.1.6 Mini Nutritional Assessment

Given that it has been specifically created and tailored for the senior population, the MNA is the most extensively used and advised research approach for determining the risk of both undernutrition and overnutrition among the elderly (Kondrup et al., 2003; Elia, 2003a; Kabagambe et al., 2001; Ocke & Kaaks, 1997). Because it is quicker and easier to complete, the MNA-SF, a condensed form of the tool MNA, is typically employed (Kondrup et al., 2003; Elia, 2003a; Guigoz et al., 2002). The MNA-SF is made up of six components, including current BMI, lack of mobility, psychological stress, presence of stress, diagnosis of neuropsychological difficulties, and weight reduction, whereas the full MNA is made up of 18 questions (Kabagambe et al., 2001; Guigoz et al., 2002; Elia, 2003a; Kondrup et al., 2003; Stratton et al., 2004). To arrive at an overall score range between 0 and 14, each of the aforementioned parameters is scored from 0 to 2 or 0 to 3. (Kondrup et al., 2003; Elia, 2003a; Guigoz et al., 2002). The MNA-SF results show whether a person is adequately fed (score of 12–14), at risk of malnutrition (score of 8–11), or malnourished (score of 0–7) (Kabagambe et al., 2001; Guigoz et al., 2002; Kondrup et al., 2003; Elia, 2003a; Stratton et al., 2004). Although MNA is frequently cited as the best choice for elderly nutritional assessment, its application is inappropriate when the elderly don't give accurate information about themselves (Kondrup et al., 2003; Elia, 2003a; Stratton et al., 2004).

3.1.7 Malnutrition Universal Screening Tool

The MUST is a nutritional screening tool that considers three main statistics: the individual's current BMI, weight loss over time, and the occurrence of an acute illness that would significantly impair their ability to consume food for a period of more than 5 days (Kondrup et al., 2003; Elia, 2003; Elia, 2003a; Stratton et al., 2004; Ranhoff et al., 2005). Its applicability extends to adults across all healthcare settings (Kondrup et al., 2003; Elia, 2003; Ranhoff et al., 2005). Individuals are classified as having a low (score of 0), medium (score of 1), and high (score of 2 or greater) risk of malnutrition based on the MUST results (Kondrup et al., 2003; Elia, 2003a; Stratton et al., 2004; Ranhoff et al., 2005). Patients with a medium risk of malnutrition should have their nutritional status periodically checked, but those with a high risk of malnutrition require rapid therapy to be started (Elia, 2003a; Ranhoff et al., 2005). Although the MUST is quick and easy to use, it is not tailored specifically for the elderly population. (Elia, 2003; Elia, 2003a; Kondrup et al., 2003).

3.1.8 Nutritional Risk Screening-2002

The NRS-2002 is a screening tool that considers an individual's current BMI (less than 20.5 kg/m^2), history of recent weight loss, any recent decrease in food consumption, and the severity of their disease (Elia, 2003; Elia, 2003a). The NRS-2002 uses a "nutritional score" and a "severity of disease score" of 0–3 each (Kondrup et al., 2003; Elia, 2003a). The scores of seniors who are 70 years of age or older are increased by one point (Kondrup et al., 2003; Elia, 2003; Elia, 2003a). This technique results in a score range of 0–7 (Kondrup et al., 2003; Elia, 2003a), with individuals scoring 0 to be considered at no risk on undernutrition, between 1 and 2 at a relatively lower risk, between 3 and 4 at medium risk and those scoring 5 and above considered to be at a high risk on undernutrition (Kondrup et al., 2003; Elia, 2003a). NRS-2002 is a potentially unreliable screening measure since, according to study findings, it is sensitive and has a low predictive value, which can occasionally result in incorrect categorization of nutritional status or risk (Kondrup et al., 2003; Elia, 2003).

3.1.9 Factors Influencing Elderly Nutrition

A complex web of elements that work on various scales has an impact on the nutritional state of the elderly. Political, social, economic, environmental, or a combination of these factors may be involved. Elderly people's health and nutritional status can be negatively impacted by a number of factors, including loneliness, economic hardships, a lack of a shared value system among family members, stressful situations that can cause tension, and a lack of family support in times of need. These factors can further lead to a person's lack of interest in eating and living, which can result in nutritional deficiencies. The health of the elderly is negatively impacted by a lack of intimate relationships with family and friends, but elderly who feel lonely are also more susceptible to health problems. Furthermore, it should be noted that elderly find it challenging to alter their long-standing eating habits, particularly those that date back to their early years. In addition to the aforementioned, cultural norms and traditions, family history, educational background, occupation, economic conditions, and lifestyle all have a significant impact on eating habits.

Undernutrition in protein energy is a known factor in the development of osteoporotic fractures in the elderly. On the definition of protein energy undernutrition in the elderly, there is disagreement, though (Perier et al., 2004). Protein-energy undernutrition is defined by one group of academics as an insufficient intake of calories and protein (marasmus-type undernutrition), while another group contends that it results from a biological stress (low-albumin malnutrition; Fig. 3.10) (Avenell & Handoll, 2003). Traditionally, patients with marasmus-type undernutrition experience a loss of body fat and muscle mass while maintaining absolutely normal serum albumin levels. The older people who live in the community or in facilities providing long-term care are more likely to have this type of weight loss. Hospitalized patients are more likely to have low-albumin undernutrition, but the cause of the bone loss that results from this shortage is still not fully understood. An older patient's general nutritional state is further hampered by the metabolic load brought on by low protein consumption as well as the results of hepatic, renal, or intestinal disease. According to Collins et al. (2005) and Osler & Schroll (1997), protein undernutrition has also been linked to an increased risk of injury in the elderly, whereas protein supplementation has been shown to be helpful in lowering negative outcomes following injury in the elderly, especially those aged 65 years or over (Bach et al., 2006; Onishi, 2004).

3.1.10 Why is Measuring Elderly Nutrition Important?

Throughout a person's lifetime, their dietary needs are always changing. This is especially true for the senior population, where these changes may be attributed to their lifestyle, their medical issues, or the natural ageing process. Over the past few decades, there has been much

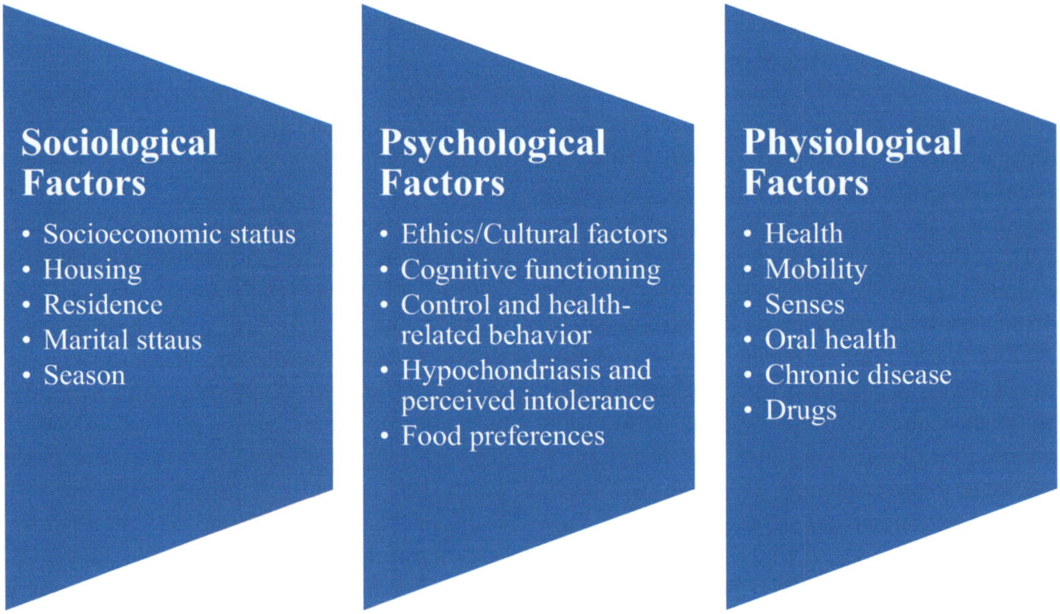

Fig. 3.10 Factors affecting the nutritional status of elderly. *Source* Adapted from Kane et al., 1995

discussion about the relevance of old age nutritional status, particularly in light of morbid illnesses like heart disease, cancer, and dementia (Natarajan et al., 1995; Ministry of Home Affairs, 2010). It is acknowledged that nutrition plays a significant role in determining the health of the elderly, particularly for those who are dealing with acute or chronic diseases (Wells & Dumbrell, 2006). In order to prevent and treat both acute and chronic illnesses, it is essential to evaluate the nutritional state of the elderly. Age-related changes in the body might affect someone's nutritional condition in one way or another. Loss of bone density, a typical issue associated with age, can increase the risk of osteoporosis. Sarcopenia is a noticeable ageing-related alteration as well. Lean muscle mass is lost as a result, which causes the body's fat percentage to rise. It is interesting that muscle loss can occur in healthy individuals as well, indicating that metabolic changes brought on by ageing make it a universal issue. The gradual loss of strength, the deterioration in functional abilities, and poor endurance may cause it to become more obvious. Additionally, this loss lowers the body's overall water content (NICE, 2010).

It needs to be understood that nutritional deficiency is not only a cause but also an aftermath of poor health (Gariballa, 2000). It can be of different types, including undernutrition, over-nutrition, or certain specific nutrient-related deficiencies. Studies suggest that nutritional discrepancies among the elderly mostly remain underdiagnosed (Whitehead & Finucane, 1997), and, thus, increased awareness pertaining to health and nutrition among the elderly is warranted. Elderly population, especially those in hospitals, are much more susceptible to developing nutritional deficiencies as compared to their middle-aged counterparts. Estimates suggest that between 2% and 16% elderly living in community settings consume diets deficient in proteins and calories and suffer from nutritional deficiencies (Tabloski, 2006). This estimate may soar up to 35% for elderly aged 65 years and above if we take vitamin and mineral deficiencies into consideration (Hall et al., 2000). Nutritional deficiencies in older adults are linked to health issues. The ramifications of the same include poor immunity, exacerbated risk of catching infections, reduction in wound healing capacity, and weak muscles, which further intensify the risk of falls and fractures (Chandra, 2002).

Nutritional inadequacies could worsen the issue by causing a loss of appetite or a loss of interest in eating altogether. Elderly who are grievously ill, and those suffering from dementia or rapid weight loss are particularly susceptible to the negative consequences of poor nutrition (Rudman & Feller, 1989). Despite there being no universally accepted definition of undernutrition or over-nutrition among the elderly, certain commonly used indicators use a meagre intake of food or a nutrient-sparse diet as a yardstick for measuring nutritional status among the elderly. The reality, however, is that nutritional inadequacies are caused by an amalgamation of factors, including physiological, psychological, and social factors. These factors manifest themselves through issues such as poor health, poor quality of diets, loss of income, alcohol addiction, lack of social contact, and depression. Such issues are especially prevalent among elderly who are hospitalized or in long-term care centres. Studies on hospitalized elderly suggest that nearly 65% of elderly patients in hospitals are suffering from some kind of nutritional deficiency (Forbes & Reina, 1970), and estimates place the prevalence of undernutrition among elderly in is hospitals and care settings between 30 and 60% (Morley, 1986). It is, therefore, crucial that there be a meticulous nutritional assessment and education related to causes and consequences of malnutrition among the elderly. This can be used as a basis for the development of relevant and encompassing policies and programs.

Active Ageing: A Call for Inter-Sectoral Policy Coordination

The World Health Organization first used the term "active ageing" in the late 1990s. It is intended to convey a broader message than "healthy ageing" and to acknowledge the variables other than health care that influence how people and populations age (Kalache and Kickbusch, 1997). The principles of autonomy, cooperation, self-respect, care, and self-contentment as outlined by the United Nations serve as the foundation for the active ageing idea. It supports a change in strategic planning that shifts the emphasis from a "needs-based" approach (which is predicated on the idea that older people are passive recipients) to a "rights-based" approach that acknowledges people's right to equality of opportunity and treatment in all facets of life as they age. It supports their ability to participate in politics and other elements of communal life with authority.

An individual's degree of diversity tends to rise with age, and older people are not one homogeneous group, according to a life course perspective to ageing. At any stage of life, interventions that promote supportive circumstances and healthy choices are essential. The primary causes of illness, disability, and mortality as people age are low nutritional status and the non-communicable diseases (NCDs) that emerge from it, particularly in developing nations. NCDs, which are essentially degenerative illnesses brought on by the poor nutritional state of the aged, are expensive for individuals, families, and the general public. However, it should be mentioned that some of the health issues caused by inadequate nutrition can be avoided or at the very least postponed. Failure to adequately prevent or manage the emergence of NCDs would have enormous negative effects on human life and society, as well as waste enormous amounts of money that could have been utilized to address the health issues that affect other age groups.

Challenges pertaining to individual and population ageing can be deterred by employing the active ageing approach to policy and program development. When different sectors, such as health, education, labour market and employment and social policies, act in tandem to support active ageing, there will indisputably be:

- reduced number of untimely deaths in the productive stages of life,
- less number of disabilities associated with long-term ailments in older ages,
- increased number of elderlies enjoying an improved quality of life as they grow older,
- ensuring increased engagement of elderly in different facets of the society such as socio-cultural, economic, and political and in both paid and unpaid roles in both family and society,
- reduced cost of treatment and care services.

Active ageing policies and initiatives recognize the value of promoting and balancing individual accountability (self-care), age-friendly surroundings, and intergenerational harmony. Families and individuals need to make persistent efforts to acquire healthy lifestyle habits from a young age, as there is an increasing need to plan for and prepare for older years. Encouraging settings are required to "make the healthy choices the easy choices" at the same time. Executing policies and programs that support active ageing in terms of improved participation and reduced care costs is beneficial economically for a number of reasons. As they age, those who maintain their health encounter fewer obstacles in their ability to work. Public policies that have encouraged early withdrawal from the labour force are primarily to blame for the parallel trend towards early retirement in developed countries. As populations get older, there will be increased pressure on legislators to change these rules, especially if more and more people live into old age in better health, or are "fit for employment." This would be crucial in reducing the rising costs associated with medical and social care expenses, as well as pensions and income security plans. The evidence from the data that is now available strongly suggests that growing old is not associated with rising public expenditures for medical care. Disability and bad health, which are frequently linked to ageing, are more expensive. It's possible that medical spending won't increase at an unprecedented rate as the population ages in better health.

Policy Response to Elderly Nutrition

It is pertinent to realize that nutritional inadequacies among the elderly are caused by a web of social, economic, and political factors, operating at varying levels. It is, thus, crucial to address all these underlying issues while formulating policies. It is advisable to ensure that national nutrition policies and action plans take cognizance of elderly as a potentially susceptible group and certain exclusive provisions are included to combat nutritional issues and food security and safety is ensured as more and more people grow old. The following major changes could be incorporated into the policy planning framework in order to tackle the growing burden of elderly nutritional deficiencies in India:

- *Creating more responsive health systems:* Health systems must respond adequately to ageing populations. Effective health interventions can help sustain an ageing person's general health as well as help them improve their emotional and physical well-being. However, only a small number of therapies have had their economic effectiveness assessed; as a result, there are worries that some of these interventions may potentially worsen patient health and raise expenses (Oxley, 2009). Healthy ageing is anticipated to have significant economic benefits because people who expect to live long and healthy lives may be more motivated to invest in their skill development because they know it will pay off in the long run, even though the impact on direct health care costs is still unknown and requires further research (Suhrcke et al., 2006). They might also be more likely to continue working. Concerns about ageing populations call for policies that balance support for the elderly with those aimed at younger generations who will gain from early intervention. Better care coordination, better management of hospital admissions, enhancing prevention, and energizing healthy lifestyles, such as boosting physical exercise or promoting healthy eating, are all possible policy outcomes. The following can be done to ensure that health systems give the necessary response:
- *Better care coordination:* Growing numbers of chronic diseases and co-morbidities are brought to light as people age, forcing senior patients to consult with a variety of service providers for both social and medical treatment. Because of this, it is becoming more and more important to integrate care across health and social sectors as well as between various levels of healthcare. There is currently a growing amount of research on the most effective treatments for chronic, complicated illnesses (Nolte & McKee, 2008). The coordination of care across locations and sectors, the promotion of self-management, the expansion of a workforce with the right mix of skills, supportive information systems, and financial structures that promote amalgamation rather than dissolution are all crucial problems (Oxley, 2009).
- *Improvising the management of hospital admissions*: The majority of the time, the decline in functional ability in older persons is continuous, but it happens gradually, with reductions accelerated by an episode of acute illness, accident, or a related event. As a result of the aforementioned, hospital admissions to institutions occur more frequently than admissions from homes. In some situations, improved rehabilitation treatments may enable elderly individuals to regain enough function to go back to their homes. Prior research has demonstrated a correlation between expert geriatric teams' assessment and post-discharge home interventions and shorter hospital stays, substantially fewer readmissions, and fewer nursing home placements (Nikolaus et al., 1999). Thus, there are significant opportunities for the expansion of such approaches, particularly in nations with underdeveloped and poorly managed geriatric services, as well as for providing more empowering interventions like podiatry and physiotherapy as opposed to surface-level program interventions like home delivery meals (in this case, improving function might enable some disabled older people to do their own cooking) (O'Neil et al., 2004). As a strategy of reducing emergency admissions, better coordination and a stronger emphasis on preventive care rather than curative care have also been promoted (Kendrick & Conway, 2006).

- *Promoting better self-care*: Increased access to technology, including computers and the internet, and improved health literacy could help patients better understand and manage their ailments and engage in more self-care (Oxley, 2009). It is important to realize that not all disabilities cause handicaps; rather, a handicap results from the interplay of a person's surroundings and their condition. Therefore, gains can be made with relatively easy interventions, such as those that help with mobility. This is especially important for developing nations, where there is a lot of room to use assistive technology more frequently (Freedman et al., 2006).
- *Augmenting preventive behaviour:* Population-based initiatives to promote health and prevent disease are unusually popular with senior citizens. The motivating strategy is primary prevention, which aims to prevent or defer disability (Daviglus et al., 2005; Gandjour & Lauterbach, 2005; Gandjour, 2009; Fries, 2005). Prevention efforts for senior persons should not be based on single illness models because this could merely result in the replacement of one cause of mortality with another, which would not yield the greatest advantages. Instead, they ought to take into account the total burden of disease over the course of the remaining lives of people who will benefit from preventative treatments (Mangin et al., 2007). Including this broad perspective in economic analyses is also essential (Gandjour, 2009).
- *Building suitable systems for long-term care:* The long-term care industry must have enough capacity to meet the health and housing needs of the senior population as a result of the population's inevitable ageing. There is a lot of room for improved service structure and coordination, which can be accomplished in the following ways:
- *Assimilating formal and informal care:* Numerous possibilities exist to support long-term care systems. Supported self-care and home-based services that would enable older persons to stay in the comfort of their own homes or a homelike environment are the ones that are most important. Systems of long-term care can benefit friends and family members so they can continue to serve and support the elderly without jeopardising their own health or financial situation. There may be certain drawbacks to relying on families for personal care (rather than assist in instrumental activities of daily living, which perhaps should be viewed as an essential component of intergenerational transfer). First of all, it might have detrimental effects on the health and well-being of family caregivers, especially women, who frequently bear the brunt of the load and may have competing goals and obligations (Evandrou, 1996). Second, it might have detrimental psychological effects on senior citizens who value autonomy and "not being a burden" (Lee, 1985).
- *Ensuring appropriate care settings:* There is evidence that social support and life satisfaction each put somewhat less stress on the health system (Roos et al., 1989). However, special measures are required to support elderly persons in maintaining their daily activities, promote ageing in place, and prevent the need for long-term institutional care (Hakkinen et al., 2008). For older persons with chronic illnesses, it is crucial to provide services that are appropriate, with care settings like home care and daycare at their core. Additionally, it is essential to integrate long-term care at various levels of service and both the social and long-term care sectors (Coyte et al., 2008).
- *Encouraging economic and social integration:* The active participation of elderly people in society can be greatly improved by employment and retirement policies. This contributes to successful and healthy ageing as well as maintaining funding options for the healthcare and pension systems (Lievre et al., 2007). The maintenance of social integration and self-esteem depends greatly on the employment (Oxley, 2009).
- *Increasing labour force participation:* Incentives for early retirement are being phased out in a number of European nations in favour of initiatives that would increase the

employment of senior individuals (Casey et al., 2003; European Commission, 2006). However, there is still a lack of evidence about the effectiveness of the policies being followed (Taylor, 2004).

- *Increasing the retirement age:* In order to ensure social integration and improved engagement among the elderly, increasing labour force participation below retirement age may not be enough. Another option is to raise the retirement age to reflect improvements in the average healthy life expectancy (Ritsatakis, 2008). According to some calculations, stabilizing the size of the working population relative to the economically inactive population would come from raising the working age by 1.2 years every 10 years together with anticipated increases in life expectancy (Oliviera et al., 2005). In a perfect world, employment and pension changes would not only help to address the anticipated effects of ageing on public budgets and economic growth but also encourage choice and support career possibilities for older employees (European Commission, 2006; Keese et al., 2006).
- *Encouraging social engagement:* Policies promoting healthy ageing must also address the issue of the elderly's ongoing social acceptance. Evidence suggests that a lack of social interaction increases the chance of developing depression and cognitive decline in the elderly, both of which are severe and expensive disabling disorders that affect older age groups (Fratiglioni et al., 2000). Participation in social activities, such as joining philanthropic or community organizations, can increase integration into society (Oxley, 2009). Additionally, this will be crucial for raising public awareness of ageism and age-related discrimination (London Department of Health, 2004).

In conclusion, it is essential to set gender-specific and quantifiable goals for improvements in elderly population health status as well as the reduction of chronic diseases, impairments, and early mortality as individuals age. It is critical to consider their preferences and opinions and to offer both men and women a continuum of care as they age. Reorienting current systems, which are currently centred on acute care, to provide an effortless continuum of care that covers disease prevention, health promotion, the appropriate treatment of chronic diseases, the equitable provision of community support, and respectable long-term and palliative care at every stage of life.

3.2 Conclusion

The United Nations Decade of Healthy Ageing (2021–2030) is an effort to improve older people's lives internationally. Given the COVID-19 epidemic, which has highlighted the gaps and weaknesses in current policies and initiatives, this is currently very important. Thus, there is a pressing need to take a coordinated effort to promote active and healthy ageing in order to ensure that older people can employ their potential to the maximum in a manner that is respectable, equitable, and wholesome. Recognizing the elderly as a vulnerable age group and developing a thorough understanding of their nutritional needs, illness patterns, dietary requirements, and the socio-economic factors at work are the most effective ways to move in this direction. The fact that older persons do not constitute a homogeneous group and that individual variability tends to increase with age must also be recognized. At all stages of life, but especially in later years, policy initiatives aimed at promoting healthy choices and enabling supportive settings are essential. The creation of an ecology that is inclusive and age-friendly must be the primary strategy. To do this, it is necessary to remove social and physical barriers and to put in place policies and programs that address the factors that influence healthy ageing. In order to provide the elderly with non-discriminatory access to quality essential health services, such as curative, palliative, safe, affordable, and efficient assistive technologies, it is important to establish a system where economic inequalities, gender biases, stigma, and discrimination are eliminated. Connecting stakeholders from many industries is urgently needed to maximize resources, share knowledge, and assist the spread of policy and practical action. Therefore, a "whole of government" and "whole of society" reaction is needed to create an ecosystem where older people, their families, and communities experience an improvement in their quality of life.

Key Findings
25%, 16% and 9% elderly in India are underweight, overweight and obese respectively
The proportion underweight and overweight are more for elderly females as compared to their male counterparts.
Edentulism is a significant risk factor for elderly undernutrition, with 74% elderly with edentulism being underweight.
The prevalence of overweight and obesity is higher in urban areas, while the prevalence of underweight is higher in rural areas.
Prevalence of food insecurity is higher among undernourished elderly, with 62% elderly facing food insecurity constraints. About 60% undernourished elderly do not have PDS card.

Factors Playing Role in Determining Anaemia Among Tribal Women in India

4

Samriddhi S. Gupte and Aparajita Chattopadhyay

Abstract

India's story of multifaceted undernutrition is not unheard of. From malnourished children to undernourished mothers, undernutrition is pervasive irrespective of age and sex. According to National Family Health Survey (2015–2016), nearly 54% of women in the reproductive age group suffer from anaemia. This number takes a new colour when seen in the light of India's diverse population. A section of society that despite decades of special treatment by the government remains marginalized and lags—geographically, socially, economically as well as in health care—behind their non-tribal counterparts. Small studies have tried to capture the snapshot of tribal undernutrition. However, the majority of studies so far have been geographically limited. This chapter attempts to analyse and understand the prevalence and determinants of anaemia among tribal women of India taking into account the dietary considerations along with other variables such as WASH indicators, autonomy indicators, etc. The study is one of the few to encompass the tribal population across the entire country and give a comprehensive result. It uses data from the fourth round of the National Family Health Survey (2015–2016) to capture the variation in prevalence and determinants of tribal anaemia. The results indicate the difference in the prevalence of anaemia among tribes and their non-tribal counterparts. Further the determinants of tribal anaemia range from socio-economic variables to dietary variables as well as autonomy variables. Factors such as wealth index, rural/urban residence, and education do have a negative association with anaemia, i.e. if these factors increase, anaemia level decreases. Other significant and less explored factors include the type of contraception usage, type of diet, access to improved sanitation facilities, and the number of birth last year. Regression-based Fairlie decomposition analysis also confirms these variables' significant contribution to anaemia status. It is worth to note that contraceptive behaviour is rarely seen as a correlate of anaemia. Thus, a single umbrella policy approach might not be the right direction to take on the way to eradicate anaemia among the tribes and thereby improve the nutritional condition of tribal women in India. A differentiated, multi-pronged approach may be the way forward taking into account the heterogeneous nature of tribes in India.

Keywords

Anaemia · Tribes · Tribal undernutrition · Diet diversity · Contraceptive use · WASH factor

A. Chattopadhyay et al., *Undernutrition in India*, Sustainable Development Goals Series,
https://doi.org/10.1007/978-981-19-8182-1_4

4.1 Introduction

India is home to almost half the tribal population of the world. Over 10 crore individuals belonging to 705 tribes are identified as Scheduled Tribe by the Constitution of India (Indian Ministry of Tribal Affairs), every tribe different from the other. These 705 tribes constitute around 8.6% (Census, 2011) with varying proportions in different Indian states. These tribes can be majorly categorized into four sections based on where they live. The categories are (a) tribal people living in Schedule V areas and tribal-dominated districts and blocks, (b) tribal population in north-east India, (c) particularly vulnerable tribal groups and (d) tribal people living outside scheduled areas (Tribal Health in India, Expert committee report on Tribal Health, 2018). India's tribal population is dispersed across the country. From a lush green village in North-east to the dunes of the West, they live in a unique physical, socio-economic, and cultural environment, isolated from the general population. These variegated settlements of the tribes are reflected in their food and dietary pattern as well as culture. Since Independence, government policies have aimed at the betterment and upliftment of the tribal community in India. However, despite every effort, tribes remain to be marginalized—geographically, economically, socially, and thus in the nation's psyche. Tribes are thought of as "semi-naked" people who live in far-away mountains or forests and are poor, lack adequate education, and health facility, and primarily depend upon local food availability (Agrawal, 2013; Chhotray, 2003; Tribal Health in India, 2018).

Various studies talk about tribal woman's status in their society. It is a common perception that tribal women have better social status as compared to their non-tribal counterparts. Studies dated as back as 1921, talk about tribal practices such as bride price instead of dowry, and lesser child marriages in north-east India which indicate a higher stature of tribal women (Furer-Haimendorf, 1943; Hutton, 1921). However, there are also studies that indicate a lower status as tribes do not have property rights for women. Taboos and discrimination by far and large exist in these communities (Dalton, 1846; Rivers, 1973). Recent literature also points towards a lower status of tribal women as they are worst hit by the prevailing disparities and discrimination and are at a great disadvantage due to illiteracy and ignorance (Ghosh, 2016). With these contradicting views that exist around the status of tribal women, a commonality that arises is her lower health status.

Anaemia, defined as a lack of sufficient haemoglobin concentration in blood, has a detrimental physical, social and economic effect (Bharati et al., 2008). Across the globe, according to World Health Organization, 1 in 3 women in the reproductive age group is anaemic. India-level estimates show around 53% of women aged 15–49 are anaemic (NFHS IV, 2015–2016). These staggering figures have a significant consequence on the low- and middle-income countries. Anaemia and Iron deficiency substantially decreases physical productivity among adults (Zimmermann & Hurrell, 2007).

One of the common types of anaemia is iron deficiency anaemia, otherwise known as nutritional anaemia. It is a major problem among women throughout the Indian sub-continent. It is aggravated in tribal and rural belts. Most of the tribes are hunters and gatherers in nature and largely depend upon nature and ecology for their sustenance (Tribal Health in India, 2018). Owing to these circumstances, the condition of anaemia becomes particularly serious among tribal women. It has a profound effect on their physical health with lower fatigue resistance and increased susceptibility to other diseases (Basu, 1993).

Policies have been formulated and programs implemented to combat this tenacious problem. National Nutrition Policy, 1993 was introduced to combat undernutrition but, the interventions are yet to reach the tribal population. They still are likely to be malnourished with an insufficient dietary energy intake (Maiti et al., 2005). India's National Iron Plus Initiative (2013), another attempt to safeguard women and children from anaemia, identifies children and pregnant/lactating women as vulnerable sections but does not say anything about tribal women.

Existing literature does point towards anaemia being widely prevalent among tribal women in India (Kamath et al., 2013). Even the women with BMI in the normal range were found to be anaemic (Choudhary & Dashora, 2015). De et al. (2006) confirmed the prevalence of anaemia among tribes of North-eastern India. It highlighted that more than half the tribal women's population of Assam had anaemia (59.82%), closely followed by Tripura and Arunachal Pradesh (57.44 and 53.77%, respectively).

A community-based study by Joshi (2011), found a 95.3% prevalence of anaemia in a group of tribal women. Balgir et al. (2003), assessed the prevalence of anaemia among two of the tribes in Odisha, namely, Bhuyan and Kharia. Bhuyan tribe had 89.9% of prevalence of anaemia, whereas Kharia showed 73.8% prevalence. Along the same lines Kamath et al. (2013) also found anaemia to be prevalent among tribes of southern India with a prevalence percentage of 55.9.

Many factors have been identified as determinants of anaemia among women. Diet plays an important part in defining the anaemia status of women. Various studies conform to this association between anaemia and dietary diversity. Women with a low dietary diversity score are more likely to develop anaemia as compared to women with higher dietary diversity (Abriha et al., 2014). These findings correspond with a study conducted in nine regions of Ethiopia (Gebremedhin et al., 2005). Poor dietary diversity has also been identified as a leading cause of mineral and vitamin deficiency which impacts the iron level and thereby the anaemia status among women (Jemal, 1999). Consumption of meat more than twice a week also shows a significant association with a lower level of anaemia among women (Abriha et al., 2014). Factors such as women's education, and standard of living play a major role in reducing anaemia. Women aged less than 25 years were more likely to be anaemic and thus age also was a significant determining factor (Bharati et al., 2008). The evidence that improved water and sanitation facility also translates to a lower prevalence of anaemia cannot be ignored. Studies have confirmed this association thus bringing it to the forefront as a determinant of anaemia among women (Chattopadhyay et al., 2019; Habyarimana et al., 2014; Nankinga et al., 2019). Food intake, workload, and reproductive factors such as type of delivery, and whether menstruating now are also identified as correlates of Anaemia (Unisa et al., 2011).

Menorrhagia, i.e. severe blood loss (abnormally heavy or prolonged bleeding) during the menstrual period was also identified as a prominent risk factor for anaemia among women (Ismail et al., 2016). Recent studies also identify the type of contraception that used to be associated with the level of anaemia among women. Usage of hormonal contraception (Pills, some IUDs, and injectables) is associated with lower anaemia levels (Haile et al., 2016). Similar findings have been supported by Gebremedhin et al. (2011) in their study pertaining to correlates of anaemia among women in the reproductive age group in Ethiopia. They also identified high parity as a risk factor. Haile et al. (2017) in a study based on the Tanzanian population also confirmed that women using hormonal contraceptives showed significantly lower odds of being anaemic as compared to the non-users. Hormonal contraceptive is known to have man-made estrogen and progestin hormones which inhibits heavy blood loss in women using such contraceptives.

Having thus established the prevalence of anaemia in various pockets of India and the roles of various factors in determining anaemia level, this study is one of its kind to bring out the prevalence and explore the determinants of anaemia among tribal women across India. The present study aims to capture pan-India diversity in the diet of tribal women as compared to their non-tribal counterparts. It further tries to examine the effect of certain parameters on anaemia status of tribal women.

The questions answered in the study are what is the level of anaemia among tribal women across India? Is there a difference in the frequency of diverse diets between tribes and their non-tribe counterparts? What are the factors that affect anaemia levels among tribes?

4.2 Data and Methods

4.2.1 Data and Sampling Design

The *Individual Record* file from the fourth round of the National Family Health Survey (2015–2016) was used for the analysis. Four rounds of the survey have been conducted so far, with the first round beginning in 1992–1993. The survey provides state and national information for India on nutrition, anaemia, fertility, the practice of family planning, maternal and child health, reproductive health, utilization, and quality of health and family planning services.

Anaemia in National Family Health Survey is characterized as a low level of haemoglobin in the blood. In the dataset, three levels of anaemia have been categorized for women. Mild (10.0–11.9 g/dl), moderate (7.0–9.9 g/dl), and severe (less than 7.0 g/dl).

Following WHO guidelines (WHO, 2012), unimproved toilet facilities were defined as pit latrines without slabs or platforms, open pits, hanging latrines, bucket latrines, or open defecation. Improved toilet facilities were defined as a flush toilet, ventilated improved pit latrine, pit latrine with a slab, and composting toilet.

An improved water source was defined as the main source of drinking water of piped connection to water supply, private and public tap, borehole, protected/dug well, protected spring, rainwater, or bottled water. All other sources were considered unimproved.

4.2.2 Statistical Analyses

Level of anaemia among tribal women of India and their non-tribal counterparts

To establish the variation in the prevalence of anaemia among tribal and non-tribal women, bivariate analysis and the descriptive statistic has been used. Chi-square statistic is used to assess the association between anaemia level and background characteristics of tribal women.

Frequency of diverse diet among tribal women.

Bivariate analysis has been done to assess the food consumption pattern among tribal women across India.

The mean score for the frequency of consumption of five food groups as categorized in the NFHS dataset, namely, milk and milk products, pulses or beans, fruits, green leafy vegetables, and non-vegetarian food, has been calculated. Individual category scores ranged from 0 to 2 with 0 being never consumed the food group and 2 being daily consuming that certain food group. The total dietary score ranged from 0 to 15 with a mean of 8.54 and a standard deviation of 2.14.

Socio-economic and demographic factors have been assessed to check their effect on the frequency of diverse diets of women belonging to tribes in India using the ordered logistic regression. The ordered categories of the dependent variable (Dietary score) are 1 = (Mean – SD) to (Mean + SD), 0 = minimum to category 1 and 3 = category 1 to maximum.

Determinants of anaemia among tribal women in India.

Adjusted and Unadjusted odds have been calculated for tribal women being anaemic by respondent's socio-economic, demographic, health, and health utilization facilities to understand the determinants of anaemia among women belonging to tribes.

Effect of selected significant parameters on Anaemia level of tribal women

Fairlie decomposition is a non-linear decomposition technique (extension of Blinder-Oaxaca decomposition) that has been implemented as the dependent variable is binary in nature (0 = non-anaemic, 1 = anaemic) to determine the contribution of the selected parameter in explaining the anaemia status. Following the Fairlie technique, the non-linear equation $Y = F(X\widehat{\beta})$ can be written as

$$\overline{Y}^A - \overline{Y}^{NA} = [\sum_{i=1}^{N^A} \frac{F\left(X_i^A \widehat{\beta}^{NA}\right)}{N^A} - \sum_{i=1}^{N^{NA}} \frac{F\left(X_i^{NA} \widehat{\beta}^{A}\right)}{N^A}] + [\sum_{i=1}^{N^{NA}} \frac{F\left(X_i^{NA} \widehat{\beta}^{A}\right)}{N^{NA}} - \sum_{i=1}^{N^{NA}} \frac{F\left(X_i^{NA} \widehat{\beta}^{NA}\right)}{N^{NA}}]$$

The aforesaid variable has been decomposed to check for the contribution of type of diet (0 = vegetarian, 1 = non-vegetarian), type of contraceptive use (1 = modern spacing method, 0 = otherwise), and number of births by respondent in the past year (0 = no birth, 1 = at least 1 birth). Other variables checked for their impact on anaemia among women are improved sanitation facility (0 = No, 1 = Yes) and if the women have met *Anganwadi worker*/ ASHA, ANM, or any other community health worker in the past 3 months (0 = No, 1 = Yes).

4.3 Results

Figure 4.1 shows the trend of anaemia among tribes and their non-tribal counterparts from the second round of NFHS to the fourth round. It is easy to notice that a high level of anaemia is prevalent for both sections of the population. However, the prevalence of anaemia among tribal women is visibly high throughout the period from 1998 to 2015. A gradual decline is observed but the prevalence remains alarmingly high. Even in the fourth round of the National Family Health Survey, more than 50% of women were reported to be anaemic belonging to both tribal and non-tribal populations.

Figure 4.2 shows the difference in anaemia levels of tribal and non-tribal counterparts. It is important to note that although a significant difference is not visible in the population that is not anaemic, tribal women are plagued with a higher level of anaemia (moderate to severe level of anaemia).

Figure 4.3 shows the proportion of women suffering from anaemia among tribal and non-tribal communities. While background characteristic show a similar level of anaemia among women belonging to tribal and non-tribal communities, type of diet and type of contraception use shows a significant difference in the prevalence of anaemia. Tribal women with a vegetarian diet show a higher prevalence of anaemia. Similarly, tribal women using pills/injections/ IUDs as a method for contraception show a lower prevalence of anaemia as compared to their non-tribal counterparts. The prevalence of anaemia also varies by sanitation facility. It is seen that not having an improved sanitation facility results in a disproportionately high level of anaemia among tribal women in comparison to other women (tribes—60.93%, others—44.77%). The vice-a-versa also holds, i.e. prevalence of anaemia is comparatively lower among tribal women who do have improved sanitation facilities as compared to non-tribal women. Another factor that shows disparity prominently is whether or not the woman has money she can decide to spend by herself. Not having such financial autonomy translates into a higher prevalence of anaemia among women belonging to tribes than to non-tribes.

There is a huge incongruence in the prevalence of anaemia among tribal women to their socio-economic characteristics. This incongruence is captured in Table 4.1. Running the bivariate analysis, it is found that the tribal women belonging to the poorest wealth quintile, living in a rural area in the northern region of India, having no education, in the age bracket of 15–24 with at least 1 birth in the past one year are affected by anaemia. These are the women who are suffering from anaemia. More than half of women who are using contraception such as pills or injectables are not anaemic as opposed to women not using or using any other method of contraception. Similarly, the prevalence of moderate to high anaemia is notable across access to improved sanitation and water facility. The women who do not have access to improved water and sanitation facility have a prevalence of

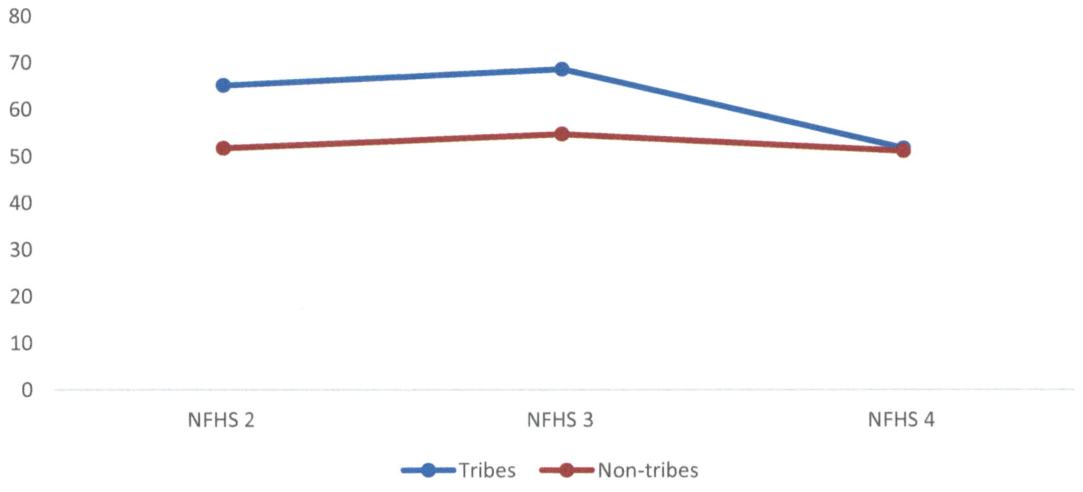

Fig. 4.1 Trend of anaemia among tribal and non-tribal women. *Source* National Family Health Survey (1998–1999, 2005–2006, 2014–2015)

Fig. 4.2 Prevalence of anaemia anong tribal and non-tribal women. *Source* Author

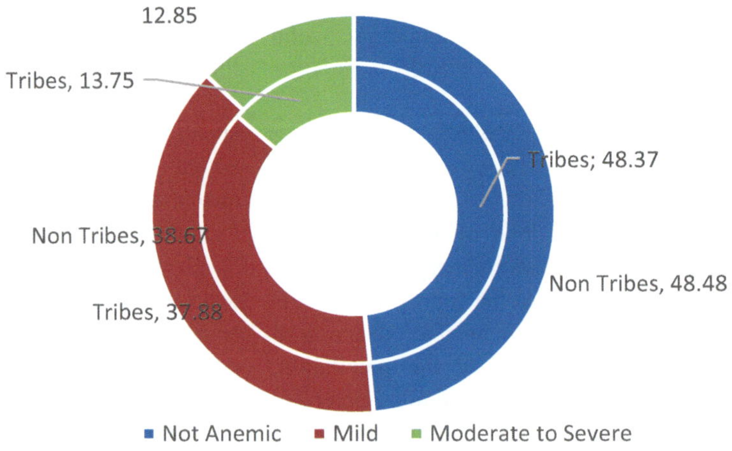

15 and 17% anaemia, higher than those who have access to improved water and sanitation facility (13 and 10%, respectively). It was seen that, while the sex of the head of the household did not show a major difference in the prevalence of moderate to severe anaemia, there was a difference in the prevalence of mild anaemia.

4.3.1 Dietary Diversity

It is safe to assume that there would be a difference in the diet pattern of people belonging to tribal communities and that of their non-tribal counterparts. Figure 4.4 tries to capture the variation in the diet pattern of tribes and non-tribes.

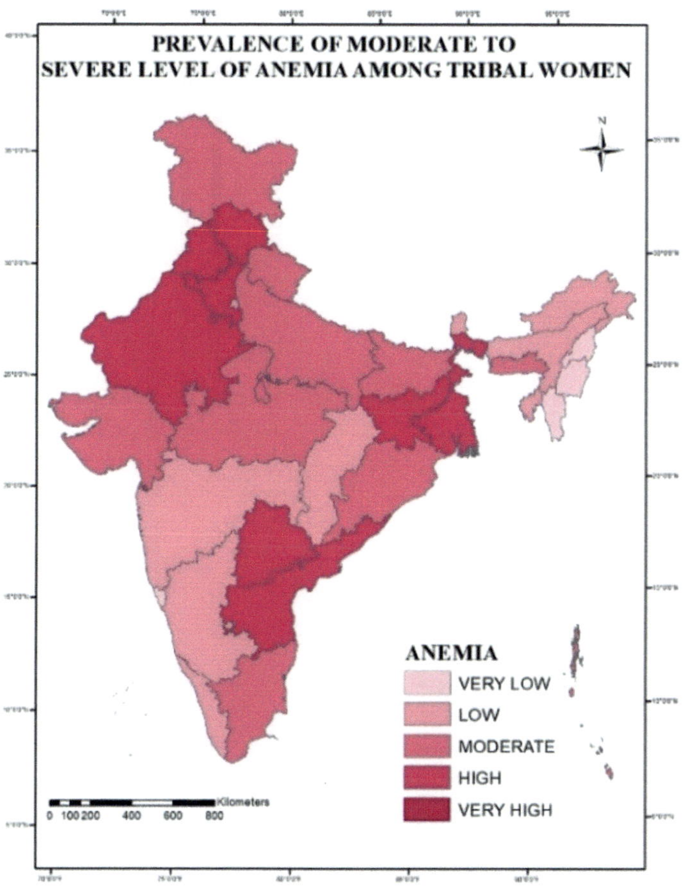

The map shows the distribution of tribal women suffering from moderate to severe anemia across various Indian states. A darker shade of the color corresponds to higher proportion of tribal women suffering from higher degree of anemia.
It can be seen that western region of India i.e. Rajasthan, some eastern parts along with two southern states show a higher prevalence of moderate to severe degree of anemia.

Fig. 4.3 Percentage of anaemic women by selected background characteristics: tribes and non-tribes. *Source* Author

It is seen that the mean dietary score of non-tribes is higher than that of women belonging to tribes. A higher dietary score corresponds to a higher frequency of diverse diets.

Similar consumption of non-vegetarian food on a weekly basis and consumption of green vegetables on a daily basis is found to be higher among the tribes. However, they significantly lag in other category food items such as fruits, pulses, beans, milk, and milk products.

The figure below (Fig. 4.5) gives the mean scores of consumptions by selected variables for tribes and non-tribes. The score ranges from 0 to 15, the higher the score, the higher the frequency of having a diverse diet.

It can be seen that for almost all characteristics, non-tribes are better off than their tribal counterparts regarding the frequency of diverse diets. As we move up the wealth quintile, the frequency of consuming a more diverse diet increases for both tribes and non-tribes, with slightly better improvement among the non-tribes. A similar pattern can be seen with upward movement in education level. Non-tribes have a better diet diversity score at all ages as compared to tribal women of the same age group. An interesting finding is that crops up is with children ever born. With an increase in the number of children ever born, the frequency of diverse diets increases for non-tribes, while, for tribes, it takes a sudden dip. Non-tribal rural women show a higher diet diversity score in comparison to rural tribal women.

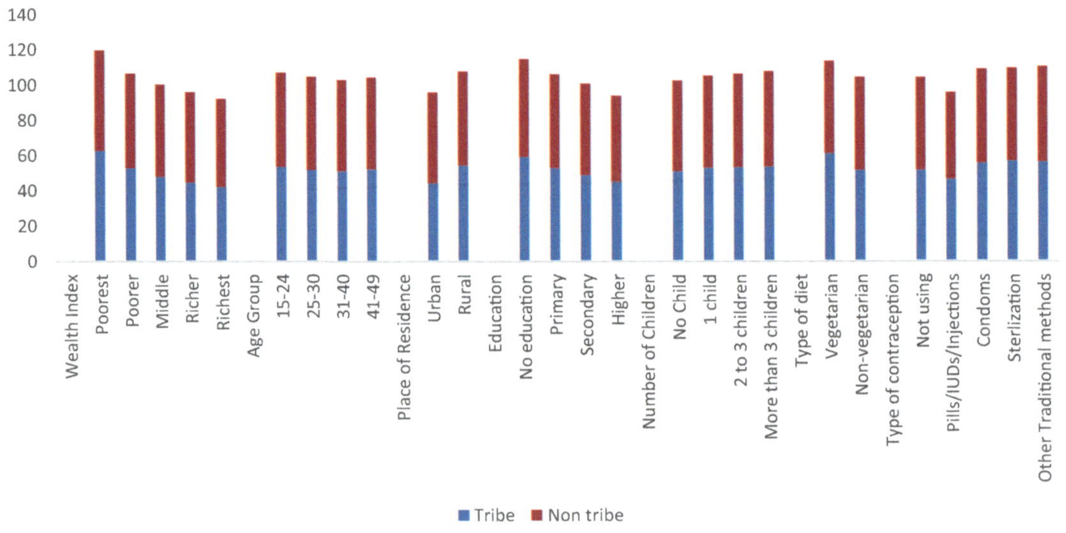

Fig. 4.3 (continued)

Table 4.1 Level of anaemia among tribal women by selected background variables, classified by its severity

Independent variables	Anaemia among tribal women (%) (*N* = 127,133)			Chi-squared (significance)
Socio-economic variables	Moderate/severe	Mild	Not anaemic	
Wealth index				0.000
Poorest	17.07	45.82	37.12	
Poorer	14.21	38.32	47.48	
Middle	11.64	33.72	54.64	
Richer	10.44	30.95	58.61	
Richest	8.98	27.81	63.20	
Level of education				0.000
No education	16.54	42.88	40.58	
Primary	13.72	38.10	48.18	
Secondary	12.10	35.38	52.52	
Higher	10.45	31.26	58.29	
Demographic variables				
Age group				0.000
15–24	14.02	39.03	46.95	
25–30	13.80	37.72	48.48	
31–40	13.25	37.01	49.74	
41–49	13.45	37.48	49.08	

(continued)

Table 4.1 (continued)

Independent variables	Anaemia among tribal women (%) (N = 127,133)			Chi-squared (significance)
Socio-economic variables	Moderate/severe	Mild	Not anaemic	
Number of children ever born				0.000
No child	12.63	36.43	50.94	
1 child	15.28	37.14	47.57	
2–3 children	13.97	38.70	47.33	
More than 3 children	13.84	38.72	47.44	
Births in last year				0.000
No birth	13.52	37.44	49.04	
At least 1 birth	16.19	42.52	41.29	
Type of contraception usage				0.000
Not using	13.89	36.60	49.51	
Pills/injections/IUDs	11.54	34.37	54.09	
Condoms	14.93	39.97	45.10	
Sterilization	13.79	42.97	43.24	
Any traditional method	13.86	41.88	44.26	
Geographical variables				
Place of residence				0.000
Urban	9.98	30.86	59.16	
Rural	14.51	39.55	45.94	
Geographical region				0.000
North	23.68	40.08	36.24	
South	15.53	37.86	46.61	
East	19.30	50.46	30.24	
West	14.24	44.55	41.21	
Central	15.72	46.51	37.77	
North-east	8.15	27.82	64.03	
Dietary variables				
Type of diet				0.000
Vegetarian	18.36	44.61	37.04	
Non vegetarian	13.20	37.05	49.75	
Consumption of dark green leafy vegetables				0.000
Never	17.10	34.43	48.48	
Weekly/occasionally	15.32	40.18	44.50	
Daily	12.23	35.67	52.10	
Dairy products (milk, curd)				0.000
Never	13.70	38.31	47.99	
Weekly/occasionally	13.75	38.56	47.69	
Daily	13.41	34.80	51.79	

(continued)

Table 4.1 (continued)

Independent variables	Anaemia among tribal women (%) (*N* = 127,133)			Chi-squared (significance)
Socio-economic variables	Moderate/severe	Mild	Not anaemic	
Pulses/beans				0.000
Never	14.23	34.12	51.65	
Weekly/occasionally	12.87	36.11	51.02	
Daily	15.34	41.28	43.38	
Fruits				0.000
Never	16.55	43.15	40.30	
Weekly/occasionally	13.64	37.98	48.38	
Daily	13.76	33.44	52.80	
WASH indicators				0.000
Improved sanitation facility				
Yes	10.3	31.19	58.78	
No	17.20	44.12	38.68	
Improved water facility				0.000
Yes	13.40	37.51	49.09	
No	15.04	39.27	45.69	
Autonomy indicator				0.000
Met any community health worker (ASHA/ANM/other) in the last 3 months				
Yes	16.57	41.99	41.44	
No	13.07	36.91	50.01	
Respondent has money that she can decide how to spend				0.000
Yes	16.41	38.34	45.25	
No	15.22	38.87	45.91	
Sex of head of the household				0.000
Male	13.73	39.14	48.13	
Female	13.80	36.34	49.86	

4.3.2 Determinants of Anaemia

Table 4.2 shows the determinants of anaemia among tribal women across India. It gives the unadjusted and adjusted odds for anaemia by selected background characteristics. The factors such as wealth, level of education, age, number of children, dietary variables, health, and health utilization factors all come to be significant in affecting the anaemia status among women belonging to tribes. However, upon adjusting for each other, only variables such as wealth index, level of education, place of residence, type of diet, dietary score, number of births in the last year, and type of contraception hold significance in determining the anaemia status of these women. With upward movement in wealth, the probability of tribal women being ananaemic decreases significantly. Similarly, higher the educational status, the lower the risk of anaemia.

While for the type of contraception currently being used, it is evident that the usage of

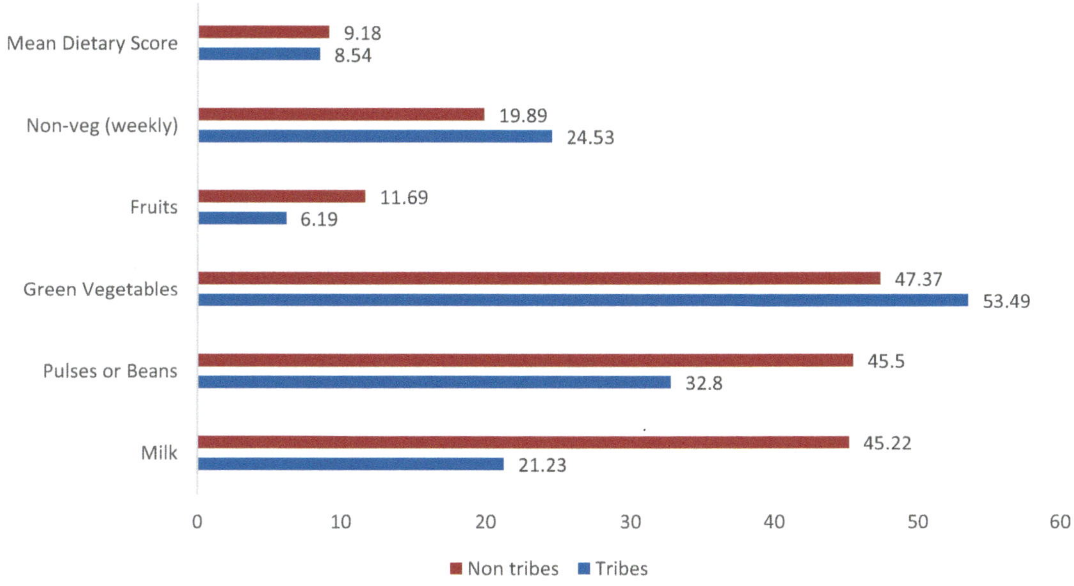

Fig. 4.4 Percentage of women consuming specific food daily and mean dietary score. *Source* Author

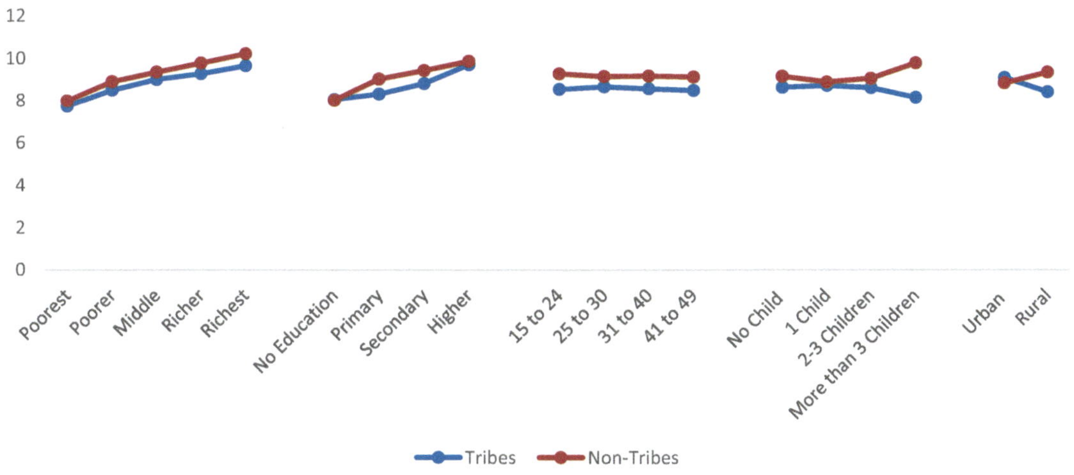

Fig. 4.5 Mean scores of frequency of consumption of diverse diet. *Source* Author

contraception such as pills, and injectable show a lower odd (0.95) than those not using, i.e. women currently using the modern spacing method of contraception have 5% lower chances of being anaemic as compared to their counterparts who do not use. A good dietary score also shows lower chances of anaemia. Women who gave birth to at least 1 child in the past 1 year were found to have 22% higher chances of being anaemic. Women belonging to rural areas have higher odds of being anaemic. In reference to the northern region of India, only women residing in

Table 4.2 Determinants of anaemia among tribal women (unadjusted and adjusted odds): India-level estimates

Independent variables	Unadjusted odds ratio (95% C.I.)	Adjusted odds ratio (95% C.I.)
Socio-economic variables		
Wealth index		
Poorest®	Ref.	Ref.
Poorer	0.700*** (0.684–0.717)	0.91*** (0.88–0.94)
Middle	0.571*** (0.5570.586)	0.83*** (0.80–0.86)
Richer	0.498*** (0.485–0.511)	0.74*** (0.71–0.78)
Richest	0.452*** (0.438–0.466)	0.65*** (0.62–0.69)
Level of education		
No education®		
Primary	0.743*** (0.717–0.769)	0.97 (0.94–1.01)
Secondary	0.639*** (0.623–0.655)	0.92*** (0.89–0.95)
Higher	0.553*** (0.528–0.579)	0.90* (0.84–0.95)
Demographic variables		
Age group		
15 to 24®		
25 to 30	0.913*** (0.887–0.940)	0.95* (0.91–0.98)
31 to 40	0.857*** (0.829–0.876)	0.92*** (0.88–0.96)
41 to 49	0.878*** (0.851–0.906)	0.94* (0.90–1.00)
Number of children ever born		
No child®		
1 child	1.131*** (1.091–1.172)	1.06* (1.01–1.10)
2–3 children	1.143*** (1.112–1.174)	1.06* (1.02–1.11)
More than 3 children	1.106*** (1.072–1.141)	1.05* (1.05–1.10)
Geographical variables		
Place of residence		
Urban®		
Rural	1.481*** (1.451–1.512)	1.11*** (1.07–1.15)
Geographical region		
North®		
South	0.699*** (0.665–0.734)	0.72*** (0.68–0.77)
East	1.197*** (1.149–1.247)	1.18*** (1.11–1.24)
West	0.881*** (0.842–0.921)	0.79*** (0.75–0.84)
Central	0.914*** (0.880–0.949)	0.83*** (0.79–0.88)
North-east	0.526*** (0.504–0.539)	0.36*** (0.34–0.38)
Dietary variables		

(continued)

Table 4.2 (continued)

Independent variables	Unadjusted odds ratio (95% C.I.)	Adjusted odds ratio (95% C.I.)
Type of diet		
Vegetarian®		
Non vegetarian	0.560*** (0.538–0.582)	0.95* (0.91–1.00)
Consumption of dark green leafy vegetables		
Not daily®		
Daily	0.75*** (0.74–0.77)	0.86*** (0.83–0.88)
Dietary score		
Low®		
Normal	0.85*** (0.83–0.88)	1.05* (1.02–1.09)
Good	0.79*** (0.76–0.82)	0.95*** (0.93–0.99)
Health variables		
Number of birth in last year		
No birth®		
At least 1 birth	1.35*** (1.30–1.40)	1.22*** (1.17–1.28)
Type of contraception currently using		
Not using®		
Pills/injections/IUDs	0.811*** (0.774–0.851)	0.95* (0.90–1.00)
Condoms	1.171* (1.069–1.283)	0.97 (0.89–1.07)
Sterilized	1.259*** (1.223–1.296)	0.91*** (0.88–0.95)
Any traditional method	1.21*** (1.14–1.29)	1.08* (1.01–1.16)
WASH indicators		
Improved sanitation facility		
No®		
Yes	0.452*** (0.44–0.46)	0.471*** (0.44–0.49)
Improved water facility		
No®		
Yes	0.873*** (0.85–0.89)	1.001 (0.93–1.07)
Autonomy indicator		
Met any community health worker (ASHA/ANM/other) in last 3 months		
No®		
Yes	1.38*** (1.34–1.42)	1.209** (1.12–1.29)
Respondent has money can decide how to spend		
No®		
Yes	1.02 (0.96–1.08)	1.07 (1.01–1.13)
Sex of head of the household		
Male®		
Female	0.943*** (0.91–0.97)	1.006 (0.93–1.08)

Note ®Reference category, C.I.: Confidence interval, *** $p < 0.01$, ** $p < 0.05$, * $p < 0.10$

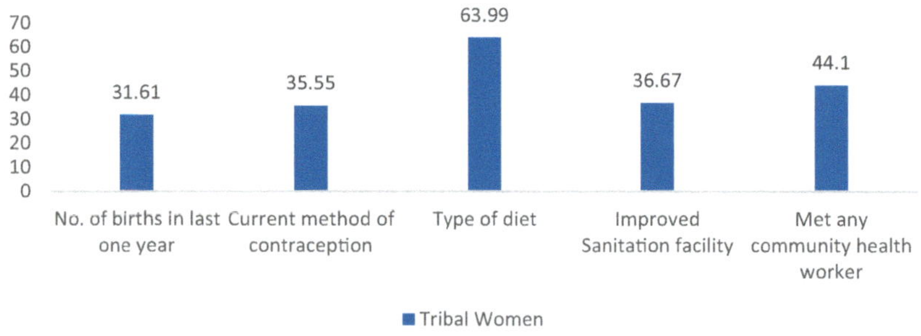

Fig. 4.6 Effect of significant parameters in determining anameia level among tribal women in India. *Source* Author

the eastern region are more likely to be anaemic (odds—1.18), the rest of the regions, i.e. western, north-eastern, southern, and central regions had slightly lesser odds of tribal women being anaemic.

WASH variables, i.e. improved water and sanitation facility also significantly reduce the likelihood of anaemia among tribal women. While the unadjusted odds of women being anaemic decrease by nearly 60% with access to improved sanitation and water facility. But, in the adjusted model, only improved sanitation facility shows a significant decline in odds of women being anaemic (nearly 60% lesser odds).

Another factor that holds significance in both adjusted and unadjusted models is whether or not the women have met any Anganwadi worker, ASHA, ANM, or any other community. It is peculiar to note that having met any community health worker in the last 3 months translates into a higher likelihood of women reporting anaemia (Fig. 4.6).

4.3.3 Contribution of Selected Parameters as Determining Factors of Anaemia Among Tribal Women

Decomposition analysis shows the percentage contribution of *type of diet (vegetarian/non-vegetarian), contraceptive use (modern spacing method, otherwise, number of births in last 1 year (0, at least 1), improved sanitation (yes, no), and met any community health worker in last 3 months (yes, no)* in determining anaemia. Fairlie decomposition of anaemia among tribal women by these variables shows that type of diet explained nearly 64% of anaemia. Contraceptive use explained nearly 35% and the number of births in the past year explained 31% of tribal women's anaemia. Improved sanitation facilities had an effect of nearly 37% on anaemia, whereas having met any community health worker showed nearly 44% impact on explaining anaemia among tribal women.

4.4 Discussion

The present study tried to establish the prevalence of anaemia in tribal women populations across India. It studied the difference in the prevalence of anaemia among women belonging to tribes and non-tribes by their socio-economic and demographic characteristics. The study also attempted to understand if there is a difference in the frequency of diverse diets among tribes and non-tribes. It tried to examine the factors that significant role in determining anaemia level among tribal women and took it a step ahead by quantifying the effect of each significant parameter on the anaemia level of women belonging to tribes of India.

Although, there is no dearth of literature on the prevalence of anaemia among women, literature on tribal women's health status is a different story. There is limited to almost no study that gives a comprehensive picture of anaemia prevalence and its correlates among tribal women of reproductive age group across India. The study finds the prevalence of anaemia to be higher among tribal women as compared to their non-tribal counterparts. While a mild degree of anaemia showed similar prevalence in both tribes and non-tribes, a moderate to severe degree of anaemia was found to be higher in tribal women's population.

The prevalence of anaemia was found to be highest among tribal women belonging to the poorest section with no education aged 15–24 and residing in rural areas of eastern and northern India. A high prevalence of moderate to severe anaemia was also found in women who consume only a vegetarian diet (not even egg). The results from the study align with the previous studies which also point towards a high prevalence of anaemia among tribal women in different pockets of India (Shrinivasa et al., 2014; Unisa et al., 2011).

The study found that a higher dietary score which corresponds to a higher frequency of diverse diet was associated with non-tribal women. Tribal women showcased a lower frequency of consuming a diverse diet.

It is interesting to note that although weekly consumption of non-veg and daily consumption of green vegetables was more in the tribal population, they lagged behind in every other category of food. Their diet was found to be significantly deficient in milk and milk products, fruits, pulses, and beans. This makes them considerably susceptible to micronutrient deficiencies such as iron, vitamin A as well as zinc (Ghosh-Jerath et al., 2016; Mittal & Srivastava, 2006). However, a higher frequency of consumption of meat and vegetables can be attributed to their proximity to the environment and forest-dwelling. of the tribes are non-vegetarian with a few exceptions and depend upon forest which provides rich bio-diverse food (Qamra et al., 2009; UNDP, 2008).

While comparing diet diversity scores for women belonging to tribes and non-tribes, it was found that non-tribes were well off in all categories of select background variables. Upward movement in wealth quintile as well as education corresponded to better diet diversity scores for both tribes and non-tribes, however, not much change was seen with a change in age groups. Existing literature does establish the importance of dietary diversity and its nutritional outcome (Agrawal et al., 2019; Mittal & Srivastava, 2006) but there is no study that draws tribe non-tribe comparison for the same.

The result from the regression analysis brings to light the determinants of anaemia among tribal women across India. While initially all the socio-economic, and demographic factors were showing a significant relationship with anaemia level among tribal women; upon adjusting them for one another, only geographic, economic, and demographic factors determined the anaemia level.

The odds ratio shows that women coming from better economic footing were less likely found to be anaemic. This association has been identified in the previous studies with the specific tribe as their study population (Bharati et al., 2008). Tribal women belonging to rural areas of the eastern region were more likely to suffer from anaemia when compared to their urban/rural counterparts in other regions of India. Studies have established the status of undernutrition among the *Santhal* tribes which are predominantly found in the Eastern regions of India (Stiller et al., 2020).

Vegetarianism is also found to be a strong predictor of anaemia among tribal women. The type of diet has not been studied as a predictor of anaemia in the tribal context previously. However, studies pertaining to non-tribe do show a strong association between vegetarianism with a higher likelihood of anaemia (Rammohan et al., 2012). Vegetarianism, although found less among tribes, is not an uncommon concept for non-tribes. Abstaining from meat consumption and not supplementing vegetarian food with iron-rich items has a serious implication on women's micronutrient and iron levels (Rammohan et al., 2012).

WASH indicators such as improved water and sanitation facility were seen to be significant predictors affecting the anaemia level among women positively. Access to improved sanitation facilities resulted in lesser chances of developing anaemia. This could be attributed to the fact that women with an unimproved source of drinking water and sanitation facility are more vulnerable to both waterborne and vector-borne diseases which might, in turn, increase the risk of anaemia. Along with this, this group of women is also at risk of various infections such as hookworm, which is another cause of anaemia under poor sanitary conditions (Chattopadhyay et al., 2019; Habyarimana et al., 2014; Nankinga et al., 2019).

Women's autonomy is a concept that is recognized as a precursor to the betterment of their lives. It is not only important as their right but also crucially linked to women's health and health-related issues (Green et al., 2019; Mistry et al., 2009; Osamor et al., 2016). Evidence suggests that access to the financial resource is essential for women to exercise this autonomy. The factor that whether or not a woman has money that she herself can decide how to spend is found to be a factor that is associated with anaemia among women. Although no significant relationship is established with particularly this factor, it was found that women belonging to households with female heads were less likely to be found anaemic. The factor of sex of the head of the household cannot directly be termed as an autonomy factor but existing literature proves that women belonging to such households enjoy better autonomy over resources (Chakrabarti, 2019).

Another significant predictor of anaemia that shows up in the study is the current method of contraception. Tribal women using modern contraception such as pills, IUDs, or injections were found to be at a lower odd of suffering from anaemia in reference to women either not using any contraception or using a traditional method. A similar association has been found in previous literature pertaining to populations of various countries. The explanation for it could be a reduction in cyclic blood loss which is often documented with the usage of oral contraceptive pills (Bahamondes et al., 2015; Gebremedhin et al., 2011). Moreover, placebo iron pills provided by some brands of contraceptives can also elevate the anaemia level among women (Gebremedhin et al., 2011). The result is also in congruence with studies conducted in Tanzania and Ethiopia (Hailie et al., 2016, 2017, Zerfu et al., 2016).

A peculiar predictor that is consistently significant in the analysis is whether or not the woman has met health workers such as Anganwadi workers, ASHA, ANM, or any other community health worker in the last 3 months. One would assume that having met any such worker, the anaemia prevalence would be less among women, however, the result indicates the opposite. It is found that women who've met such workers report and have a higher likelihood of being anaemic. Evidence is not easily available to support the finding. The possible reason is that as they met the health worker, they are aware of their anaemia level. It is important for future research to explore this association among tribal women.

To take a step ahead and quantify the contribution of each significant variable in explaining the anaemia level among tribal women in India, decomposition analysis was used. The regression-based decomposition analysis highlighted that while the type of diet had the significant impact on anaemia, i.e. it explained 64% of anaemia, factors such as whether met community health workers, improved sanitation facilities, current contraception use, and the number of births in last year also significantly impacted anaemia among women belonging to tribes. These factors accounted for 44, 37, 35, and 32% of change in the anaemia prevalence of women belonging to tribes.

4.5 Conclusion

Policies and programs aimed at betterment and safeguarding the interests of the tribal community can be found in abundance, and significant feat has been achieved by equalizing the level of anaemia among tribes and non-tribes. However, the level itself is quite high. Further, Indian tribes are a heterogeneous group with diverse cultures. But the point of commonality that holds true for all tribes across the Indian subcontinent is that they have poorer health indicators, a higher burden of mortality and morbidity, and limited access to healthcare facilities. These tribes live in isolated rural hamlets in geographically remote locations where factors like illiteracy, lack of improved sources of drinking water, sanitation facility, and lack of accessibility to nutritious food make them vulnerable to various deficiencies and diseases. This is compounded by lack of health facilities or access to health facilities, discriminatory practices, lack of awareness about the importance of diverse food, and micronutrient deficiencies.

There are various studies with limited geography but these are enough to show a holistic picture of tribes. Hence, the present study aimed at capturing this snapshot of tribal women's anaemia level in comparison to the non-tribes across India. It is widely accepted that women suffer from anaemia due to multiple causes, some of them being immediate causes such as frequency of consumption of diverse diet or number of births given by the woman in last 1 year, underlying causes such as wealth index, educational level, age, and basic causes such as geographic region, place of residence, etc. In recent times, an association between hygiene and sanitation is also asserted as an important factor that determines anaemia levels among women.

The present chapter establishes that tribes have a lower frequency of consuming a diverse diet as compared to non-tribes and this corresponds with a higher level of anaemia among tribal women. Type of diet was found to be a significant predictor of anaemia among tribal women. It also contributed considerably to explaining anaemia level. At the same time, the number of children born to the woman in the past year and the current method of contraception also contribute significantly to anaemia levels. A component of WASH practice, i.e. access to improved sanitation facility significantly impacted anaemia among tribal women and an improved sanitation facility was associated with a lower risk of anaemia.

It is important to note that since poor health indicator of the tribes has been a persisting concern over the years, government policies have been implemented but those are critically addressed to just the immediate causes such as diet and are not sufficient to address the larger issue of poverty or unmet need for contraception among others. There is a compelling need to take measures in order to assimilate the fragmented tribes into a similar socio-economic, and demographic profile as that of non-tribes. A differentiated, multi-pronged approach across concerned ministries is needed to tackle the persevering problem of not just anaemia among tribal women but the multifaceted problem of undernutrition among tribes.

The study has certain limitations such as the dataset for the National Family Health Survey does not categorize the tribal population by name of the tribe. Hence, a precise picture of different tribes cannot be drawn. Aspects of the study have not been studied previously in a tribal context; hence, it is difficult to ground the found result in any existing literature.

Key Findings
Higher prevalence of anaemia among tribes belonging to the eastern and northern regions of India.
Non-tribal women show a higher frequency of diverse diets than their tribal counterparts.
While anaemia level is found to be higher among the tribal population, consumption of meat as well as green leafy vegetables is also found to be more in the tribal community as compared to non-tribes.
Type of diet, number of births in the previous year, type of contraceptive use, access to an improved sanitation facility, and whether or not met any community health worker are found to be significant predictors of anaemia among tribal women.
Using modern spacing methods also known as hormonal contraception such as pills/IUDs /injectable reduces the chances of being anaemic.
Access to improved sanitation facilities significantly reduced the chances of women suffering from anaemia.
Having met any community health worker showed an association with women's anaemia status.
The factors that contributed (increasing to decreasing order) to explaining anaemia are as follows: type of diet (64%), access to improved sanitation facilities (37%), the current method of contraception use (35%) and the number of births in last year (32%).
A differentiated, multi-pronged approach to tackle anaemia is the need of the hour as there are multiple causes of anaemia among tribal women.

Understanding Anaemia in Tribal Children and Women with Special Focus on Nagaland, Maharashtra, and Odisha

5

Samriddhi S. Gupte, Aparajita Chattopadhyay, and Akancha Singh

Abstract

Anaemia is one of the major hidden problems that affects both old and young alike. Although anaemia is more of a manifestation of iron deficiency than disease itself, it reduces vitality among old and has detrimental impact on children's children and physical development. Pocket studies in India have confirmed the prevalence of anaemia among tribal women and children who bear the harshest brunt of the problems due to their physical, geographic, economic, and environmental isolation. This evidence is, however, limited to particular districts or tribes. There is a dearth of pan-India literature. The present study aimed at giving a snapshot of the prevalence of anaemia among women and children across India with special focus on Nagaland, Odisha, and Maharashtra to bring out the regional disparity in prevalence and predictors. The result shows the regional disparity in not only prevalence of anaemia but also predictors of anaemia in various states. Along with type of diet given to children or consumed by women, the use of modern (hormonal) contraception such as pills, injections, and IUDs among women also come out as significant predictors of anaemia. Hence, it can be said that an umbrella approach may not work to tackle the problem of tribal anaemia and there is an urgent need for differentiated, multi-pronged approach at the grass root level with tribal culture at its focal point.

Keywords

Anaemia · Tribal women · Tribal Children · Nagaland · Maharashtra · Odisha · Hormonal contraception · Post-partum amenorrhea

5.1 Introduction

Among micronutrient-induced deficiency, anaemia is the common form of morbidity. Anaemia, however, is a manifestation and not a disease per se. One of the primary causes of anaemia is undernutrition and iron deficiency makes up a bulk of this undernutrition. Iron deficiency is a prevailing nutritional disorder across the globe. According to WHO estimates, one in every three women is anaemic globally (WHO). Over 40% of the under-5 children share the same fate. In developing countries, such as India, these numbers are exacerbated ly due to the prevalence of malaria and worm infections (Slotzfus & Dreyfuss, 1998). Currently in India, iron deficiency anaemia exerts high toll on women in the reproductive age group and children under 5 years of age. India ranks 170 out of 180 with regard to women and children's anaemia (Global Nutrition report, 2016). Anaemia is a major

A. Chattopadhyay et al., *Undernutrition in India*, Sustainable Development Goals Series,
https://doi.org/10.1007/978-981-19-8182-1_5

health problem that plagues old and young alike. From reducing vitality among both old and young, it has dire implications on child's cognitive development (Kotecha, 2011). More often than not, anaemia is a hidden deficiency with not very overt symptoms (IDPAS, 2001).

There is ample evidence that shows predominance of anaemia in various tribes and regions of India. Scheduled tribes, essentially live in socially, economically isolated areas with distinct culture, food, and dietary pattern in itself (Laxmaiah et al., 2007). Given the exclusion of tribes from formal education, proper healthcare practices, and their dependence on primitive agriculture for food, anaemia is not unheard of in various tribes across India (Maiti et al., 2005). The trend of anaemia among tribal women and children is declining gradually but the proportions remain alarming nonetheless (India State-Level Disease Burden Initiative Undernutrition Collaborators, 2019). Various region-specific studies show the prevalence of anaemia across India. While anaemia among tribal women and children of Kerala range from 78.3% to nearly 96% (Rakesh, 2017), anaemia status of women in eastern India, such as the state of Odisha remains 74% (Rokade et al., 2020; Agrawal, 2013). North-eastern states do slightly better in this context with Assam at 59.82%, Arunachal Pradesh at 53.77%, and Tripura at 57.45% (De et al., 2006).

These variations not only arise from the variation in geographical regions that they inhabit but also due to distinct cultural differences in each tribe which in turn leads to differences in food consumption. Gond tribe, for instance, which is found predominantly in central India (parts of Chhattisgarh, Madhya Pradesh, and Maharshtra) have *kodo* and *kutki* millets as their staple food and are also meat-eaters (The Indigenous Colour of India—The Indian Tribes, 2019). Bhil tribes (found predominantly in Madhya Pradesh, Gujrat, and parts of Maharashtra) have cereals and pulses as their staple food with seasonal vegetables and fruits. Consumption of milk is rare in this tribe while consumption of meat is seen to be a matter of prestige and, thus, is reserved for special occasions along with wheat and rice (Qamra et al., 2009). The food habits of tribes belonging to North-Eastern India are different from rest of the tribes in their pattern of meat consumption. Staple food for these tribes is rice or millets, vegetables flavoured with fish and species and pork or bird meat. The Naga tribe of north-east consume dogs, fish, crabs, and spiders along with pork, beef, pigeon, and other bird meat (Food Consumption Patterns of North Eastern Communities, 2015).

One of the crucial components of Sustainable Development Goals is health for all. However, it may not be possible to fully attain it if more attention is not paid to the vulnerable groups such as tribal women and children. Hence, it is of utmost importance to understand the regional differences in anaemia among tribal women and children and to identify their predictors.

The chapter aims to understand the prevalence of anaemia among tribal women and children across India and the regional disparity that exists. It also aims to identify the predictors of childhood anaemia and anaemia among tribal women with special focus on three different states—Nagaland, Maharashtra, and Odisha—to bring out the regional difference in underlying causes of anaemia. The chapter tries to explore the dimension of diet diversity among women and what determines the frequency of consumption of diverse diet. Finally, it aims to understand the impact of selected predictors on anaemia level of tribal women belonging to the three selected states.

5.2 Data and Sampling Design

The Individual Record and Kids Record file from the fourth round of the National Family Health Survey (2015–16) was used for the purpose of the analysis. Four rounds of the survey have been conducted so far, with the first round beginning in 1992–93. The survey provides state and national information for India on nutrition, anaemia, fertility, the practice of family planning, maternal and child health, reproductive health, utilization and quality of health, and family planning services.

Anaemia in the National Family Health Survey was characterized as low level of haemoglobin in blood. In the dataset, three levels of anaemia had been categorized for women and children as Mild (10.0–11.9 g/dl), moderate (7.0–9.9 g/dl), and severe (less than 7.0 g/dl).

5.3 Statistical Analyses

5.3.1 Under-5 Children

5.3.1.1 Level of Anaemia Among Tribal Children

To understand the distribution of anaemia among tribal children across India, bivariate and descriptive statistics were used. Similar analysis has been done to showcase the association of various food group consumption with anaemia among children. The five food groups used were non-vegetarian food, milk and milk products, pulses and beans, fruits or fruit juices, and dark green leafy vegetables. Anaemia level was measured against the consumption of food groups by children.

Bivariate statistic was used to establish the difference among three selected states, i.e. Nagaland, Maharashtra, and Odisha in terms of varying degrees of anaemia. The three states were selected based on ranging prevalence of tribal anaemia. Nagaland was a lower order state, whereas Odisha was a higher order in terms of prevalence of anaemia, while Maharashtra lied in the middle.

Logistic regression was applied to determine the predictors of anaemia among the tribal population across India and among three selected states.

5.3.2 Women

5.3.2.1 Prevalence of Anaemia

Bivariate analysis and descriptive statistics have been used to establish the prevalence of anaemia, diversity in frequency of food consumption among women belonging to varying socio-economic, geographies, and demographic groups. Mean score for the frequency of consumption of five food groups as categorized in the NFHS dataset, namely, milk and milk products, pulses or beans, fruits, green leafy vegetables, and non-vegetarian food had been calculated. Individual category's score ranged from 0 to 2 with 0 being having never consumed the food group and 2 being daily consuming that certain food group. Total dietary score ranged from 0 to 15 with a mean of 8.54 and standard deviation of 2.14.

5.3.2.2 Determinants of Anaemia Among Tribal Women Belonging to Three Selected States

In order to look at determinants of anaemia among tribal women, determinants of frequency of diet diversity are understood using the ordered logistic regression. Further, regression analysis had been used to understand the predictors of anaemia among tribal women belonging to three selected states.

5.3.2.3 Effect of Selected Significant Parameters on Anaemia Level of Tribal Women

In order to understand the varying determinants and their contribution to explaining anaemia in each selected state, Fairlie decomposition, a non-linear decomposition technique (extension of Blinder-Oaxaca decomposition) had been implemented as the dependent variable was binary in nature (0 = non-anaemic, 1 = anaemic) to determine the contribution of selected parameter in explaining the anaemia status.

Following the Fairlie technique, the non-linear equation $\mathbf{Y} = \mathbf{F}(\mathbf{X}\hat{\beta})$ can be written as

$$\overline{Y}^A - \overline{Y}^{NA} = \left[\sum_{i=1}^{N^A} \frac{F(X_i^A \hat{\beta}^{NA})}{N^A} - \sum_{i=1}^{N^{NA}} \frac{F(X_i^{NA} \hat{\beta}^A)}{N^A}\right] + \left[\sum_{i=1}^{N^{NA}} \frac{F(X_i^{NA} \hat{\beta}^A)}{N^{NA}} - \sum_{i=1}^{N^{NA}} \frac{F(X_i^{NA} \hat{\beta}^A)}{N^{NA}}\right]$$

The aforesaid variable had been decomposed to check for the contribution of type of contraceptive use (1 = modern spacing method, 0 = otherwise) and number of births by respondent in the past year (0 = no birth, 1 = at least 1 birth).

5.4 Result

5.4.1 Anaemia Among Tribal Children

Table 5.1 shows the per cent distribution of tribal children in accordance to various socio-economic, demographic, and geographical characteristics. It can be seen that percentage of children suffering from anaemia decreased with the increase in wealth ladder. A higher percentage of tribal children living in the northern region of India was seen to be anaemic as compared to other regions of India. Anaemia was seen to be more prevalent among tribal children belonging to rural areas rather than urban.

Figure 5.1 depicts the prevalence of anaemia among tribal children across India based on their food consumption pattern. It can be observed that there was a difference in the prevalence of anaemia among children who were given dark green leafy vegetables or non-vegetarian food and the children who weren't given these food groups. Children who consumed these food items

Table 5.1 Percent distribution of anaemia among tribal children by various socio-economic and demographic characteristics—India-level estimates

Socio-economic characteristic	Not anaemic	Mildly anaemic	Moderate to severely anaemic
Wealth quintile			
Poorest	35.56	28.92	35.57
Poorer	46.95	26.04	27.01
Middle	53.43	24.45	22.12
Richer	58.97	21.99	19.04
Richest	63.66	20.16	16.18
Demographic variables			
Age of child			
0 to 1	34.02	26.36	39.62
1 to 2	35.03	26.69	38.28
2 to 3	46.67	25.93	27.40
3 to 4	51.60	26.42	21.98
4 to 5	56.29	25.54	18.17
Geographical variables			
Place of residence			
Urban	57.18	22.48	20.35
Rural	43.75	26.80	29.45
Geographical region			
North	25.92	23.57	50.51
Central	33.34	29.58	37.08
East	30.21	32.35	37.44
North East	64.23	21.64	14.13
West	37.89	31.86	30.24
South	39.79	27.46	32.75

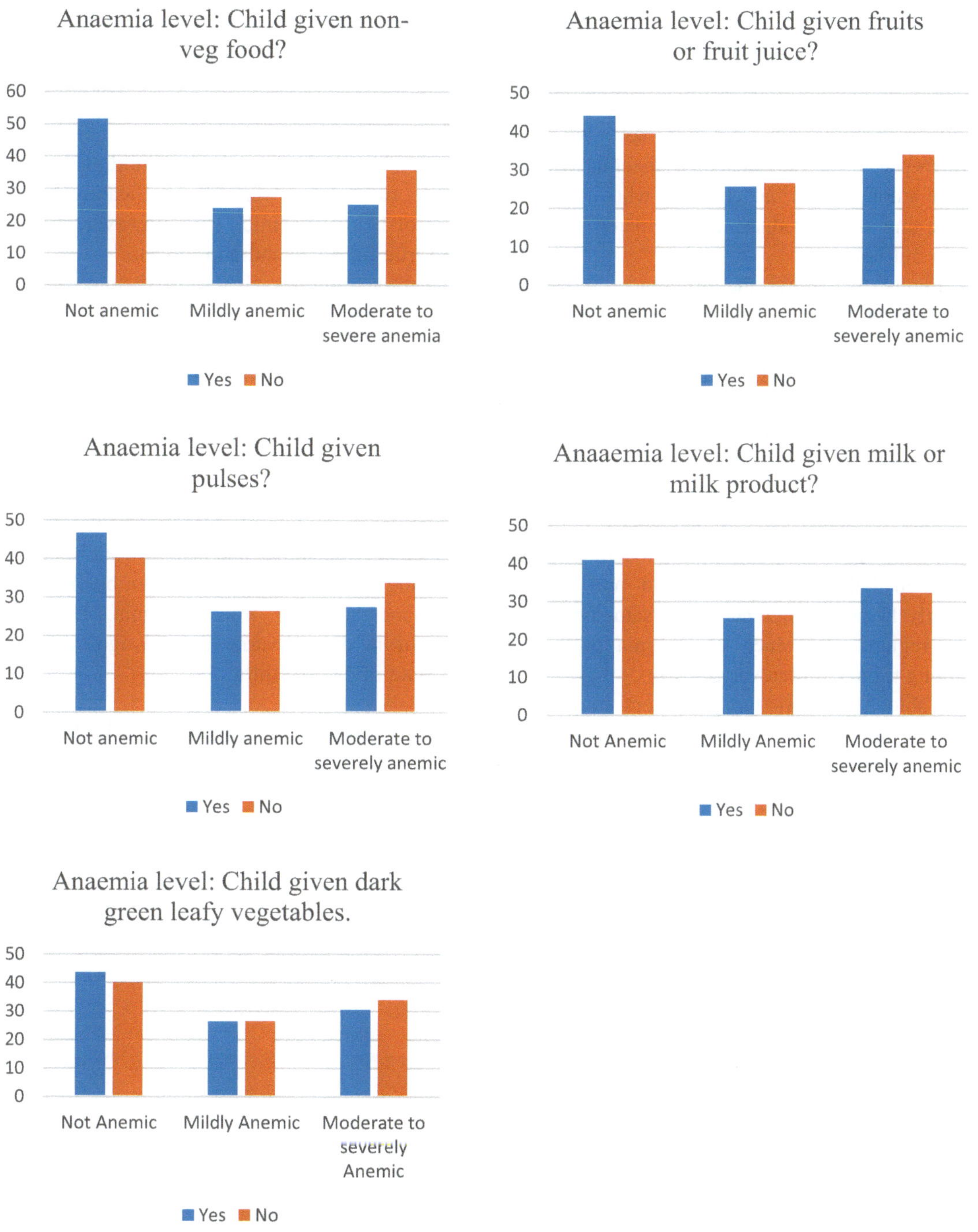

Fig. 5.1 Prevalence of anaemia among children based on their food consumption: India-level estimates

were less suffering from anaemia as compared to their counterparts who did not consume those food items. A slight difference may be noticed among children who consumed pulses/beans or fruits and those who did not. An observable difference in the prevalence of anaemia was not seen among the tribal children who consumed milk and milk products as compared to those who did not.

Figure 5.2 shows the difference in varying degrees of anaemia between India and three selected states. As the figure shows, Nagaland had the least percentage of anaemia-affected children, whereas Odisha had the highest. Among the three selected states, a higher percentage of tribal children belonging to Odisha were affected by moderate to severe degrees of anaemia. There was also a huge difference in the percentage points of moderate to severe degree of anaemia among children belonging to Nagaland and Odisha. Nearly 19-point difference in the same brings out the regional difference in anaemia prevalence among tribal children very clearly.

Table 5.2 shows the predictors of anaemia among children belonging to tribes across India and of three selected states, i.e. Nagaland, Maharashtra, and Odisha.

For both India and Nagaland, the odds of children being anaemic decreased with an increase in wealth status. However, wealth did not show a significant association with anaemia level in Maharashtra and Odisha. Age of the child was seen to be a significant predictor of anaemia in all three states as well as pan-India. The odds of a child being anaemic were higher at an early age as compared to later stages of childhood. Place of residence played a significant role in predicting anaemia in tribal children of Maharashtra and across India. Children belonging to rural areas were at significantly higher odds of being anaemic. This, however, did not hold true for Nagaland and Odisha.

Dietary variables also showed some significant association with anaemia status of children across India. Consumption of non-vegetarian food is associated with significantly lower odds (0.56) of children being anaemic across India and in Nagaland and Odisha. Children being given pulses, beans or fruits showed lower odds of suffering from anaemia pan-India, whereas consumption of milk and milk products or dark green leafy vegetables had a significant impact in lowering the odds of tribal children belonging to Nagaland suffering from anaemia. However, none of the dietary variables held significance in the state of Maharashtra.

5.4.1.1 Anaemia Among Tribal Women

Figure 5.3 shows the prevalence of varying degrees of anaemia among tribal women belonging to India and three selected states. Anaemia in women also followed a similar pattern as that of anaemia in children. Tribal women belonging to Nagaland had the least prevalence of anaemia with barely 6% of them suffering from moderate to severe anaemia, while tribal

Fig. 5.2 Prevalence of anaemia among tribal children belonging to three selected states of different regions

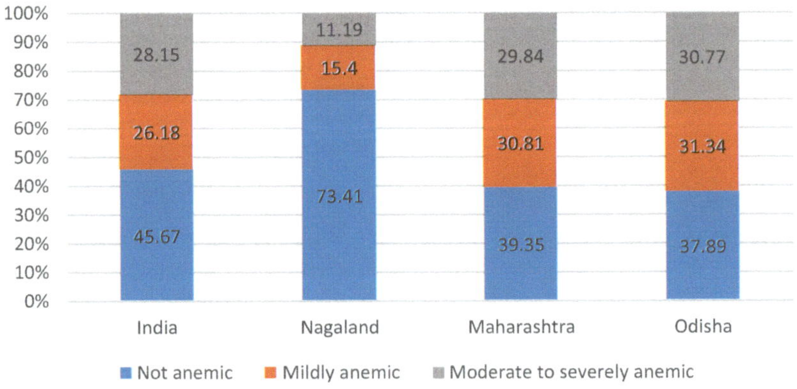

Table 5.2 Predictors of anaemia among tribal children—India and selected states: Results from logistic regression

Socio-economic characteristic	India	Nagaland	Maharashtra	Odisha
Demographic variables				
Age of child				
0 to 1®				
1 to 2	0.460** [.428, .495]	0.34** [.27, .43]	0.56* [.36, .86]	0.36** [.26, .49]
2 to 3	0.229**[.208, .252]	0.12** [.09, .16]	0.31** [.17, .56]	0.31** [.19, .50]
3 to 4	0.202** [.185, .220]	0.13** [.10, .17]	0.26** [.15, .43]	0.17** [.12, .25]
4 to 5	0.160** [.146, .176]	0.11** [.08, .16]	0.24** [.13, .42]	0.14**[.09, .021]
Geographical variables				
Place of residence				
Urban®				
Rural	1.070* [.998, .1.16]	0.87 [.67, 1.12]	1.06* [.80, 1.65]	0.91 [.60, 1.38]
Dietary variable				
Non-veg food item				
No®				
Yes	0.565** [.525, .608]	0.84* [.77, .94]	0.70 [.41, 1.19]	0.73* [.53, 1.00]
Pulses and beans				
No®				
Yes	0.988* [.908, .1.07]	1.09 [0.84, 1.42]	1.22 [.64, 2.30]	0.75 [.50, 1.13]
Milk and milk products				
No®				
Yes	1.18 [1.11, 1.26]	0.71* [.56, .88]	1.03 [.69, 1.54]	0.90 [.65, 1.24]
Fruits				
No®				
Yes	.959* [.908, 1.07]	.97 [.77, 1.23]	.79 [.53, 1.78]	1.24 [.91, 1.67]
Dark green leafy vegetables				
No®				
Yes	.898** [.838, .962]	.95* [.85, 1.09]	1.30 [.82, 2.07]	.89 [.67, 1.19]

*Note: ® Reference Category, C.I: Confidence Interval, ** p<0.01, * p<0.10 Source*: Authors.

women belonging to Odisha had the highest prevalence among the three selected states with nearly 17% suffering from moderate to severe anaemia.

Figure 5.4 shows the distribution of women consuming various food groups' daily and non-vegetarian food on weekly basis. The mean dietary score of women belonging to tribes residing in Nagaland was higher than the national score (8.9 and 8.54, respectively). A higher dietary score was indicative of more frequent consumption of various food groups that was a better diversity in diet. Highest per cent of weekly consumption of non-vegetarian diet was found in Maharashtra whereas Odisha had the highest share of women who consumed green vegetables and pulses/beans on a daily basis. Daily consumption of milk was found to be highest among women residing in Nagaland and least in those residing in Odisha.

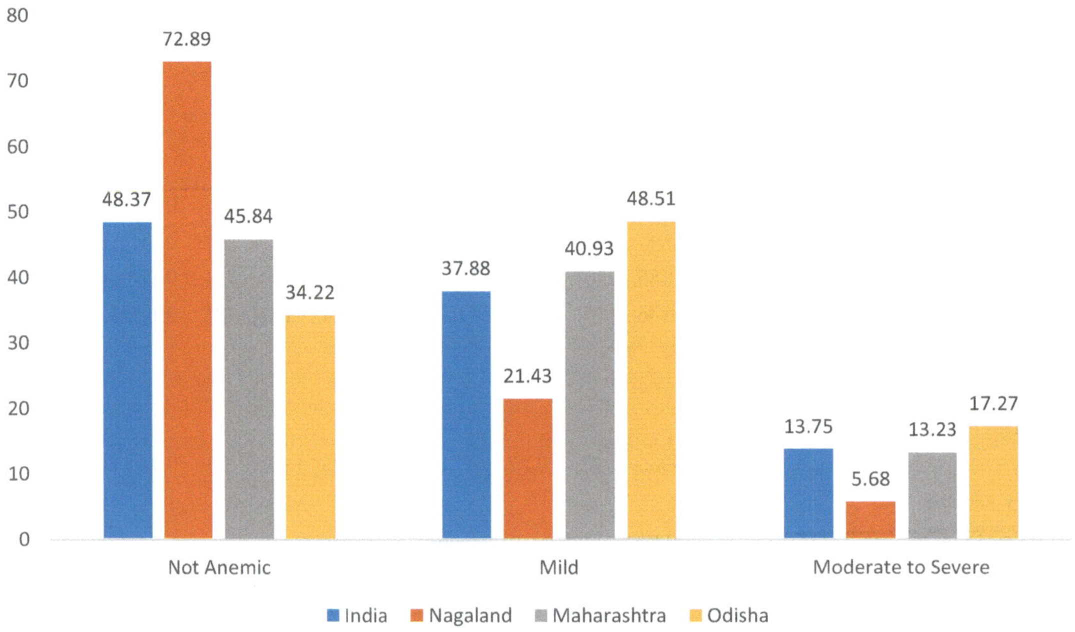

Fig. 5.3 Prevalence of anaemia among tribal women: India and selected states

Table 5.3 shows the determinants of frequency of diverse diet for women belonging to tribes of the three selected states. Wealth was a predominant determinant that held significance for all the three states. Though all states showed a positive change in the frequency as we climb up the wealth ladder, the variation was vast in Odisha. Tribal women belonging to upper wealth index had 9 folds higher chances of consuming a diverse diet. Slightly lesser variation can be seen in Nagaland (sevenfold) and the least variation was seen in the lowest and upper wealth quintile in Maharashtra.

Another factor that significantly determined the frequency of diverse diet consumption was the educational level of the tribal women. A higher educational level concurred with a better diversity in diet.

Factors such as age, geographical location and number of children held significance for two out of three states. It was seen that women residing in rural areas had lower odds of diet diversity as compared to their counterparts in urban areas for the states of Nagaland and Odisha. Having children increased the odds of diet diversity among tribal women of Maharashtra and Odisha as compared to women of these states with no children. However, with an increase in the number of children, it showed a declining trend. Odds of higher frequency of dietary diversity showed a peculiar trend. For Nagaland, the odds of better dietary diversity are highest in the age group 31–40 while other age groups (25–30 and 41– 49) had higher odds than the reference age group, i.e. 15–24. Contrary to Nagaland, in Maharashtra as age increased the odds of tribal women having a better dietary score diminished.

Table 5.4 talks about the predictors of women's anaemia in different states. As the table suggests, each state has a different set of predictors of anaemia.

While wealth, education, number of children, number of births in last 1 year and current method of contraception use were seen as

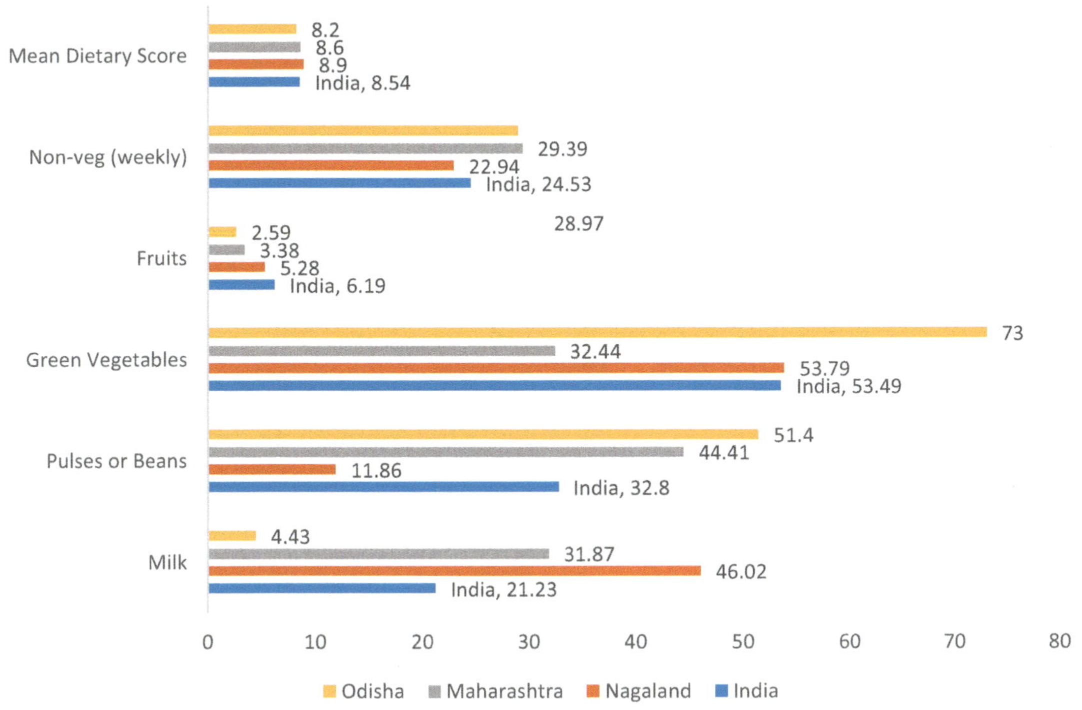

Fig. 5.4 Frequency of diverse diet among tribal women—daily consumption of various food groups: India and selected states

determinants of anaemia in women belonging to tribes of Nagaland, the same pattern is not followed by Maharashtra or Odisha.

For Odisha, the number of births in the last 1 year held the significance in determining anaemia level (women who had at least one birth in the past year were at a higher risk of being anaemic) followed by dietary variable such as consumption of non-vegetarian food and consumption of dark green leafy vegetables- better consumption of these food items leads to less likelihood of anaemia.

Current contraception practice, followed by wealth index, was seen to be a predictor of anaemia among tribal women belonging to Maharashtra. It was seen that women who use modern contraception (hormonal contraception such as IUDs, Pills, or Injections) had significantly lower odds of being anaemic as compared to their counterparts who did not use contraception.

Figure 5.5 explains the contribution of significant predictor of anaemia for respective states. Decomposition analysis gave the impact of the selected significant variable on respective state's anaemia level. For Nagaland and Maharashtra, current contraception practice was used as decomposing variable, whereas, for Odisha, the number of births in the last 1 year had been used. Movement from any other method of contraception to modern (hormonal) contraception resulted in a decrease in anaemia level among women belonging to tribes residing in Nagaland and Maharashtra, whereas change in the number of births in last 1 year from no birth to at least 1 birth resulted in an increase in anaemia level among tribal women of Odisha.

Table 5.3 Determinants of diverse diet among tribal women belonging to selected states: Result from ordered logistic regression

Independent variables	Odds ratio (Nagaland)	Odds ratio (Maharashtra)	Odds ratio (Odisha)
Socio-Economic variables			
Wealth index			
Poorest®			
Poorer	1.43*** (1.21–1.68)	1.51*** (1.28–1.79)	1.73*** (1.54–1.95)
Middle	2.28*** (1.91–2.73)	1.92*** (1.59–2.32)	2.63*** (2.18–3.18)
Richer	3.71*** (3.05–4.52)	2.96*** (2.36–3.73)	4.80*** (3.66–6.27)
Richest	7.29*** (5.85–9.09)	4.47*** (3.28–6.07)	9.93*** (6.94–14.21)
Level of education			
No education®			
Primary	0.89 (0.75–1.06)	1.01 (0.83–1.23)	1.79*** (1.54–2.09)
Secondary	1.11 (0.96–1.29)	1.20* (1.01–1.43)	2.22*** (1.95–2.54)
Higher	1.69*** (1.38–2.07)	1.88*** (1.35–2.61)	3.16*** (2.28–4.38)
Demographic variables			
Age group			
15 to 24®			
25 to 30	1.20* (1.04–1.38)	0.72* (0.59–0.89)	1.07 (0.92–1.25)
31 to 40	1.34*** (1.17–1.55)	0.79* (0.64–0.97)	1.10 (0.94–1.28)
41 to 49	1.29* (1.10–1.52)	0.792* (0.62–0.99)	1.12 (0.95–1.34)
Number of children ever born			
No Child ®			
1 Child	1.09 (0.93–1.27)	1.04 (0.84–1.30)	1.38*** (1.18–1.60)
2-3 Children	1.11 (0.97–1.28)	1.38* (1.13–1.69)	1.36*** (1.17–1.58)
More than 3 children	0.88 (0.75–1.04)	1.25* (0.96–1.63)	1.18* (0.98–1.41)
Geographical variables			
Place of residence			
Urban ®			
Rural	0.77*** (0.69–0.86)	1.01 (0.83–1.23)	0.72*** (0.61–0.85)

*Note: ® Reference Category, C.I: Confidence Interval, *** p<0.01, * p<0.10* | Dependent Variable = Dietary Score.
0 = Minimum to (Mean – Std.Dv.)
1 = (Mean – Std. Dvn.) to (Mean + Std. Dvn.)
2 = (Mean + Std. Dvn.) to Maximum

5.5 Discussion

The present study sought to understand the prevalence of anaemia among tribal women and children across India and the regional disparity that exists. It also tried to identify the predictors of childhood anaemia and anaemia among tribal women with special focus on three different states- Nagaland, Maharashtra, and Odisha- to bring out the regional difference in underlying causes of anaemia. Aspect of diet diversity and determinants of frequency of consumption of diverse diet were also explored. Finally, it aimed to understand the impact of selected predictors on anaemia level of tribal women belonging to the three selected diverse states. There are studies that talk about tribal women and children's anaemia; however, all of these are geographically limited to a certain region or state. There is

Table 5.4 Predictors of anaemia among tribal women belonging to selected states: Results from regression analysis.

Independent variables	Nagaland	Maharashtra	Odisha
Socio-Economic variables			
Wealth Index			
Poorest®			
Poorer	0.75*** (0.64–0.87)	0.95 (0.80–1.12)	1.04 (0.93–1.16)
Middle	0.62*** (0.52–0.73)	0.83*(0.68–1.01)	0.91 (0.77–1.07)
Richer	0.60*** (0.50–0.73)	0.69* (0.54–0.87)	0.95 (0.73–1.24)
Richest	0.48*** (0.38–0.61)	0.57* (0.41–0.79)	0.99 (0.68–1.44)
Level of education			
No Education®			
Primary	0.90 (0.76–1.05)	1.00 (0.82–1.21)	0.94 (0.82–1.08)
Secondary	0.86* (0.75–0.99)	0.94 (0.78–1.12)	0.96 (0.85–1.08)
Higher	0.78* (0.63–0.96)	0.97(0.69–1.37)	0.76* (0.56–1.03)
Demographic variables			
Age Group			
15 to 24®			
25 to 30	0.90 (0.78–1.04)	0.95 (0.76–1.19)	1.03 (0.89–1.20)
31 to 40	0.89 (0.77–1.02)	0.92 (0.73–1.16)	1.15* (0.99–1.34)
41 to 49	0.90 (0.77–1.07)	0.82 (0.63–1.06)	1.21* (1.02–1.44)
Number of children ever born			
No Child ®			
1 Child	1.06 (0.90–1.25)	1.10 (0.86–1. 42)	0.94 (0.83–1.08)
2-3 Children	1.14* (0.98–1.32)	1.17 (0.91–1.52)	0.89 (0.99–1.05)
More than 3 children	1.10 (0.93–1.30)	0.85 (0.62–1.15)	0.87 (0.71–1.05)
Geographical variables			
Place of residence			
Urban ®			
Rural	0.97 (0.87–1.09)	0.84 (0.68–1.04)	0.85* (0.73–0.99)
Dietary variables			
Type of diet			
Vegetarian ®			
Non vegetarian	0.82 (0.74–0.92)	0.93 (0.78–1.11)	0.74* (0.57–0.96)
Consumption of dark green leafy vegetables.			
Not daily ®			
Daily	0.96 (0.88–1.06)	1.05 (0.88–1.24)	0.88* (0.78–1.00)
Dietary score			
Low®			
Normal	1.00 (0.85–1.17)	1.10 (0.91–1.33)	1.02 (0.87–1.18)
Good	0.94 (0.76–1.18)	1.16 (0.84–1.59)	0.96 (0.75–1.23)

(continued)

Table 5.4 (continued)

Independent variables	Nagaland	Maharashtra	Odisha
Health variables			
Number of birth in last year			
No Birth ®			
At least 1 birth	1.27* (1.08–1.48)	1.03 (0.78–1.36)	1.52*** (1.26–1.83)
Type of contraception currently using			
Not using ®			
Pills/Injections/IUDs	0.92* (0.76–1.11)	0.63* (0.36–1.07)	0.99 (0.83–1.18)
Condoms	1.19 (0.70–2.00)	0.88 (0.57–1.35)	0.91 (0.64–1.29)
Sterilized	0.81 (0.67–0.99)	0.78* (0.64–0.96)	1.07 (0.93–1.23)
Any traditional method	1.09 (0.85–1.39)	0.58* (0.33–1.02)	0.99 (0.84–1.17)

*Note: ®Reference Category, C.I: Confidence Interval, *** p<0.01, * p<0.10*

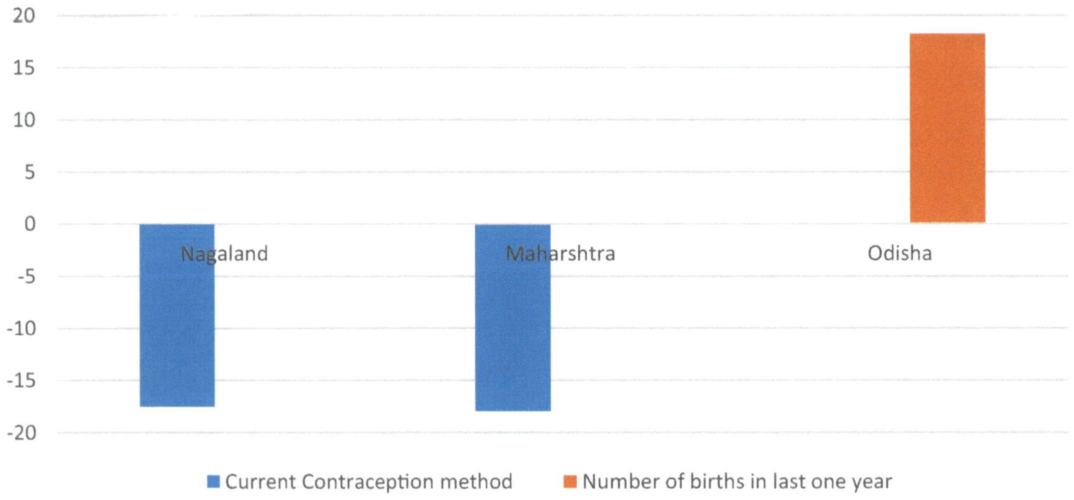

Fig. 5.5 Contribution of significant parameter in explaining anaemia for women belonging to respective states: Results from Fairlie decomposition analysis

minimal evidence of an all-inclusive study that encompasses pan-India prevalence and predictors of women and child anaemia among tribes.

5.5.1 Childhood Anaemia

The present study found a higher prevalence of anaemia among tribal children belonging to northern region (Chandigarh, Haryana, Himachal Pradesh, Jammu and Kashmir, Delhi, Punjab, Rajasthan, and Uttarakhand) of India. More than 50 percent of children belonging to tribal regions of north are found to be severely anaemic. As compared to 14 percent of children being severely anaemic in the north-eastern region, it is a staggering number. Hence, it can be said that there exists a huge regional variation in the prevalence of anaemia across different tribal populations. While there is no specific study that brings out this difference, it can still be seen evidently through different pocket studies (De et al., 2006; Rakesh, 2017). A study on children aged 12–23 months living in New Delhi reported 79.2 percent anaemia prevalence (Houghton et al., 2019). The regional difference is significantly visible when the three selected states are taken into consideration. The state of Nagaland shows prevalence of severe anaemia as low as 11%, whereas, in the state of Odisha the prevalence surpasses the national prevalence of severe anaemia among tribal children (31% Odisha, 28% India).

An age-dependence is also found in prevalence of anaemia among children. The study finds that prevalence of anaemia is higher in younger children. It is believed that iron requirement are highest at the age of 7–12 months due to rapid growth, hence, the critical Hb levels at lower age. Given the higher prevalence of iron deficiency anaemia during the first 1000 days and its implications such as cognitive impairment and physical deficits, it is of utmost importance to identify, intervene, and prevent iron deficiency anaemia at an early age (Burke et al., 2014). Higher prevalence was also found among tribal children residing in rural areas and belonging to economically disadvantageous groups.

Prevalence pattern is also found to be varying based on food groups consumed. Prevalence of severe anaemia is found to be lowest among children who were given non-vegetarian food items such as meat, fish or eggs. Similar results have been found in studies conducted outside the geographical boundaries of Indian subcontinent. Vegetarian dietary habit is associated with a higher prevalence of iron deficiency anaemia (Pawlak & Bell 2017). There is evidence of vegetarian diet being associated with higher prevalence of anaemia among pediatric age group at India level as well (Naik&Venkatesha, 2019).

The present study goes beyond difference in prevalence of anaemia for tribal children in three selected states to understand the predictors of anaemia in these states along with India-level predictors. It is found that different states have disparate predictors of anaemia among tribal children. While existing literature establishes a higher index of poverty (Goswami & Das, 2015), lack of diverse diet (Stiller et al., 2020) as common predictors of anaemia among children, the results from the present study show that it doesn't hold true for all states alike. Wealth index is found to be a significant determinant at India level as well as for Nagaland. It doesn't come across as significant for Maharashtra or Odisha. Similarly, dietary pattern is seen to be a significant determinant of anaemia for tribal children living in the state of Nagaland and Odisha as well as proves to be a determinant at national level but not so much in case of Maharashtra. However, age group of children is found to be a common predictor of anaemia among tribal children belonging to India as well as specifically for selected three states. Child's age is reported as a determinant of anaemia by a few other studies as well (Pasricha, et al., 2010). Authors have reported younger age to be associated with higher likelihood of anaemia (Adish et al., 1999; Ray et al., 2016; Chandra et al., 2002). This could be attributed to incompleteness of weaning practices, exclusive breastfeeding for a longer duration or top feeding with liquid/diluted diet.

5.5.2 Anaemia Among Women

The present study notices a similar pattern in regional prevalence of anaemia among tribal women as is observed among tribal children. Nagaland has the least prevalence of anaemia among tribal women while Odisha has the highest. This finding is supported by pocket studies that have been conducted at different time points (see, Kamath et al., 2013; Kumud & Priyanka, 2020; De et al., 2006). This variation could be attributed to difference in food habits. It is known that north-eastern region of India is predominantly non-vegetarian. The study does find tribal women from Nagaland to have a higher frequency of consumption of diverse diet. There is an undoubted association of diet diversity with prevalence of anaemia as has been established by not only domestic studies but also through studies globally (Delil et al., 2018). The study found that factors such as wealth, number of children ever born, and place of residence, i.e. whether living in an urban or rural area determines the diet diversity. While it is observed that wealth and place of residence have a direct relationship with high frequency of diet diversity, i.e. as the wealth increases so does the frequency of consumption of a diverse diet. Tribal population residing in urban areas have a better dietary diversity than their rural counterparts. It is a common notion for people to believe that rural population would have a better dietary diversity given their involvement in agriculture and their close proximity to nature. However, previous studies have proven it wrong (GSS, 2015; Ayensu et al., 2020). This maybe because urban dwellers might have better nutritional knowledge that is needed for selection, preparation, and consumption of a diverse diet.

The study found that although the same factors also determine prevalence of anaemia among tribal women but they aren't uniform across India. It is seen that, while economic status, i.e. wealth index, number of children in the last 1 year and type of current contraception act as predictors of anaemia for tribal women residing in Nagaland, the same doesn't hold true for either Maharashtra or Odisha. Method of current contraception comes across as a significant predictor of anaemia in Maharashtra ,while the number of births in last 1 year strongly determine anaemia in tribal women of Odisha. There are a number of studies globally that talk about the association of hormonals contraceptive (modern contraceptive) such as pills/IUDs/injections with a reduced risk of anaemia (Haile et al., 2017; Gebremedhin et al., 2018; Teshale et al., 2020). These studies point towards the use of hormone-coated IUDs that reduce the likeliness of anaemia (Wilunda et al., 2013). It is also to be noted that prevention of iron anaemia is a known non-contraceptive benefit of oral contraception (Mishell 1993). However, this association is yet to be explored in detail in Indian context. This study is one of the few to talk about effect of hormonal contraception on tribal women's anaemia level.

Similarly, another important factor that determines anaemia level among women residing in Odisha is number of births in past one year. It is seen that women who had given birth to at least one child in the past one year were more susceptible to being anaemic. There is evidence that postpartum amenorrhea causes anaemia (Bodnar et al., 2005; Bodnar et al., 2001), however this association, has by far and large, not been studied for India.

The study finds that current method of contraception i.e. use or non-use of modern hormonal contraception explained nearly 18% of anaemia in both the states of Maharashtra and Nagaland and at least one birth in the last year corresponded with explaining 18% of anaemia among tribal women of Odisha.

5.6 Conclusion

Prevalence of anaemia is fluctuates with region and state. While Nagaland reported least prevalence, Odisha had a significantly higher prevalence of anaemia among both women and children. This varying prevalence may be attributed to differences in diet pattern and food consumption. While diet can be said to play an important role in determining anaemia level among women and children, it cannot be classified as sole predictor. The predictors that determine anaemia also vary from tribe to tribe. Wealth index, level of education does play their part but predictors such as current method of contraception use among women take the forefront in determining anaemia for Nagaland and Maharashtra. A significant predictor for Odisha comes out to be number of births in the last 1 year. It was found that non-dietary factors such as type of contraception use and number of births in the last 1 year also play an important role in determining anaemia among tribes. Although, the percentage contribution of such factors in explaining anaemia differs with tribes.

Hence, it is imperative to not have an umbrella approach while dealing with anaemia among tribal women and children. Given, the range of causes and determinants of anaemia, it is important to pin-point the root cause and to try to tackle it for different tribes. It is of utmost importance to curate state-specific interventions to combat alarmingly high rates of anaemia among some tribal women and children. The healthcare services must reach the tribal areas. Along with an increased accessibility and affordability of various food groups, it is crucial to spread nutritional awareness among these tribes.

The study has certain limitations such as dataset for National Family Health Survey does not categorize the tribal population by name of the tribe. Hence, a precise picture of different tribes cannot be drawn.

Key Findings:
Along with prevalence of Anaemia being alarmingly high among tribal women and children, it fluctuates with region – Northern region of India showing higher prevalence than the rest.
One factor that determines anaemia among tribal children residing in all of the selected states (Nagaland, Maharashtra and Odisha) is age of the child – younger the child, higher likelihood of being anaemic.
Diversity in consumption of diet plays an important role in determining anaemia level among women – non-vegetarianism is associated with lower likelihood of anaemia.
Wealth index, educational level come out to be significant determinants of better diet diversity.
Determinants of anaemia among tribal women cannot be pin-pointed to single factor – they differ from tribe to tribe.
Apart from dietary factors, non-dietary factors such as type of contraception used (hormonal or other), whether given birth to at least one child in the last one year, also play a crucial role in determining anaemia among tribal women.
It is important to curate state specific interventions to tackle anaemia among tribal children and women – an umbrella approach might not work given the range of predictors of anaemia.

The Role of Inequality in Determining Nutrition: Explaining the Gujarat Paradox

6

Akancha Singh and Aparajita Chattopadhyay

Abstract

One of the industrialized states with concomitantly high rates of urbanization and economic development, Gujarat is one of the fastest growing states among the bigger Indian states. The incidence of poverty in Gujarat is lower than that in India in both rural and urban areas. The impact of the sustained economic growth on health and nutrition outcomes in Gujarat has been far from satisfactory. For an economically prosperous state, Gujarat continues to perform poorly in standard nutrition indicators. This chapter tries to understand this paradoxical relationship between economic development and child undernutrition indicators. It further explains the inequality in child undernutrition in Gujarat and identifies that socio-economic status of households explains more than half of the inequality that is prevalent in child undernutrition in Gujarat. The findings suggest that an improvement in wealth status of households is more beneficial for those children who are already relatively healthy.

Keywords

Inequality · Gujarat · India · Decomposition · Economy · Development · Stunting

6.1 Introduction

6.1.1 Development, Economy, and Nutrition

A recurring hurdle to achieving economic and human development goals globally is the high rates of undernutrition and child mortality (Accorsi et al., 2005; Koblinsky et al., 2008; Adjiwanou & LeGrand, 2014; Ezeh et al., 2014; Singh, 2014; Bishai et al., 2016; Anele, 2017; Cha, 2017). An important predictor of child mortality and morbidity, chronic undernutrition posits both long-term and short-term challenges. While the short-term challenges are obvious, the long-term consequences include cognitive impairment, and impeded opportunities for upward mobility in both educational and professional spheres (Fulhan et al., 2003; Kar et al., 2008; Martins et al., 2011; Cursick & Georgieff, 2016). The relationship between economic growth and child nutrition has interested remarkable research and donor attention during the last two decades (Martorell, 1996; Ali & Goudar, 2014; Vollmer et al., 2014; Bershteyn et al., 2015; Biadgilign et al., 2016; Hurley et al., 2016; McGovern et al., 2017). There has been abundant evidence to elucidate the fact that economic growth may be necessary but is defi-

A. Chattopadhyay et al., *Undernutrition in India*, Sustainable Development Goals Series,
https://doi.org/10.1007/978-981-19-8182-1_6

nitely not a sufficient condition for improvement in nutrition situation among children (Mary, 2018). Another set of evidence suggests that the largest contributors to reductions in child stunting are deworming initiatives, IFA supplementation, and immunization (Buisman et al., 2019). It is important to note that the only way economic growth can decisively reduce poverty is if the income distribution is constant over time, otherwise economic growth can lead to the furthering of inequalities in a plethora of ways, the pertinent examples being access to basic amenities such as health, education, and technology (McGovern et al., 2017). In light of recent evidence on the relationship between child nutrition and economic consequences in adulthood, it can be concluded that when improvements in national income are aimed at reducing gender inequalities, improving women's status, water and sanitation facilities, and children's diets, only then is economic growth effective in improving children's nutritional status (Beker, 2016).

Despite the momentous decline in maternal and child undernutrition in India since the 1990s, undernutrition remains the crucial risk factor for disease and death in not just children under 5 years of age but all age groups in India. Research suggests that disability adjusted life years (DALYs) for undernutrition is the highest in those states that are economically not well-off or have low socio-demographic index (India State-Level Disease Burden Initiative Undernutrition Collaborators, 2019). The DALYS for undernutrition in children under the age of 5 years are predominantly because of premature mortality. Despite the proportional share of maternal and child undernutrition to the total DALY burden across all age groups in India has fallen substantially from 36.5% in 1990 to 17.3% in 2017, it is still the important and leading risk factor for health loss (India State-Level Disease Burden Initiative undernutrition Collaborators, 2019). This becomes especially more pertinent because although, in 2017, the population of 1.38 billion in India constituted nearly 18% of the global population, yet India shouldered nearly 25.4% of the total burden of global DALYs attributable to maternal and child undernutrition in 2017 (Institute for Health Metrics and Evaluation; 2018). In 2017, undernutrition was the important risk factor among under-five children in Indian states (India State-Level Disease Burden Initiative undernutrition Collaborators, 2019).

6.1.2 Economic Growth and Undernutrition

There is a seething debate in the literature on whether the impact of improvements in the economic indicators of a country manifest themselves in simultaneous improvements in nutritional status of children (Ruel et al., 2013; Alderman et al., 2014; Vollmer et al., 2014a, b; Smith & Haddad, 2015; O'Connell & Smith, 2016; Vollmer et al., 2016). This debate is important because it stresses on the need to aid poor-centric growth policies targeted at reducing undernutrition with direct nutritional investments. Additionally, given the scarcity of resources, it is also pertinent that resources are spent in a diversified manner. A lack of consensus can easily be established by the wide range of estimates provided by empirical literature. For instance, findings from a recent research by Ruel et al. (2013) suggest that with a 10% increase in GDP per capita, there is a 6% reduction in child stunting. These findings concur with those of other studies (Smith & Haddad 2015; O'Connell & Smith 2016). There is also evidence to suggest that there are chances for the contribution of economic growth to be even be higher (i.e. a 7.3% reduction in child stunting would be the result of a 10% increase in GDP per capita) (Mary, 2018). Another set of contrasting evidence suggests that there is a very small quantitative relationship between economic growth and child undernutrition (Vollmer et al., 2014a). Studies conducted in Sub-Saharan Africa have also found that economic growth has limited positive impacts on the odds of being stunted (Harttgen et al., 2013).

Amelioration in the health status is considered a spin-off of economic growth and of improvements in per capita income. History suggests that with industrialization and increased economic growth, there has been betterment in the health status of people. Thus, it is obvious that the people living in the developed economies enjoy better health status as compared to their counterparts in the developing economies. However, it will be incorrect to assume that the relationship between per capita income and health status is always direct. While some countries have a relatively better public health scenario at lower levels of economic growth, others have dismal public health scenario despite impressive levels of income and development. Samuel H. Preston first brought this hypothesis to the fore in his pioneering work "The Changing Relation between Mortality and Level of Economic Development" (Preston, 1975). He argues that at low levels of per capita income, improvements in income are associated with immense advancements in life expectancy, but at as the income levels plateau at a relatively high level, this increased income has little ramifications for life expectancy. In other words, if the relationship between per capita income and life expectancy is hypothesized to be causal, then there are diminishing returns to income as far as life expectancy is concerned. Talking about demographic indicators and economic growth, Angus Deaton, further extending the hypothesis given by Preston, elucidates that while economic growth is the key to poverty reduction, there is no conclusive evidence to prove that it will automatically lead to health improvements in the absence of appropriate conditions. Summarily, he concludes by saying that it is actually the growth of real income that has ramifications on demographic indicators (life expectancy, infant and child mortality in his case), factoring in the importance of determinants such as education and the quality of life in general that have important bearings for both health and growth (Deaton, 2001, 2006) (Fig. 6.1).

It is often stipulated that urbanization leads to an improvement in the health status of the general population because urban areas tend to have better health facilities than rural areas in developing countries. Additionally, due to improved access to pertinent information in urban areas, child mortality and fertility rates are lower in urban areas as compared to rural areas (Murthi et al., 1995). But, even in developing countries with high per capita incomes, urban environmental conditions are quite poor and industrialization is causing serious pollution. As a consequence of the above, the overall urban health status is low, particularly among the poorer households.

6.1.3 Nutrition-Related Aspects of SDGs

Although SDG2 ("End hunger, achieve food security and improved nutrition and promote sustainable agriculture") is the sole SDG that visibly lays emphasis on nutrition as the core area, it is crucial for working on all the SDGs in tandem in order to achieve SDG2. It is, therefore, conspicuous that nutrition is a fundamental element for achieving other SDGs (Table 6.1) and achieving other SDGs is imperative for achieving the nutrition goal on the other. Lack of nutrition can be attributed to myriad socio-economic factors, encompassing lack of food security attributable to poverty and war (SDG 1). Estimates suggest that nearly 800 million individuals worldwide are suffering from hunger that is caused by poverty (FAO et al., 2018). SDGs 4 and 8 dealing with education, decent work, and economic growth can also be linked to improved diet quality. Despite the absence of strong evidence suggesting causal inference (preferred consumption of low-quality foods (energy-dense and nutrient-poor) by lower socio-educational classes may be due to lack of accessibility to, and/or non-affordability of, higher quality foods, among other factors), diet quality is still a significant determinant of educational attainment and working conditions (Jacobs et al., 2019). Dietary choices are also crucial for the maintenance of good health and well-being (SDG 3). The double burden of undernutrition is manifested in, not only nutritional deficiencies (leading to an increased risk of infectious diseases) but also overweight/obesity (leading to an escalated risk of non-communicable diseases). This becomes particularly pertinent as a pandemic of

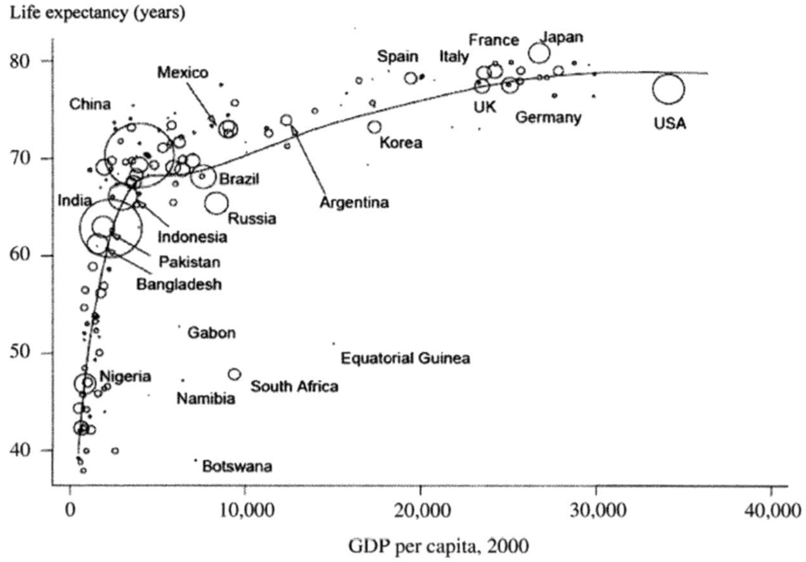

Fig. 6.1 The Millennium Preston Curve. *Source* Based on Deaton (2000)

enormous proportions is wreaking havoc on approximately 4 billion people residing in both developing and developed countries (NCS-RisC, 2017).

Nutrition, as a component, is a part of SDGs both via direct and indirect pathways. It is an important component of SDG 11, dealing with rural and urban environments, in the sense that rise in BMI in rural areas accounts for more than 50% of the rise in BMI globally in the last 3 decades. This further stresses on the need for creating health-sustaining environments, especially around housing developments (NCS-RisC, 2019). Other than that, the 5th and 10th SDGs (gender equality and reducing inequalities, respectively) also correlate strongly with nutrition. Additionally, especially in economically laggard countries, the females work in farms and fields. They are also often the ones taking charge of household chores such as cooking, cleaning, and taking care of their families and communities. It is this household-based knowledge that can be used to improve nutrition and create healthier communities and societies (ISS FANSAA et al., 2018). In addition to the above, there are environment-related SDGs that are impacted by food production and consumption practices (water and sanitation, clean and affordable energy, industry, sustainable communities, responsible consumption, climate and life on land and below water). The process of food production, ranging from irrigation practices to fertilizer usage, is associated with greenhouse gas emissions, release of toxic gases such as nitrogen and phosphorus, depletion of water resources, and loss of biodiversity (Smetana et al., 2019). Another food-related aspect that has ramifications for the environment is food wastage. With nearly 930 million tons of food being wasted globally, food that has not been consumed accounts for about 8–10% of global greenhouse gas emissions (UNEP, 2021). It is, thus, clear that both policymakers and end-product consumers will have to come together to make the SDGs a reality. It is also important to ensure that food production and consumption practices are sustainable and healthy so that the global food systems become an agent in aiding the achievement of such substantial and ambitious changes.

6.1.4 The Gujarat Paradox

Gujarat is one of the important industrialized states of India with persistently high rates of economic growth and urbanization. As per a new series of data on the Gross State domestic

Table 6.1 Nutrition-related aspects of sustainable development goals

Sustainable development goals	Linkages with nutrition
SDG1: No poverty	Poverty restricts access to adequate food intake and makes it difficult to attain nutritional recommendations
SDG2: Zero hunger	Unsustainable food production causes undernourishment
SDG3: Good health and well-being	Healthy and sustainable nutrition may lead to a reduction in premature mortality, including death due to NCDs
SDG4: Quality education	Malnutrition impairs learning ability, while improved awareness may lead to healthy and sustainable food choices
SDG5: Gender equality	Empowering women leads to an improvement in their quality of life and nutritional status; better nutrition improves learning outcomes, which, in turn, is manifested in better job opportunities
SDG6: Clean water and sanitation	Access to safe drinking water and sanitation may reduce undernutrition
SDG7: Affordable and clean energy	Reducing dependence on fossil fuels will lead to a reduction in greenhouse gas emissions and environmental pollution, and ensure food security
SDG8: Decent work and economic growth	Improvement in economic conditions may improve nutrition security
SDG9: Industry, innovation and infrastructure	Affordable access to technologies and infrastructure is essential for agriculture development and food security
SDG10: Reduced inequalities	Inequalities create disparities in income and access to food, health, and educational infrastructure
SDG11: Sustainable cities and communities	Expansion of settlements into rural area increases demand for food, creates competition for already scarce food and water resources, and increases dependence on food items purchases
SDG12: Responsible consumption and production	Sustainable solutions for food production and access to water are required for meeting the nutritional needs of a rapidly growing global population. This is important because inefficient food production causes greenhouse gas emissions and soil degradation
SDG13: Climate action	Climate change impacts global food production and food security in addition to impeding access to freshwater resources
SDG14: Life below water	Aquaculture leads to a reduction in hunger and improvement in nutritional status
SDG15: Life on land	Change in pattern of land use causes degradation of soil quality, simultaneously leading to a reduction in biodiversity and food production, and impaired access to fresh water
SDG16: Peace, justice and strong institutions	War also leads to malnutrition and death due to impediments in food supplies and impaired access to food
SDG17: Partnership for the goals	Partnership between diverse sectors, various stakeholders, and governments is needed in order to achieve the goals

Source Grosso et al. (2020)

product of states with its base year as 2011–12 and published by the Central Statistics Office in 2015–16, Gujarat, after Jammu and Kashmir, is the state that has the highest rate of growth among the other bigger Indian states. According to the India Human Development Report, 2011, proportion of population below poverty line in Gujarat is lower than India's figure in both rural and urban areas. The impact of this sustained economic growth on health and nutrition outcomes has, however, not been up to the mark. An exception can be made in the area of improvement in the proportion safe deliveries, where Gujarat has fared remarkably well. For an economically puissant state, Gujarat's performance in definitive nutritional indicators remains extremely deficient. Data from the fourth round of the National Family Health Survey, 2015–16 show that among all the states and UTs, Gujarat ranks 29, 34, and 32 in terms of childhood stunting, wasting, and underweight, respectively. This reckons prompt policy attention as undernutrition at a scale so massive can have adverse impact on the sustainability of economic development through different pathways. The state has earned the sceptical distinction of being the only economically prosperous state to be in the top 10 states that have the highest percentage of childhood stunting in India. It is also important to note that the proportion of undernourished children also shows a considerably high variation between districts within Gujarat. The proportion of child wasting is particularly high in districts such as the Dangs, Jamnagar, Junagadh, Kachchh, Narmada, Panchmahal, and Valsad. Similarly, districts that report a high stunting prevalence are Anand, Bhavnagar, the Dangs, Kheda, Narmada, Sabarkantha, and Surendranagar (NFHS-4, 2015–16). There is, thus, an imminent need to identify the high-burden districts as well as worse performing talukas from the other districts for corrective action.

Gujarat, like India, has made massive strides towards improvement in the health status of its population. In India, the crude death rate (CDR) has declined from 27.4 in 1951 to 6.2 in 2018 (Gowarikar, 1993; SRS, 2018) and the IMR has dramatically reduced from the estimated 200–225 per 1000 live births at the time of independence to 32 in 2018 (Visaria & Visaria, 1994; SRS, 2018). The decline in IMR is primarily due to the decline in the neo-natal mortality (NNM), added benefit of the widespread immunization programs in the country. Gujarat's performance is better than that of India (Table 6.2). Nearly all the crucial demographic indicators such as crude birth rate, crude death rate, maternal mortality rate, life expectancy at birth, and total fertility rate are lower in Gujarat when compared to India's estimates (Table 6.2).

What is more surprising is that Gujarat's performance is worse than that of Kerala, a state which is economically worse off when compared to Gujarat. Estimates from the latest round of Sample Registration System (2018) suggest that Gujarat is lagging far behind of Kerala as far as reaching the health achievements of Kerala reconcerned. For instance, infant mortality rate and neo-natal mortality rate in Gujarat are about four times that in Kerala. The total fertility rate in Gujarat is also greater than that in Kerala (Table not shown). Among the major states in India in 2018, Gujarat can be placed in the middle on important indicators of health status. It ranked 14th with respect to crude birth rate and 16th with respect to crude death rate out of 29

Table 6.2 Health status indicators in Gujarat and India

Indicators	Gujarat	India
Crude birth rate	19.7	20
Crude death rate	5.9	6.2
Infant mortality rate	28	32
Maternal mortality rate	75	113
Life expectancy at birth	68.7	67.9
Neo-natal mortality rate	19	23
Post-natal mortality rate	19	22
Under-five mortality rate	31	36
Gross fertility rate	70.1	70.4
Total fertility rate	2.1	2.2
Sex ratio	866	899

Source Sample Registration System (2018)

states and union territories. It is in fact surprising that the tribal-dominated Tripura and non-urbanized state of Sikkim were doing better than Gujarat with respect to these two indicators of health. Even among the 15 large states, Gujarat was in the middle, 7th in crude birth rate, 6th in crude death rate and infant mortality rate, and 9th in life expectancy at birth in 2018 (SRS, 2018).

With respect to neo-natal mortality, the state ranked 16th out of 29 states surveyed by the NFHS. As per the latest round of SRS, the state ranked 11th with respect to infant mortality rate (as per the NFHS data Gujarat ranked 17th in infant mortality rate and 18th in under-five child mortality). Studies suggest that 17 out of 26 districts in Gujarat are likely to miss the SDG target 3 pertaining to neo-natal mortality (Bora & Saikia, 2018). Though different surveys give different estimates of child health indicators in Gujarat, it is evident that there have been improvements over time. Such improvements, however, have been far from satisfactory. Another state that is Gujarat's parallel in terms of economy and urbanization is Maharashtra. However, its performance is far better in terms of child health and nutrition as compared to Gujarat. The economically not so developed north-eastern states of India too are doing much better than Gujarat in child health, not to mention Kerala which is showing the best results with respect to health indicators (IIPS, 2016). As per the National Goitre Control Program, goitre is endemic to Gujarat (Nutritional Foundation of India 1983, as quoted by Ali 1992). Additionally, prevalence of vitamin A deficiency and resulting blindness is also the highest in Gujarat as compared to other Indian states (IIPS, 2016).

Eleven districts of the state have endemic prevalence of goitre due to iodine deficiency (Table not shown). Among these 11 districts, all the districts have a substantial proportion of tribal population except four districts, namely, Amreli, Mehsana, Kheda, and Surendranagar. Three districts out of the 11 surveyed—Dangs, Valsad, and Bharuch—have severe iodine deficiency disorder (IDD). The districts of Gujarat which have a considerable proportion of tribal population and moderate prevalence of IDD are Dangs, Sabarkantha, Surat, and Panchmahals. It, therefore, appears that the tribal population in the state suffers undernourishment and special attention with regard to nutrition is required to improve health status of this section of Gujarat's population (Yadav & Pandey, 2018). In addition to the above, despite varying estimates of maternal mortality rate from different sources, it could be concluded that though there have been substantial improvements in maternal health over time, the improvements have been far lesser than the desirable amount. Also, on the whole, discrimination against female children and women continues due to socio-economic conditions, which is reflected in higher death rates of female children as compared to their male counterparts (Fig. 6.2).

The case of Gujarat becomes peculiar because although it is an economically well-off states, yet maternal, nutritional, and neo-natal diseases constitute a massive proportion of DALYs for children under-five years of age (Table 6.3). Additionally, although its burden has declined from 36.1% in 1990 to 14.6% in 2017, Under-nutrition is still the largest contributor to DALYs in the state of Gujarat (Table 6.3). It is, therefore, especially pertinent to understand the major factors responsible for the persistently high rates of child undernutrition in Gujarat (Figs. 6.3 and 6.4).

6.1.5 Gujarat: A Critical Look

In the developed countries, quite high proportion of the GDP is spent by the general public sector on health. Altogether, in established market economies, nearly 5.6% of the GDP was spent by the general public sector on health in 1990. In such developed countries, about 3.5% GDP was spent by the private sector, including the household sector, cumulatively taking the entire tally of health expenditure to around 9.2% of the GDP. Collectively also as individually, (except the US) the government's burden within the health sector was above the private burden. This was true for Sub-Saharan African countries, Latin America, Caribbean and west Asia, and

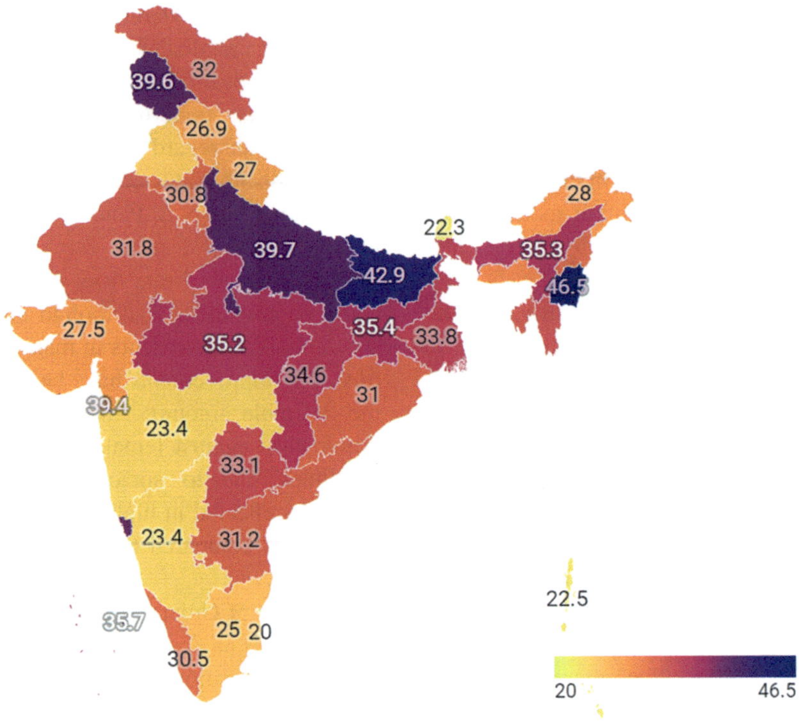

Fig. 6.2 Choropleth Map showing child stunting rates in India. *Source* Made by authors based on NFHS-5 (2019–21)

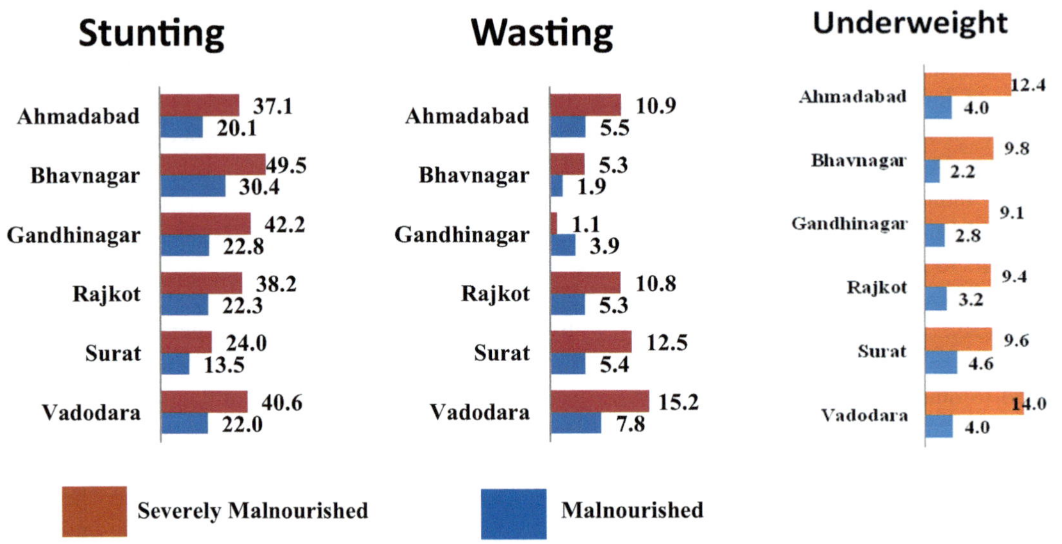

Fig. 6.3 Prevalence of child Undernutrition across the six administrative divisions in Gujarat. *Source* Based on Comprehensive Nutrition Survey in Gujarat, 2014

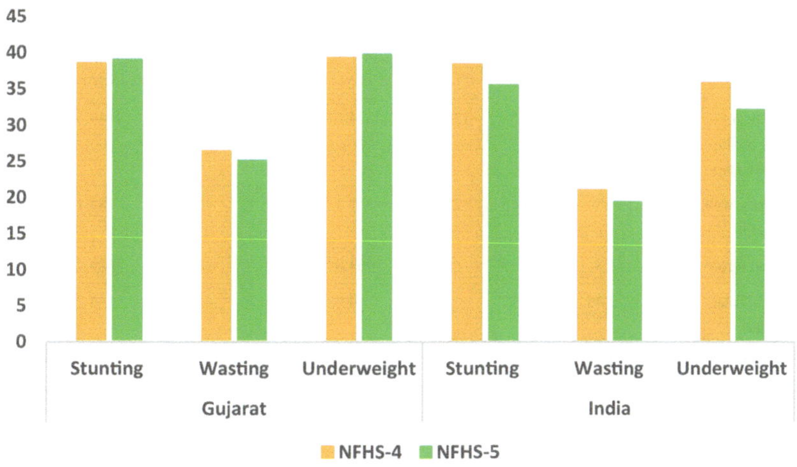

Fig. 6.4 Nutritional status of children in India and Gujarat, 2015–16 to 2019–21. *Source* NFHS-4, 2015–16 and NFHS-5, 2019–20

Table 6.3 Contribution of top 10 risks to DALYs number ranked by number of DALYs, 1990–2016, Gujarat

Risk factors (1990)	Risk factors (2016)
1. Malnutrition[a] (36.1%)	1. Malnutrition[a] (14.6%)
2. WaSH[b] (11.3%)	2. Dietary risks (10.4%)
3. Air pollution (10.2%)	3. Air pollution (9.1%)
4. Dietary risks (4.7%)	4. High blood pressure (9.0%)
5. Tobacco use (4.4%)	5. Tobacco Use (6.2%)
6. High blood pressure (4.0%)	6. High fasting plasma glucose (5.8%)
7. High total cholesterol (2.2%)	7. High total cholesterol (5.4%)
8. High fasting plasma glucose (2.1%)	8. Alcohol and drug use (4.0%)
9. Alcohol and drug use (2.1%)	9. Occupational risks (3.1%)
10. Occupational risks (2.1%)	10. Impaired kidney functions (2.7%)
11. Impaired kidney functions (1.3%)	11. WaSH[b] (2.6%)

Note The percent figure in bracket next to each risk is DALYs from that risk out of total DALYs

Note [a]Malnutrition in child and maternal malnutrition; [b]WaSH is unsafe water, sanitation, and handwashing

Source India State-level Disease Burden Initiative (2017)

countries of the previous socialist block, whereas in Asian countries, except China, private sector's involvement has always been above the general public sector within the healthcare system (World Bank, 1993). In Gujarat, within the mid-1980s, about 8% of the entire budget was allocated to the health sector within the state (Mahadevia, 2000). By mid-1990s, the proportion decreased to about 6%. Within the previous couple of years, once more, there's a rise during this share, but not reaching the extent that was within the mid-1980s. In terms of the proportion of NSDP, the expenditure on health sector was already very low within the 1980s (2.16% in 1986–87) and it has come down gradually since then. A disturbing aspect is that, as a percent of development expenditure, on the revenue also as capital account, the allocation to health sector had declined for a decade (1987–96). In 1997–98, one can observe slight increase within the proportion of the entire budget also as NSDP spent on health (Mahadevia, 2000).The proportion of net state domestic product spent on health care in Gujarat has remained dismal over the years, with increase in the ensuing years being only marginal. Although India, as a whole,

Table 6.4 Budgetary provisions for health care in Gujarat

Sectors	2006–07 (Acc)	2007–08 (Acc)	2008–09 (Acc)	2009–10 (Acc)	2010–11 (Acc)	2011–12 (Acc)	2012–13 (Acc)	2013–14 (Acc)	2014–15 (Acc)	2015–16 (RE)	2016–17 (BE)
Medical and public health (crores)	1017.92	1195.5	1393.92	2624.61	2620	2852	4144.59	4489.1	5688.3	6541.5	7230.1
Family welfare (crores)	133.38	183.45	211.77	339.32	394.6	481.2	485.14	597.51	681.55	869.18	923.69
Total (crores)	1151.3	1378.95	1605.68	2963.94	3014	3333	4629.73	5086.7	6369.9	7410.7	8153.8
% in Total budget	2.48	3.1	3.05	4.03	4.18	4.21	4.73	4.85	5.42	5.53	5.37
% in SDP	0.41	0.42	0.44	0.69	0.58	0.55	0.65	0.63	0.71	0.75	0.75

Source Jethmalani (2018)
Acc—Actual Estimates, RE—Revised Estimates, BE—Budgeted Estimates

spends a negligible 1.28% of its GDP on health, this figure is still greater than the 0.72% of GDP that Gujarat spends on health (Table 6.4). Concern and expenditure for health are spread across variety of ministries and departments. Ideally health sector expenditures should include five important heads: (a) medical and public health, (b) family welfare (including family planning), (c) water system and sanitation, (d) nutrition, and (e) child and handicapped welfare. Reddy and Selvaraju (1994) have done this categorization which has been adopted for analysing healthcare expenditures.

6.1.6 Impact of COVID-19 on Health Scenario in Gujarat

The socio-economic review for the financial year 2020–21 states that at least eight Gujarat government schemes, pertaining to nutrition and health, remained suspended or lacked funds owing to closure of faculties and Anganwadi centres (AWCs) due to the COVID-19 pandemic (Ghosh, 2021). It further adds that the mid-day meal (MDM) scheme, which provides a cooked meal to students of primary and upper primary classes, benefitted a mean of 39.97 lakh children of 34,307 primary schools within the fiscal year 2019–20. However, during the lockdown, which saw the closure of faculties and Anganwadi centres, the cash was disbursed as food security allowance under the scheme. Gujarat, which implemented the scheme in 1984, was the second state within the country to launch MDM. Nearly 50% of the sanctioned budget (549 crores) was distributed to nearly 51 lakh beneficiaries of 32,731 primary schools as food security allowance for the fiscal year 2020–21 (Ghosh, 2021). The estimates mentioned are till December last year.

In December 2020, the Indian Institute of Management, Ahmedabad, in collaboration with UNICEF, conducted a survey across 375 urban families in Ahmedabad which found that families were unable to obtain mid-day meal benefits or payment as an alternative of it (Ghosh, 2021). The report was also taken into cognizance by the High Court of Gujarat. After the government had claimed that the sample size for the survey was too small, the court had disposed of the matter while observing that despite strenuous efforts made by the state government, there were families that had to face hardships during the pandemic, especially during the lockdown. The report also states that these four important schemes related to nutrition of students saw no expenditure during the pandemic due to shutting down of schools. These include the "Tithi Bhojan" scheme that involves the area people sponsoring food for youngsters on different occasions. Reports suggest that during the fiscal year 2019–20, nearly 41 lakh students in Gujarat benefitted from the above-mentioned scheme and a contribution amounting to nearly Rs. 19 crore was collected.

6.1.7 Welfare Schemes in Gujarat

The "Anna Sangam Scheme", which provides 60 kg of free food grain to oldsters of tribal girl students up to class 8 who register attendance above 70%, also remained suspended during the pandemic. The "Sukhadi Project", a fortified sweet aimed towards enhancing calorie and protein intake, and "Dudh Sanjivani Scheme", which provides 200 ml of flavoured milk 5 days every week in anganwadis, saw no spending in 2020–21 fiscal. For the "Dudh Sanjivani Scheme", a mean of 13.07 lakh beneficiaries was covered during 2019–20. Additionally, the report states that owing to the closure of schools due to COVID-19, of the funds allotted for several schemes in the state for the fiscal year 2020–21 could not be used. A take-home meal provision of a "third meal of a 50-gram laddoo", aimed towards improving the nutrition level among registered, moderate, and underweight children under the Integrated Child Development Services (ICDS) scheme, too remained suspended due to the closure of AWCs. The sweet is given aside from the morning snacks and afternoon meal at AWCs for 6 days every week. During the fiscal of 2019–20, a complete of 71,306 beneficiaries were covered under this scheme.

Not only children, pregnant women and lactating mothers, too, lost out on nutritional benefits from government schemes due to the pandemic. The Poshan Sudha Yojana that aims to scale back the prevalence of undernutrition, micronutrient deficiencies, and improve the nutritional status of pregnant women and lactating mothers and pregnancy outcomes saw no beneficiary in 2020–21 due to the closure of AWCs against the entire 24,665 women who had benefitted from the scheme in 2019–20. The beneficiaries under this scheme are provided a day with one meal, iron vitamin Bc tablets, and calcium tablets at the AWC. Infant and Young Child Feeding training (IYCF), a health department intervention that appears at continued breastfeeding and infant nutrition to scale back infant death rate, too, was halted. The SER report states also that owing to the closure of training centres as a precautionary measure due to contain the pandemic, infant, and child feeding training for the year 2020–21 could also not be done (Ghosh, 2021).

Along with nutrition, screening activities to work out health status in children—either school-going or those aged up to 5 years—took successful. Screening program for severe acute malnourished (SAM) children up to 5 years of age, under the "Kuposhan Mukt Gujarat Mahabhiyan", saw 40.56 lakh being screened by field-level workers during 2019–20 of whom 3.46 lakh (8.53%) children were identified as suffering from severe acute undernutrition. However, in 2020–21 (until December 2020) a complete of 31.62 lakh children were screened of the targeted 49.48 lakh children. Among those who were screened, nearly 1.66 lakh (5.25%) children were identified as suffering from severe acute undernutrition. In addition to the above, regular health department schemes were also affected severely (Ghosh, 2021).

6.1.8 Why Is It Important?

Due to the lack of consensus on the magnitude of impact of economic growth on improvements in nutritional status of children and its policy implications, there is a need to revisit the relationship between economic growth and child nutritional indicators. There are a very few studies that account for the reverse causality between economic growth and reductions in child undernutrition. This could be a source of bias in the estimates of these studies. Economic growth and nutrition have a less linear and sloppier relationship than that between economic growth and poverty. It is so because increase in GDP may not have a proportional impact on child nutrition indicators because of its complexity and additional eccentric socio-economic reasons (cultural factors, diet quality, and health behaviour). Thus, it may not be suitable to draw parallels between poverty and child nutrition. In the following sections, we aim to explain the relationship between economic growth and child nutrition using Gujarat as a case study and nationally representative data from India. The ultimate agenda of the statistical analyses that follows is to identify the reasons for the anomaly that exists in Gujarat and identify policy implications to solve this puzzle.

6.1.9 Data and Sampling Design

We used the Kids Recode File from the fourth round of the National Family Health Survey (NFHS-4) for the purpose of analysis. The National Family Health Survey (NFHS), conducted by the International Institute for Population Sciences, is a large-scale survey conducted in rounds in a representative sample of Indian households. Three rounds of the survey have been conducted since the initial round in 1992–93. State- and national-level information on health and demographic characteristics of the population are provided by the survey.

6.1.10 Study Population and Sample Size

The unit of the analysis is children under-five years of age. In case of missing data or inadmissible height and weight information, the particular case was excluded (defined as ±6 standard deviations WHO growth standards; WHO, 2006) resulting in a sample size of 259,627 for India and 7730 for Gujarat. To facilitate with existing studies, the age group taken into consideration for the analysis is 0–59 months, as compared to the 24–36 months' partial life range used in selective studies. Stunting, wasting, and underweight are measured using height-for-age (HAZ) scores, weight-for-height (WHZ) scores, and weight-for-age (WAZ) scores, respectively. Stunting, wasting, and underweight are expressed as HAZ, WHZ, and WAZ scores, respectively, below minus 2 variance units from the median of a reference population as devised by WHO (WHO Multicentre Growth Reference Study Group, 2006; World Health Organization, 2010).

6.1.11 Outcome Variable

The outcome variable, a representative of children's nutritional status, was measured by height-for-age (HAZ scores), weight-for-age (WAZ scores), and weight-for-height (WHZ scores). These measures are optimum because they are suggestive of nutritional inadequacies at the lower tail of the distribution. Thus, those children whose height-for-age, weight-for-age, and weight-for-height are more than two standard deviations below the median of the international reference population for children of the same gender are considered stunted, underweight, and wasted, respectively. The data for child stunting, wasting, and underweight is taken from the Kids file. The HAZ, WAZ, and WHZ scores have also been used to create a stunting, underweight, and wasting variables, respectively, wherein 0 means the child is not stunted, underweight, and wasted and 1 means otherwise.

6.2 Statistical Analyses

6.2.1 Determinants of Child Undernutrition in Gujarat

We measure the nutritional status as z-scores of height-for-age (stunting). The z-scores method propounded by WHO that have been taken from child population from countries, such as Brazil, Ghana, India, Norway, Oman, and the USA (WHO, 2006), have been followed. Based on previous literature (WGO, 1997), z-scores for the purpose of this analysis have been defined as

$$\text{z score} = (\mathrm{x_i} - \mathrm{x_{median}})/\sigma^{\mathrm{x}}$$

where xi is height of the *i*th child, xmedian is the median height from the reference population of the same age and gender, and σx is the standard deviation from the mean of the reference population. We assume that the z-scores for the reference population are normally distributed. Binary logistic regression was used to establish the relationship between child stunting and background characteristics of both the parents. The binary category (1 = Child is Stunted, 0 = Child is not Stunted) for each respondent is related to a bunch of categorical independent variables, X, by a logit function

$$\log\mathrm{it}[\mathrm{P}(\mathrm{Y}=1)] = \beta_0 + \beta_1\mathrm{X} + \varepsilon$$

The parameter β0 estimates the log odds of the child being stunted for the reference group, while β1 estimates the maximum likelihood, the differential log odds of the child being stunted associated with a set of predictors X as compared to the reference group and ε represents the residuals in the model.

6.2.2 Decomposing the Socio-Economic Inequality in Child Undernutrition

The widely applied concentration index and its decomposition (Wagstaff, 2005; Wagstaff, Paci & Van Doorslaer, 1991; Wagstaff & Watanabe, 2000) has been used to estimate the wealth-based inequality in childhood undernutrition in the state of Gujarat and the main causes behind this inequality. The concentration index is instrumental in assessing the socio-economic inequalities that are prevalent in child health outcomes (Kakwani et al., 1997; O'Donnell et al., 2008). A measure of inequality, the concentration index is defined as twice the area between the line of equality (45° line) and the concentration curve. In case of no inequality, the concentration index is zero. A negative concentration index signifies disproportionate concentration of the variable in question among the poor and a positive value signifies pro-rich inequalities.

$$C = \frac{2}{\mu}[\sum_{i=1}^{n}(Yi) \qquad (6.1)$$

where Yi is the child health indicator of the ith individual, Ri is the fractional rank of the *i*th individual (for weighted data) in terms of the index of household economic status, and μ is the (weighted) unconditional mean of the health variable of the sample.

By using Wagstaff et al. (2003) method, socio-economic inequality in stunting, wasting, and underweight among the under-five population of Gujarat has been decomposed into its determinants. This helps in estimating the contribution of these determinants to the inequality in child undernutrition.

In the following ordinary least squares model, the variable of interest (Yi) is linked to a set of covariates (Xki):

$$\mathrm{Yi} = \alpha + \sum + \varepsilon i \qquad (6.2)$$

where ε is an error term, given the relationship between Yi and Xki in the equation, the concentration index (C) for y can be written as

$$\sum \frac{\beta kxk}{\mu} Ck + \frac{GCe}{\mu} = Cy = \frac{GCe}{\mu} \qquad (6.3)$$

Decomposition analysis has been carried out based on previous literature (Wagstaff et al., 2003; Hosseinpoor et al., 2006; O'Donnell et al., 2008).

6.2.3 Understanding the Differential Impacts of Wealth on Child Undernutrition: Quantile Regression

The advantage of using quantile regression is that it helps to understand the impact of a set of covariates on different sections of the dependent variable, as opposed to the simple linear regression that gives the mean value. This is beneficial because it helps to offer a more comprehensive picture of the impact of asset ownership on child nutrition. Quantile regression provides us with a parameter that explains the marginal effect of explanatory variables on a specified quantile of the dependent variable. It also ensures comparability of estimated coefficients from various quantiles. Based on the anthropometric structure, children at the left tail (poor health) of the distribution may have a negligible response to changes in the explanatory variable as compared to their counterparts at the median or right tail of the distribution. The quantile regression equation is specified as follows:

$$Yi = \alpha(\tau)_0 + \alpha(\tau)_1 Ai + \alpha(\tau)_2 Xi + \varepsilon(\tau)_i$$

where τ indicates the specified quantile. The model is estimated at 10th, 25th, 50th, 75th, and 90th quantiles.

6.3 Results

6.3.1 Nutritional Status of Children by Background Characteristics

While nearly 38% female children have height-for-age scores below −3SD, the percentage is 39% for male children. The gap increases when only children −2SD are considered. It is seen that more children of higher birth order are stunted. While only 13% first-born children have height-for-age scores below −2SD, the figures go up to 29% for children who are of order 6 or above. The figures are even higher when we consider height-for-age scores below −3SD. While only 12 and 31% children, respectively, have height-for-age scores below −2SD and −3SD in urban areas, the figures increase to 18 and 41%, respectively, for rural areas. While 27 and 53% babies whose birth size is very small have height-for-age scores below −2SD and −3SD, respectively, the percentage is comparatively lesser for those babies whose birth size is average or bigger. As the educational level of mothers increases, the percentage of children who have height-for-age scores below −2SD and −3SD decreases. With the increase in mother's BMI, the percentage of children stunted decreases. Also, with the increase in wealth quintile, the percentage of children who have height-for-age scores below −2SD and −3SD decreases (Table 6.5). Nearly 38% of children in India are stunted. Bihar (48%), Uttar Pradesh (46%), Jharkhand (45%), Meghalaya (44%), and Madhya Pradesh (42%) are the states in which the prevalence of stunting is among the highest.

6.3.2 Determinants of Nutritional Status of Children in Gujarat

Table 6.6 shows the odds of a child being stunted given the background characteristics of the mother and father. Since asset ownership is our main variable, we analyse the impact of asset ownership on child stunting first. The children of those females who are in the highest category of asset ownership are least likely to be stunted, that is, the odds of children being stunted decreases as mothers move higher in the category of asset ownership. Thus, the children whose mother owns all the four assets are 0.9 times less likely to be stunted as compared to children of those mothers who do not own any asset at all. A female child is 0.9 times less likely to be stunted as compared to a male child. The odds of children being stunted increase with the increase in the birth order of children. Thus, the children who are of order 10 and above are 1.3 times more likely to be stunted than those children who are of order 0–3. The children of mothers having the highest level of education are 0.5 times less likely to be stunted than those of mothers having no education. Children of mothers who smoke are 1.8 times more likely to be stunted than their counterparts whose mothers don't smoke. The odds of children being stunted decreases with the increase in height of mothers. Those females who justify wife beating are 1.04 times more likely to have stunted children than those who do not. Just like mothers' education, the odds of children being stunted decreases with the increase in the educational qualification of fathers. Thus, children whose fathers are in the higher category of education are 0.7 times less likely to be stunted than those whose fathers have no education at all. Talking about the geographical regions, children belonging from the Central, Eastern, and Western states are 1.4, 1.2, and 1.3 times, respectively, more likely to be stunted than those

Table 6.5 Height for age scores of children by background characteristics in Gujarat—2015–16

Background characteristics	Height for age		
	Percentage below −2SD	Percentage below −3SD	Number of children
Age in months			
<6	9.5	20.1	17644
6–8	9.0	20.2	11529
9–11	11.9	25.9	10746
12–17	16.6	38.2	21941
18–23	22.0	46.9	22242
24–35	18.6	42.7	44060
36–47	17.1	43.2	46775
48–59	15.8	40	44859
Sex			
Male	16.9	38.9	113804
Female	15.6	37.9	105992
Birth interval (months)			
First birth	13.0	33.4	81837
<24	21.7	46.9	34860
24–25	19.4	43.4	41684
36+	15.5	36.9	54099
Birth order			
1	13.0	33.4	81387
2–3	16.4	39	101091
4–5	23.5	48.9	22744
6+	28.8	55	7367
Residence			
Urban	12.0	31	60124
Rural	17.9	41.2	159671
Size at birth			
Very small	26.9	52.8	5854
Small	20.0	45.1	19089
Average or larger	15.5	37.1	184569
Mother's schooling			
No schooling	24.8	50.7	64878
<5 years complete	18.5	45.3	10331
5–7 years complete	16.0	39.8	35.34
8–9 years complete	13.3	35.5	36016
10–11 years complete	10.5	29.7	23701
12 or more years complete	8.7	23.8	40970
Religion			
Hindu	16.4	38.3	172360
Muslim	17.1	39.8	36847

(continued)

Table 6.5 (continued)

Background characteristics	Height for age		
	Percentage below −2SD	Percentage below −3SD	Number of children
Christian	12.4	29.9	4488
Sikh	7.2	23.4	2826
Buddhist	16.4	43	1659
Jain	4.9	19.1	242
Others	17.5	42.5	1374
Caste			
Scheduled Caste	19.0	42.8	48359
Scheduled Tribe	19.7	43.8	22748
OBC	16.4	38.7	96364
Others	11.9	31.2	30431
Mother's BMI			
Underweight	20.5	45.8	53296
Normal	16.2	38.2	128515
Overweight	9.4	27.1	31763
Wealth index			
Poorest	25.7	51.4	35578
Poorer	18.3	43.5	48758
Rich	13.5	36.5	43642
Richer	10.6	29.2	39941
Richest	7.9	22.2	31877

Footnote 2SD includes children who are below −3 standard deviations (SD) from WHO Child Growth Standards population median

children who belong to the northern states (which is the reference category).

6.3.3 Inequality in Child Undernutrition in Gujarat

Table 6.7 shows the concentration indices for child undernutrition indicators. The concentration indices for stunting, wasting, and underweight are negative −0.17, −0.06, and −0.16, respectively, for Gujarat. All the indices are significant at 1% level of significance. This result stresses on the fact that the children belonging to the lower socio-economic strata in Gujarat share a significantly higher burden of undernutrition. This fact is further underpinned by the concentration curves shown in Fig. 6.5. The concentration curves for stunting and underweight coincide with each other which is suggestive of the fact that the inequality in these two domains of child undernutrition is quite similar. Inequality in wasting is relatively less pronounced in Gujarat (as is the case with all of the states for which table has not been shown) and the concentration curve also shows the same thing. This indicates that poverty and inequality in income distribution have a more pronounced effect on chronic nutritional deprivation as compared to acute health conditions. The fact that all the concentration indices are statistically significant amply stresses upon the fact that the prevalence of higher rates of both chronic and acute nutritional deprivation in children is well rooted in the overall levels of socio-economic inequality (Wagstaff & Watanabe, 2000).

Table 6.6 Odds ratio of child stunting based on mothers' background characteristics in Gujarat

Mother's asset ownership	Odds ratio	95% confidence interval
Basic asset index (ref. no assets)		
1	0.925**	(0.868, 0.986)
2	0.904*	(0.851, 0.962)
3	0.897	(0.885, 1.030)
4	0.857*	(0.783, 0.938)
Characteristics of the Child		
Sex of the child (ref. boy)		
Girl	0.917*	(0.879, 0.957)
Birth order (ref. 0–3)		
4–9	1.088	(1.024, 1.156)
10–15	1.324	(1.128, 1.144)
Mother's characteristics		
Level of education (ref. no education)		
Primary	0.921**	(0.859, 0.987)
Secondary	0.740*	(0.696, 0.786)
Higher	0.486*	(0.437, 0.542)
Mother smokes (ref. no)		
Yes	1.838*	(1.256, 2.690)
Mother's height (ref. 950–1450)		
1451–1650 cms	0.484*	(0.454, 0.516)
1651–1840 cms	0.218*	(0.171, 0.277)
1842–2052 cms	0.566**	(0.358, 0.892)
Frequency of listening to radio (ref. not at all)		
Less than once a week	0.956**	(0.870, 1.050)
At least once a week	0.962**	(0.765, 0.892)
Al every day	0.879	(0.778, 0.994)
Frequency of watching television (ref. not at all)		
Less than once a week	0.881**	(0.811, 0.957)
At least once a week	0.826**	(0.765, 0.892)
Al every day	0.745**	(0.704, 0.788)
Attitude towards wife beating (ref. no)		
Yes	1.041	(1.00, 1.09)
Father's characteristics		
Father's educational level (ref. no education)		
Primary	0.949	(0.881, 1.023)
Secondary	0.815*	(0.764, 0.869)
Higher	0.657*	(0.595, 0.724)
Geographic regions (ref. north)		
Central	1.392*	(1.307, 1.484)
East	1.150*	(1.072, 1.232)
North East	0.857*	(0.792, 0.930)
West	1.286*	(1.177, 1.403)
South	1.042	(0.955, 1.136)

The notation * is $p < 0.01$, ** is $p < 0.05$; Sample is children of married mothers ($n = 7730$)

Table 6.7 Concentration indices for stunting, wasting, and underweight, India and Gujarat, 2015–16

	Stunting (CI) index value	Wasting (CI) index value	Underweight (CI) index value
India	−0.16***	−0.06***	−0.16***
Gujarat	−0.17***	−0.06***	−0.16***

* $= p \leq 0.01$, ** $= p \leq 0.05$

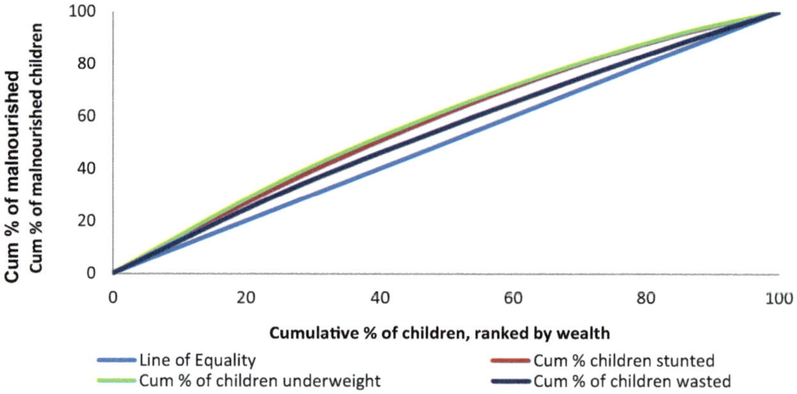

Fig. 6.5 Concentration curve of stunting, wasting, and underweight in Gujarat, 2015–16

6.3.4 Decomposition of Concentration Indices

Figures 6.6a, b show the results of the decomposition. As evident from the figures, wealth-based inequality in child undernutrition can be majorly explained by determinants at the household level, with the wealth index alone accounting for more than 50% of the total inequality. This pattern, however, is not followed by wasting. For wasting, mother's BMI is the largest contributor (29%), followed by caste (18%), wealth index, place of residence, and safe stool disposal, all contributing nearly 13% each to the inequality in child wasting. Wealth also affects inequality through the indirect effects of other proximate determinants of inequality. For both stunting and underweight, wealth is the single largest contributor to the inequality with wealth index contributing nearly 78 and 69%, respectively, to the inequality in child stunting and underweight. Mother's BMI is also a significant variable for underweight as it contributes nearly 15% to the inequality in underweight. This helps us in concluding that household economic status alone contributes to the observed inequality in child nutritional status in Gujarat, with the contribution of other factors being less pronounced. The tables show that stunting was more concentrated among children belonging to poorest and poorer wealth quintiles, children residing in rural areas, whose families did not practice safe stool disposal, and who did not have immunization. The fact that the decomposition model is robust can be adjudged from the near-zero contribution of the residual (O'Donnell et al., 2008).

6.3.5 Differential Impacts of Wealth on Child Undernutrition in Gujarat

Quantile regression facilitates an understanding of the impact of a set of explanatory variables on different sections of the dependent variable distribution, compared to ordinary linear regression, which provides estimates at the mean, which can offer a more comprehensive idea of the impact of female asset ownership on the nutritional status of their children. The quantile regression parameter explains the marginal effect of an explanatory variable on a particular quantile of the dependent variable. Coefficients estimated with linear regression do not portray these

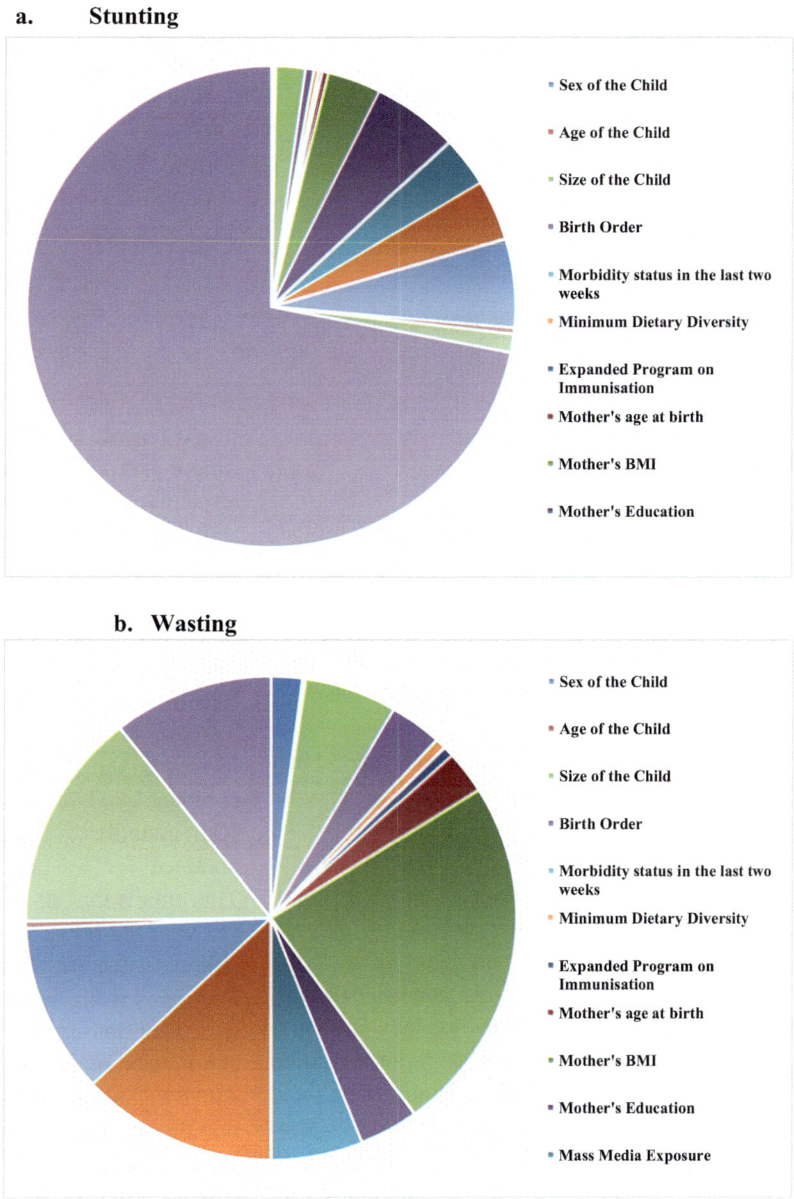

Fig. 6.6 Decomposition of inequality in Child Nutrition Indicators in Gujarat **a** Stunting, **b** Wasting

differences. Specific portions of the kid nutrition Z-score distributions are analysed using quantile multivariate analysis. Table 6.8 shows the quantile regression estimates for the wealth index. This table, again, stresses on the importance of the economic situation of the households in determining the nutritional status of the children. Results for stunting indicate that a one-unit increase in the asset index score at the median increases the HAZ score by 27.4 points as compared to 37.5 and 35.7 points at the 75th and 90th quantiles, respectively. Similar results are obtained for wasting and underweight as well. This entails that an improvement in the economic status of the household is more beneficial for the children who are already relatively healthy. Another point that comes through from this table is that the economic conditions of the household are more crucial for the long-term nutritional status of the child, as is evident from the greater coefficients obtained for stunting (Fig. 6.7).

Table 6.8 Summary of quantile regression estimates for wealth quintiles in Gujarat

Wealth index coefficients for HAZ scores	Quantile				
	0.10	0.25	0.50	0.75	0.90
Wealth index	*Stunting*				
	22.57*	26.05*	27.41*	37.48*	65.67
Wealth index	*Wasting*				
	13.64**	14.71*	15.77**	16.40*	46.91
Wealth index	*Underweight*				
	25.83*	25.95*	28.61*	31.16*	53.74

The notation * is $p < 0.01$, ** is $p < 0.0$. Sample is children of married mothers (n = 7730)

6.4 Discussion

The results from logistic regression are a clear indication towards the fact that the prevalence of child stunting decreases with mother's ownership of asset. Mother's background characteristics such as her education, attitude towards wife beating, and height are also important determinants of child health.

The findings of this chapter also show that though the per capita income of the state may be high, the socio-economic inequalities that persist are equally high. These inequalities, in fact, are the major contributors towards the alarmingly high levels of child undernutrition in Gujarat. With wealth explaining more than half of the inequalities that persist in child undernutrition, it provides ample evidence to explain the high levels of the latter. The fact there is more inequality in child stunting points towards the fact that socio-economic inequality has more serious repercussions for the long-term health of the child. It is also established that household level accounts for the observed wealth-based inequality in child undernutrition indicators, with household wealth alone accounting for more than 50% of the total inequality. This pattern, however, is not followed by wasting. For wasting, mother's BMI is the largest contributor (29%), followed by caste (18%), wealth index, place of residence, and safe stool disposal. Wealth also affects inequality through the indirect effects of other proximate determinants of inequality. For both stunting and underweight, wealth is the single largest contributor to the inequality with wealth index contributing nearly 78 and 69%, respectively, to the inequality in child stunting and underweight.

The quantile regression estimates for the wealth index stress on the importance on the economic situation of the households in determining the nutritional status of the children. Results for stunting indicate that a one-unit increase in the asset index score at the median increases the HAZ score by 27.4 points as compared to 37.5 and 35.7 points at the 75th and 90th quantiles, respectively. Similar results are obtained for wasting and underweight as well. This entails that an improvement in the economic status of the household is more beneficial for the children who are already relatively healthy.

It is well established in literature that increased autonomy of women over their assets can be advantageous for their economic security and bargaining power within households. Additionally, it also has positive ramifications for the well-being and health of their children. However, barring few studies from selected developing countries (Allendorf, 2007; Menon et al., 2014), there is a negligible evidence to support this assertion, owing to the limited availability of sex-disaggregated large-scale datasets on asset ownership in developing countries. This study adds to this limited pool of evidence by explaining the impact of mothers' asset ownership on the health of their children, using a unique and representative dataset from India. Since gender mainstreaming has amassed popularity in recent decades, it becomes especially pertinent to

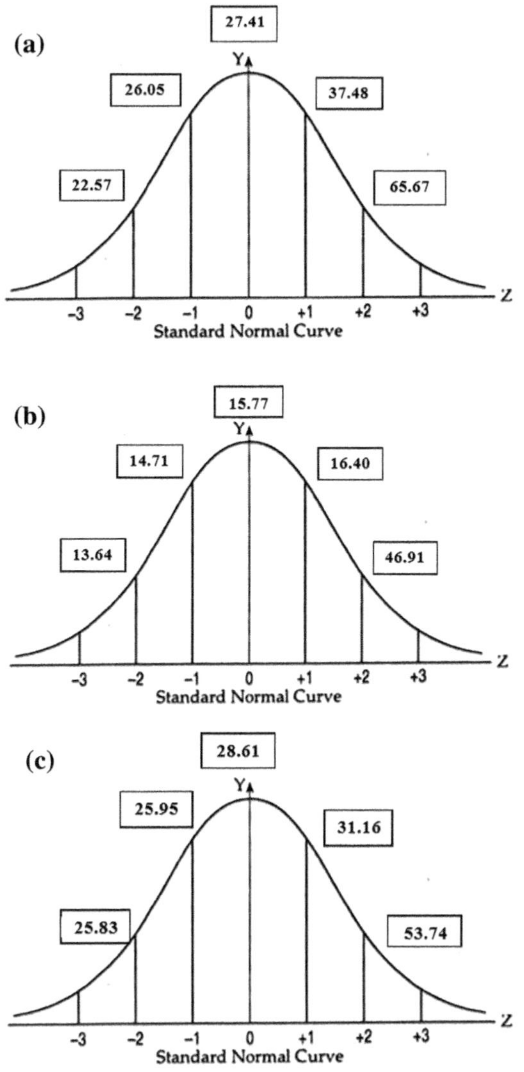

Fig. 6.7 **a** Impact estimation of household wealth index on different quantiles of child's height-for-age scores in Gujarat. **b** Impact estimation of household wealth index on different quantiles of child's weight-for-height scores in Gujarat. **c** Impact estimation of household wealth index on different quantiles of child's weight-for-age scores in Gujarat

evaluate the economic advantages of women's asset ownership. There are examples to support this hypothesis, such as the conditional cash transfer (CCT) programs like Oportunidades in Mexico (subsequently renamed Prospera) and Bolsa Familia in Brazil. Both these programs were initially designed to portray the advantages of resources being concentrated in the hands of women. Generally structured as cash distributions made to a certain section of the population subjective to fulfilment of certain conditions, conditional cash transfers often lead to increased school enrolment of children and hospital visits for vaccinations and health check-ups. Since their inception, these programs are now being increasingly used in developing countries as a poverty reduction tool, emphasizing the effectiveness of targeted interventions. However, it is important to understand that cash transfers are not a permanent solution and the need of the hour is to have strategies in place to ensure productive and income-generating activities for women (Buvinić & Furst-Nichols, 2016).

Researchers have always bene intrigued with the co-existence of economic growth and dismal child nutrition consequences in India. The prominent contributor to wasting health emergency in South Asia, India is also performing dismally as far as child stunting is concerned (UNICEF, 2013). However, it is crucial to note that these estimates are based on data that is over a decade obsolete. Hence, although these estimates pin point the neediest sections of India, the causes behind this co-existence of economic growth and child undernutrition are still perplexing and warrants explanation. Recent evidence also suggests that it is imperative to accord special importance to nutrition-sensitive policies and interventions with a targeted approach and with priority being given to all forms of nutritional disadvantages. It is also equally important to address not just the immediate but also the underlying causes of undernutrition, thus creating an enabling environment for improved nutrition and health (Maternal & Child Nutrition Series, Lancet, 2013).

India's policy focus has been towards addressing child undernutrition for a long time now. This has been ensured through channelling a gamut of policies such as the Integrated Child Development Scheme launched in 1975, the National Nutrition Policy 1993, the Mid-Day Meal Scheme for school children 1995, and the National Food Security Act 2013 (GOI, 1993; GOI, 2015). What is, however, worrisome is that despite enormous magnitude of resources and efforts, the prevalence of stunting, wasting, and underweight among children under the age of 5 years still remains considerably towards the higher end. A marker of chronic undernutrition, stunting is caused due to a typical intermingling of complex socio-economic, behavioural, and environmental factors. It is no surprise that its prevalence is the highest in the least developed states of India. The prevalence of wasting is what is intriguing. A marker of acute undernutrition, child wasting still remains highest in some of the developed Indian states, the prime example of such a state being Gujarat.

The decline in stunting is usually chaperoned by a short-lived increase or dormancy in wasting and, thus, achieving concomitant reductions in stunting and wasting could prove to be cumbersome (Sachdev, 2018; India State-Level Disease Burden Initiative UndernutritionCollaborators, 2019). The abnormally high rates of child undernutrition in India as compared to its Sub-Saharan counterparts could be attributed to low female autonomy, son preference, and lack of hygienic practices (Smith et al., 2003; Spears, 2013; Jayachandran & Pande, 2017). The current research has corroborated these findings from researches and this shows that similar trends are being observed across Indian states as well.

The need of the hour is to supplement nutrient-based intervention with more encyclopaedic and all-encompassing policies engineered towards combatting the important determinants of children's nutritional status are needed to expedite the cutback of growth failure of children in India, which was also one of the key ideas envisioned in the National Nutrition Mission (GOI, 2019). In order to facilitate the life-cycle approach and effectively address the broad determinants of child nutrition, it is important to target individual indicators and act for their improvement. These changes encompass efforts aimed at provision of clean drinking water, reduction in open defecation rates, women empowerment and education, enhancement of agricultural productivity and food security, and nutrition-sensitive agricultural interventions, coupled with synchronized actions by different actors such as governments, stakeholders, investors, and policymakers (Swaminathan, 2001; Smith et al., 2003; Black et al., 2013; Bhutta et al., 2013; Ruel et al., 2013; Das et al., 2004; Thow et al., 2016; Shankar et al., 2017).

The health area that needs changing the mindset is women's health. Women's health has got to be improved not only to ensure improved health and survival of youngsters and reduction of increase rates but also for women themselves and to enhance the general health status of the society. Till now, women's health has been viewed from the attitude of maternal health through immunization and birth control programs. Women constitute half the population. In Gujarat, as observed, health of female children is neglected, which is reflected in high death rate among the girl children as compared to their male counterparts. In other words, socio-cultural change is extremely pertinent to address women's health as their basic rights and ameliorate their overall health. The primary step towards that would be increasing female literacy. Improvement in female literacy also will significantly reduce fertility and infant death rate rates. Thus, there is a plethora of effort that needs to go into ensuring optimal health for women. For ensuring health for all, it is necessary that utilization of public healthcare facilities improves. For this, quality of public health facilities must be improved. A replacement experiment of participation of non-governmental organizations (NGOs) in running public facilities has been initiated. However, these are at the best at pilot stage. These experiments need to be either scaled up or government on its own initiative has got to improve the standard of public facilities.

Health may be a broad concept and health status may be a function of an outsized number of things. Expenditure by government on public facilities affects health status. Industrialization, urbanization, and economic process, it is hypothesized, bring about improvements in health status. This might, however, not always be the case, as is observed in the case of Gujarat. States like Kerala and Tamil Nadu, which are far behind Gujarat in terms of those three dimensions of development, are far before Gujarat with reference to health status. The problems discussed above, which emanate from the biased or lop-sided development process of the state, are outside the purview of the health department. While these issues are understood and addressed, it's time that health is viewed in reference to the general growth process of Gujarat to form health for all reality within the near future.

6.5 Conclusion

This chapter discusses the extent of undernutrition among children under-five years of age and the linkages between socio-economic inequality and child nutrition. The results highlight the central role played by economic growth in influencing nutritional outcomes. One of the crucial findings of the chapter suggest that, despite years of rapid advancements made in all sectors, it is still the poor and deprived section of the society that shoulders the disproportionate burden of undernutrition and socio-economic inequality still remains the important contributor in determining the nutritional status of children. The case of India becomes even more aberrant because its fleet-footed economic advancements have not yet manifested themselves into unequivocal improvements in public health, especially in the case of child undernutrition. The findings of this chapter are a clear indication of the fact that though the per capita income of the state may be high, the socio-economic inequalities that persist are equally high. These inequalities, in fact, are the major contributors towards the alarmingly high levels of child undernutrition in Gujarat. With wealth explaining more than half of the inequalities that persist in child undernutrition, it provides ample evidence to explain the high levels of the latter. Gujarat serves as a case study for the importance of all-round development, further stressing on the need for providing amenities and services to the disadvantaged sections of the society, along with economic advancements to ensure optimal nutritional consequences.

One way to ensure this could be to ensure that India's "growth-mediated" programs to better its public health scenario are chaperoned by a "support-led" idea that places focus on acquiring panoramic knowledge of the mechanism and structural factors that influence undernutrition. To conclude, it is essential to envision future policies in a way that the poverty-nutrition nexus, along with myriad social and economic factors, are adequately acknowledged. Additionally, policies should also encompass the intricacies between social and economic development as a precursor to curtailing rising levels of undernutrition and inequality in the country.

Key findings
Kerala and Gujarat serve as interesting policy examples. Despite having identical poverty rates, their performances in child nutrition indicators are miles apart, with stunting and wasting prevalence in Kerala being far lower than that in Gujarat.
In Gujarat, factors at the household level account for the observed wealth-based inequality in child Undernutrition indicators, with household wealth alone accounting for more than 50 percent of the total inequality.
Results for stunting indicate that a one-unit increase in the asset index score at the median increases the HAZ score by 27.4 points as compared to 37.5 and 35.7 points at the 75th and 90th quantiles, respectively. Similar results were obtained for wasting and underweight as well.
The inequalities, in fact, are the major contributors towards the alarmingly high levels of child under-nutrition in Gujarat.
However, an improvement in the economic status of households is more beneficial for those children who are already relatively healthy.
Gujarat, thus, needs a slew of strategic policies that adequately acknowledge the existence of socio- economic development as a precursor to mitigating undernutrition and inequality in the prevalence of the same.

Zero Hunger, Food Security, and Nutrition: Where Are We and What's the Way Forward

7

Akancha Singh and Aparajita Chattopadhyay

Abstract

This chapter tries to understand the current status of food and nutrition security in India based on data and reports released at national and international levels. India has made concerted efforts to convert the Sustainable Development Goals (SDGs) into action plans to warrant access to sufficient and nutritive food. Food systems in the country have been transformed based on imminent priorities and capabilities in order to fulfill, particularly, the Goal 2 of the 2030 that aims to "end hunger, achieve food security, and promote sustainable agriculture". There are, however, crucial gaps, and it is the need of the hour to channel sustained efforts to conquer these obstacles. The indispensables envisage a phased and multi-pronged approach engaging various sectors that increase the reach of nutrition and health programs for women and children, and more targeted agricultural investments. Elderly in India also face food insecurity, though the issue is less highlighted. Targeted investments in agriculture are particularly important as it could pave the way for greater accessibility to food, thus, ensuring food security and expediting advancements in attaining the SDGs.

Keywords

Food security · SDG2 · Zero hunger · Nutrition · India

7.1 Introduction

Presently, 1 in 9 people, an estimated 820 million people globally, are either hungry or undernourished, with these numbers surreptitiously rising since 2015, especially in countries of Asia, Africa, and Latin America (FAO, 2019). Estimates suggest that approximately 113 million people across nearly 53 countries experience acute hunger, as a consequence of a combination of factors such as conflict and lack of food security, climate shocks, and economic consternation (Food Security Information Network, 2019). Concomitantly, globally, about 33% of the adult population is either overweight or obese, with rapid increase in such trends being observed in recent times (Ng et al., 2014). Although latest trends in data reveal some scattered headway towards selected global goals, 2025, including maternal, infant, and young child nutrition (MIYCN) indicators (WHO, 2014) and goals pertaining to diet-related NCDs (WHO, 2013), no country worldwide has managed to overturn the rapidly soaring trend in overweight and obesity. Additionally, despite the fact that there has been a 10% global relative decline in childhood stunting from 165.8 million in 2012 to 149 million in 2018, advancement towards global nutrition targets has been painfully slow or vacuous (WHO, 2020).

Perseverating at alarmingly high levels, undernutrition exists with stark differentials both

A. Chattopadhyay et al., *Undernutrition in India*, Sustainable Development Goals Series,
https://doi.org/10.1007/978-981-19-8182-1_7

between and within countries and among individuals of different socio-economic strata. To address these multifarious issues, global leaders asseverated a far-sighted vision for a global community that strives to "leave no-one behind" by committing itself to the Sustainable Development Goals (SDGs) (UN, 2018). The idea is to achieve a world that is free from all forms of hunger, deprivation, and nutritional inadequacies (UNGA, 2015). Soon after the SDGs appeared, the United Nations (UN) Decade of Action on Nutrition 2016–2025 articulated the target of eliminating all forms of nutritional discrepancies by 2025 with the intention of attaining universality of food and nutrition security (UNGA, 2016; WHO, 2017).

India presents a potentially uncommon example in the development of models and apparatuses by which sustainable ways could be put to use to address nutritional needs. In 2020, India stood at 94th position out of a total of 107 countries in the Global Hunger Index (GHI) (Table 7.1). Jointly published by Concern Worldwide and Welthungerhilfe, the Global Hunger Index ranks countries' nutritional status based on indicators of undernutrition, stunting, wasting, and child mortality indicators (von Grebmer et al., 2021). India's reduction in rates of undernutrition has been painstakingly slow when compared to its recent fleet-footed economic growth and this is precisely what puts it behind its poorer neighbours despite ranking above some of the world's poorest nations (Banerjee, 2014). It is well established in literature that India is still grappling with nutrition and food security issues. Nearly 39% of under-five children were stunted in India in 2016 (von Grebmer et al., 2020). Stunting is a strong indicator of chronic malnourishment in children and pregnant women, and a primarily irrevocable condition ultimately paving way for reduced physical and mental development (Jeyaseelan et al., 2016).

The intermingling of different factors makes the issue of deprivation and undernutrition more complex in India. It is also because nutritional status of children is determined by a plethora of factors such as dietary diversity, disease conditions, wash practices, and maternal autonomy (Bhutta, 2015). Owing to the above factors, amelioration in dietary intake alone will be inadequate to tackle challenges posed by undernutrition and hunger. It cannot, however, be denied that dietary improvement forms an indispensable component that works in tandem with other social and health indicators, especially sanitation. Research states that India is going to face increased hardships on nutrition and health fronts in the coming decades, mainly because of unchecked population growth and resources being scarce. India is enroute to become the world's most populated nation overtaking China, with its population expected to increase to 1.6 billion by 2050 from the current population of 1.26 billion (UN, 2015). What is more worrisome is that India has also been highlighted as one of the ecologically fragile nations, prone to precipitous impacts of climate change, water scarcity, and declining soil fertility through land degradation (Roberts, 2001).

This chapter tries to make an assessment of advancements (or lack of it) that India and its states have achieved in curtailing poverty rates, promoting food security and ensuring improved nutritional outcomes. It delineates the nutrition policies of India and all the states and explores the opportunities that they have in meeting, in particular, the SDG on zero hunger.

7.2 Zero Hunger in India: Where Do We Stand?

With an SDG score of 61.9, India ranks 117 among 166 countries globally (Sachs et al., 2020). Due to its colossal population, India accounts for a substantial share of global SDG performance gaps. To elaborate on the above points, India alone represents nearly 24% of the total achievement gap on SDG 2 (Zero Hunger). In addition to the above, the world would be 27.4% closer to achieving the SDG target on undernourishment if India eradicated undernourishment (currently

Table 7.1 Global hunger index ranks of major South Asian nations, 1990–2020

Country	Rank (2020)	Score								
		1990	1995	2000	2005	2015	2017	2019	2020	2021
China	1–17*	25.1	23.2	15.9	13.2	8.6	7.5	6.5	<5	<5
Thailand	48	28.4	22.3	17.6	13.6	11.9	10.6	9.7	10.2	11.7
Vietnam	61	44.6	38.8	30.3	24.6	14.7	16.0	15.3	13.6	13.6
Nepal	73	44.5	40.3	36.9	31.6	22.2	22.0	20.8	19.5	19.1
Sri Lanka	64	31.3	29.7	27.0	25.9	25.5	25.5	17.1	16.3	16.0
Bangladesh	75	52.2	50.3	38.5	31.0	27.3	26.5	25.8	20.4	19.1
India	94	48.1	42.3	38.2	38.5	29.0	31.4	30.3	27.2	27.5

Source von Grebmer et al, 2020, 2021

*The 17 countries with 2020 GHI scores of less than 5 are not assigned individual ranks, but rather are collectively ranked 1–17. Differences between their scores are minimal

GHI Severity Scale				
≤ 9.9 low	10.0–19.9 moderate	20.0–34.9 serious	35.0–49.9 alarming	≥ 50.0 extremely alarming

14.5% of the Indian population) (Sachs et al., 2020).

As per the NITI Aayog, there have been improvements in India's composite score from 60 in 2019–20 to 66 in 2020–21, suggesting substantial progress in India's journey towards achieving the SDGs. However, there are still two goals, namely, Goal 2 (zero hunger) and Goal 5 (gender equality) that warrant added scrutiny, as the total score for India for these goals is below 50 (NITI Aayog, 2021). The progress in attaining SDG 2 (zero hunger) is measured using seven indicators. These indicators are proportion of beneficiaries covered under National Food Security Act (2013), prevalence of stunting, prevalence of underweight, percentage of women aged 15–49 who are anaemic, percentage of adolescents aged 10–19 who are anaemic, annual production of rice and wheat per unit area, and gross value added (in constant prices) in agriculture per worker (NITI Aayog, 2021). According to the latest SDG India Index report published by NITI Aayog, Kerala and Chandigarh are the top performers among the states and the UTs, respectively. The category of Front-runners (score: 65–99) included seven states and four union territories. The aspirants category consisted of 11 states and 2 union territories (Score < 50) (NITI Aayog, 2021).

As per latest estimates of the World Bank, an important aftermath of the pandemic is the huge numbers of people (71 million) who will be pushed into poverty globally (World Bank,2020). As per the definition of Food and Agricultural Organization, food security is achieved when "all people, at all times, have physical and economic access to sufficient safe and nutritious food that meets their dietary needs and food preferences for an active and healthy life" (FAO, 1996). The above definition outlines four crucial facets of food security, namely, food availability, access (physical and economic), food utilization, and the cohesion of the above-mentioned components over an extended period. The UN has foreboded that the world is facing an imminent food emergency. As per World Food Program estimates, COVID-19 could lead to an estimated 130 million people facing food insecurity, in addition to the 820 million who were already food insecure as per the estimates given by State of Food Insecurity in the World Report, 2019 (United Nations, 2020). It, therefore, comes as no surprise that the outbreak of COVID-19 has already had an immensely negative impact on all

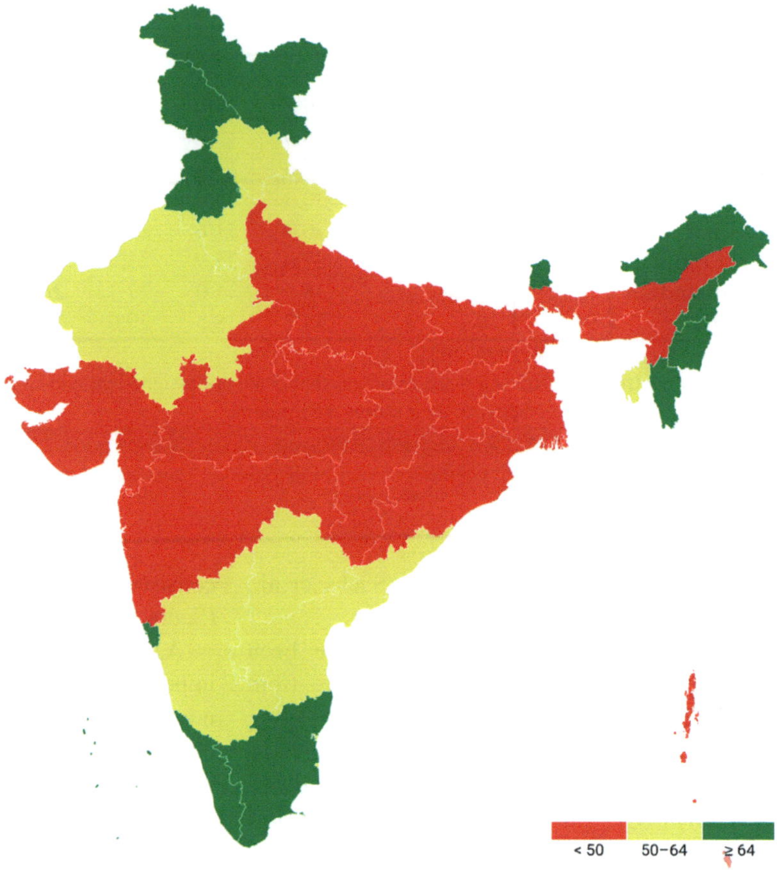

Fig. 7.1 Performance of states/UTs in SDG2 (Zero Hunger), 2020–21. *Source* Based on NITI Aayog, 2021

four dimensions of food security in India. An additional consequence of the pandemic has been the increased disruptions in food systems caused by both external and personal aspects, which include ease of geographical access, affordability, serviceability, and significance (United Nations System Standing Committee on Nutrition, 2020). The implications of the pandemic on *Zero Hunger* are manifested in the SDG scores of India and the states. It is, therefore, no surprise that the states are either off-track or struggling to meet the targets set by SDG2. Figure 7.1 shows the current status of states in achieving SDG2. The states in red are the *Aspirants,* which are lagging behind heavily. The ones in yellow and green are *Performers* and *Front Runners*, respectively. These are the states that are performing rather satisfactorily in achieving SDG2.

7.3 Food Security Among Older Adults in India: Evidence from Longitudinal Ageing Study in India

A comprehensive analysis of food insecurity warrants going beyond the conventional definition of hunger. This approach shows that nearly 1.3 billion people, or 17% of the global population, has experienced food insecurity at moderate levels. This implies that even though they are not necessarily suffering from hunger, they do not have uninterrupted access to sufficient food and this places them at an increased risk of declining health and nutritional inadequacies (FAO, 2019). The latest Global Hunger Index report marks India's hunger levels as "serious", ranking it as

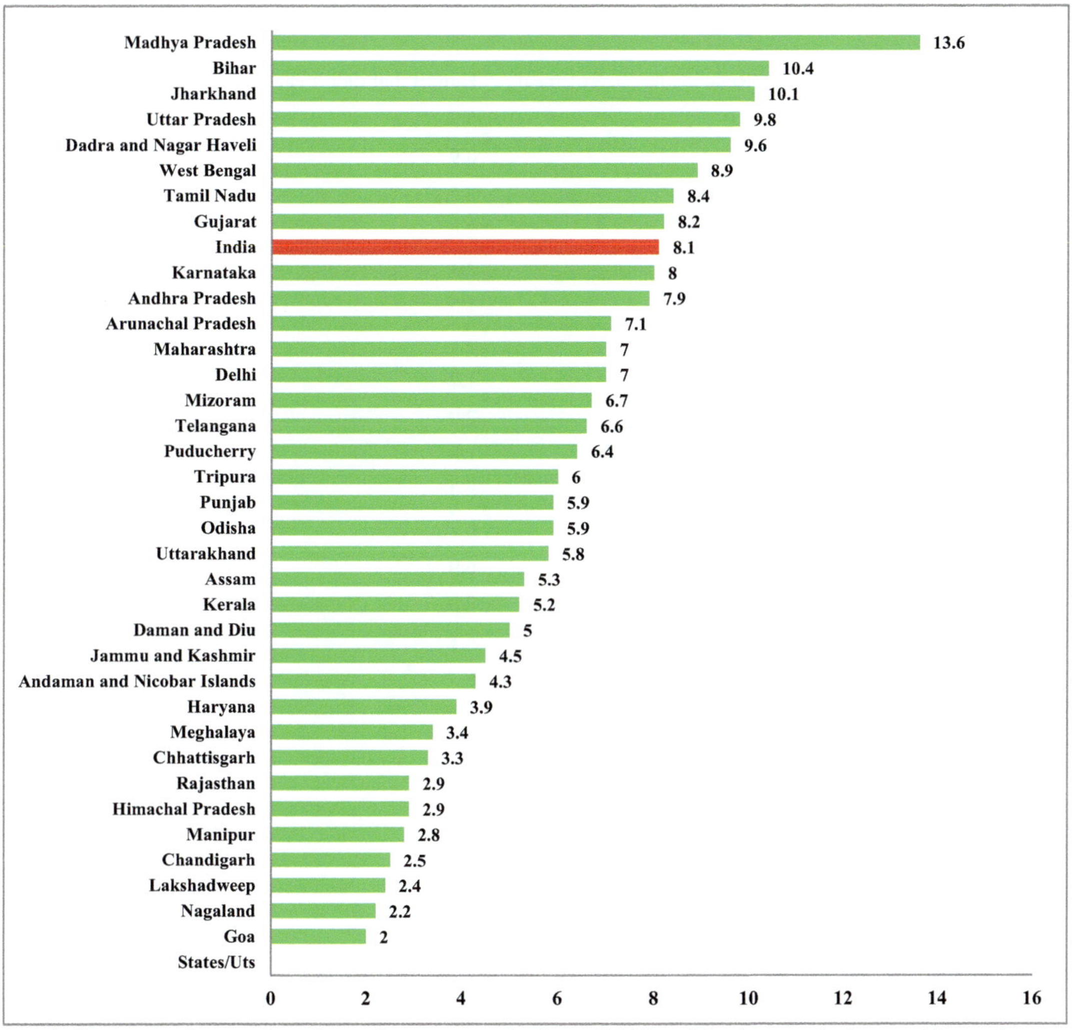

* Including spouse irrespective of age; Severe constraint in availability of food means in the past 12 months, household members had to reduce the size of meals, were hungry but did not have enough food, did not eat food of their choice, or did not have food for a full day because food was unavailable.

Fig. 7.2 Percentage of older adults age 45 and above who reported severe constraint in household food availability, India. *Source* Based on Longitudinal Ageing Study in India, 2017–18

101 out of 116 countries as far as food security is concerned (Grebmer et al., 2021).

Figure 7.2 shows the state-wise proportion of older adults experiencing constraints in food availability in India. As per the data, 8.2% older adults aged 45 years and above reported disrupted availability of food in the last 1 year, wherein they were either forced to consume less, skip meals despite being hungry, or went a whole day without eating because of unavailability of food. About one-tenth of older adults in Madhya Pradesh (14%), Bihar (10%), and Jharkhand (10%) reported disrupted food availability.

Cross-state variation of food insufficiency is shown in Table 7.2. States/UTs whose prevalence of household food insecurity is higher than

Table 7.2 Percentage of older adults who experienced food insufficiency at household, states/UTs, LASI Wave 1, 2017–18

States/UTs	Reduced the size of meal	Hungry but didn't eat	Didn't eat for whole day
India	6.0	5.3	3.8
Chandigarh	1.3	0.9	1.2
Delhi	3.9	3.5	3.1
Haryana	2.8	2.6	1.3
Himachal Pradesh	1.3	2.1	1.3
Jammu and Kashmir	3.5	1.5	0.8
Punjab	4	3.1	1.7
Rajasthan	2.2	1.7	1.1
Uttarakhand	3.6	2.9	2.7
Chattisgarh	1.5	1.8	1
Uttar Pradesh	10	8.2	6.8
Madhya Pradesh	7.7	6.2	5.7
Bihar	8.2	6.9	6.2
Jharkhand	8.4	7.8	4.7
Odisha	5.1	4.1	2.1
West Bengal	8	6.4	3.8
Arunachal Pradesh	6.1	1.9	(0.3)
Assam	4.4	2.3	1.5
Manipur	1.5	1.9	1.3
Meghalaya	1.6	2.3	0.8
Mizoram	5.1	4	3.7
Nagaland	2.1	0.7	(0.4)
Tripura	5.4	4.9	2.9
Dadra and Nagar Haveli	7.3	3.7	4
Daman and Diu	4.3	2.8	2.7
Goa	0.9	1.4	0.7
Gujarat	5.6	4.6	4.1
Maharashtra	4.6	4.4	3.6
Andaman and Nicobar Islands	3.3	3.3	1.1
Andhra Pradesh	4.7	5.3	3.9
Karnataka	5	5.6	2.3
Kerala	3.6	2.9	1.7
Lakshadweep	1.2	0.7	0.7
Puducherry	5.1	5	3.2
Tamil Nadu	5.8	6.3	4.1
Telangana	5.1	3.5	2.7

Cases in parentheses () mean less than 5 unweighted cases in the numerator or 25 unweighted cases in the denominator
Source Longitudinal Ageing Study in India, 2017–18

the national average (6%) are Dadra and Nagar Haveli (7%), West Bengal (8%), Bihar (8%), Jharkhand (8%), Uttar Pradesh (8%), and Madhya Pradesh (10%). About 6% of older adults skipped meals despite being hungry in of the eastern and central states. The proportion of older adults who did not eat for a full day is less than 5% in the states/UTs, except for Bihar (6%), Uttar Pradesh (6%), and Madhya Pradesh (7%).

India figures show that while 6% older adults decreased their meal size, 5% skipped meals despite being hungry because of insufficient food and 4% skipped meal for a whole day because of unavailability of food in the past year. While none of these indicators vary significantly across age and sex, conspicuous differentials can be observed by place of residence, wherein 7% older adults in rural areas decreased their meal size, 6% skipped meals despite being hungry because of insufficient food, and 5% skipped meal for a whole day because of unavailability of food in the past year. Similarly, food insecurity varied vastly for different living arrangements, wherein 14% older adults living alone reduced their meal size, 14% were hungry but did not eat, and 10% did not eat for a full day. Additionally, food insecurity was also found to be negatively proportional to wealth quintile and education (Table not shown).

Food insecurity constitutes a major public health dilemma and it serves as a useful criterion for measuring health and well-being because of its direct linkages with poor health, improper dietary intake (consumption of fast foods, lack of fruits and vegetables in diet), impoverishment, mental health, and social capital (FAO, 1996). Whatever little evidence that is available on food insecurity among older adults points out towards the factors that place them at a greater risk than the general population are low incomes, limited mobility, and poor health. Elderly facing food insecurity are at the risk of facing myriad problems that limit their ability to be nutritionally secure or avail benefits from social security and food-based programs. Food insecurity will aggravate existing health, economic, and emotional issues for elderly who are already vulnerable due to deteriorating health and increased dietary requirements (Lee & Frongillo, 2001). The need of the hour is, thus, an inclusive, multidisciplinary approach that targets nutritional requirements among the elderly and puts adequate redressing and treatment mechanisms in place (Wells & Dumbrell, 2006).

7.4 Linkages Between Poverty, Food Security, and Nutrition

There is abundant evidence to suggest that people across the globe who live in poverty, concomitantly grapple with food insecurity, lack of education, health care, and other indispensable needs (Ortiz-Ospina & Roser, 2019). As per the latest estimates of The World Bank, 2020 saw the falling into poverty of approximately 40–60 million people, with their incomes falling below 1.9 USD per day (Lanker et al., 2021). As a result of the above, it is estimated that global poverty rates could escalate rapidly to nine percent in 2020, which is nearly an increase of 0.4% from 2019 (Lanker et al., 2021). This is the consequence of a plethora of factors including the burgeoning burden of global population and the ensuing paucity of already scarce resources.

There was marked escalation in the global incidence of poverty in the first half of the twentieth century, coupled with contemporaneous upsurge in both industrialization and an increase in population. However, in the decades following the 1970s, there has been a continuous decline in poverty rates. Researchers are of the opinion that there will be a reversal in this pattern of downfall in poverty rates in the coming years and a marked increase in poverty will be observed (Ortiz-Ospina & Roser, 2019). Indeed, South Asia's share in global poverty has rapidly escalated from 27 to 33% between 1990 and 2013, faring better than only Sub-Saharan Africa, which accounts for nearly one half of the global poor (Patel, 2018). Despite a consistent decline in the absolute numbers of population of people living in poverty in South Asia by nearly 148.8 million during the decade following the 1990s, its poverty rate is still higher than East Asia, Central Asia, Eastern Europe, Middle East, North America, and the Pacific (Deyshapppriya, 2018).

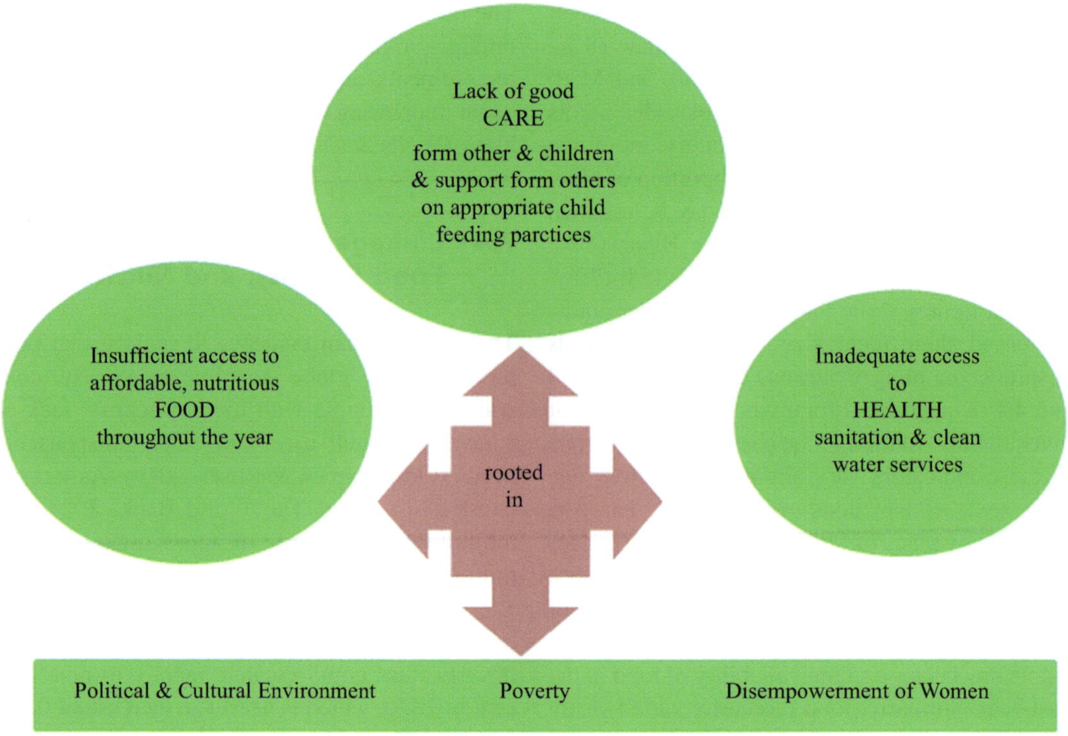

Fig. 7.3 Schematic representation of factors causing malnutrition. *Source* Authors

In Asia, urban poverty has become quite conspicuous in recent years. In what has been referred to by scholars as "urbanization of poverty", countries around the world experienced a surge in the proportion of poor people between 1990 and 2008. This was also the time when a rapid increase in urbanization was also being observed (Mathur, 2014). In developing countries in Asia, such as in India, Bangladesh, and other South Asian countries, the increase in rates of urbanization has been concomitant with the growth of slums (Mathur, 2014), retrograding living conditions, intensifying food insecurity, and severe health risks owing to alarmingly high levels of pollution (Fig. 7.3). As per the latest estimates given by UN-Habitat, the countries of Asia house nearly 60% of the global slum population. What is, however, more concerning is that these estimates exclude a vast chunk of population that lives in slum-like conditions and is still not officially categorized as such (UNICEF, 2020).

Researchers suggest myriad different approaches to deal with food and nutrition insecurity. These approaches can be crudely placed into two categories, namely, direct nutrition-sensitive interventions and indirect approach targeting different sectors (Bezanson & Isenam, 2010). The former thrives on the relationship between food security and nutrition. These approaches acknowledge the inter-woven relationship between hunger and nutritional deprivation and encompass programs and policies directly targeted at improving the nutritional status of the population. The latter targets nutritional deprivation through multiple channels. It deals with the basic and underlying causes of undernutrition, including multiple factors such as income security, agricultural production, women's status, maternal education (Gillespie & Haddad, 2003; Alderman & Headey, 2017; Spears et al., 2013; Gulati et al., 2012), and wash practices and their impact on prevention of infectious diseases (Headey et al., 2019; Gulati et al., 2012; India

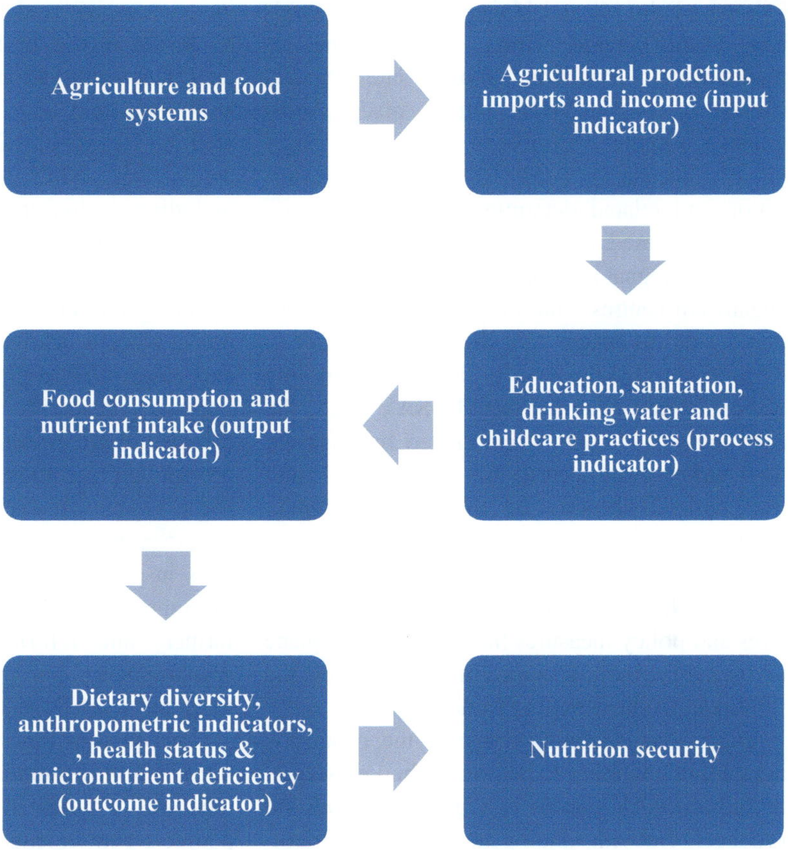

Fig. 7.4 Linkages between food security and nutrition security. *Source* Adapted from Pinstrup-Andersen and Watson (2011), Babu et al. (2016)

State-Level Disease Burden Initiative Undernutrition Collaborators, 2019; Deaton & Dreze, 2009, UNICEF, 1998). This approach also cuts across different departments and programs, with the aim of synchronizing nutritional policies with other programs to improve food and nutrition security (Gulati et al., 2012, Thow et al., 2016). One example could be how assimilating nutrition-related policies with agriculture can create a diverse and nutritious food basket and encompassing such policies in the school curriculum can lead to improved nutrition for school-going children. This approach is multi-pronged and beneficial because of the increased coordination and compliance between different departments and sectors to address the basic and underlying causes of undernutrition (Bezanson & Isenam, 2010, Fears et al., 2018) (Fig. 7.4).

7.5 Policy Initiatives in India

A near fivefold increase in India's food grain production from 50 million tons in 1950–51 to about 250 million tons in 2014–15 has made India a net food exporter and nulled its reliance on imports. The doubling farmers' income by 2022 program launched in 2016 aims to boost productivity by eliminating bottlenecks in productivity, particularly in areas dependent on rainfall. Under the aegis of Ministry of Agriculture, a target had been made to increase India's gross irrigated area from 90 million hectares to 103 million hectares by 2017. To channelize efforts for this, programs such as the National Food Security Mission, Rashtriya Krishi Vikas Yojana (RKVY), the Integrated Schemes on

Oilseeds, Palm oil and Maize (ISOPOM), Pradhan Mantri Fasal Bima Yojana, the e-marketplace, irrigation, soil, and water-harvesting program were put in place. Additionally, initiatives have been put in place since last two decades to tackle the issue of undernutrition and related determinants. These include the school-based mid-day meal program, ration supply to pregnant and lactating mothers through anganwadi centres, and targeted public distribution system to ensure subsidized food supply to those living below poverty line. Through the National Food Security Act (NFSA), 2013, the right to food is being strengthened by ensuring food and nutrition security for the vulnerable and marginalized sections of the society. Indian health policymakers were significantly involved in the stipulation of the Sustainable Development Goals (UN, 2017a, 2017b). A number of initiatives and policy measures have been put in place to underline India's commitments towards the fulfilment of these goals (Table 7.3).

Despite its declining share in the economy, agriculture continues to be one of the key sectors in India, which makes it a global agricultural producer. Notwithstanding the fact that agricultural productivity in the semi-arid tropical regions of the country is severely constrained by water scarcity and recurring droughts, India holds the record of having the world's largest area under cultivation of food crop such as rice and wheat and cash crops such as cotton. It is also the largest global producer of milk, spices, and pulses (NITI Aayog, 2017). Limitations, including environmental degradation and weather-related disaster risks, mar India's attempts at attaining food security. Schemes like doubling farmers' incomes by 2022 have been put in place to address the grievances of farmers and ensure that coping mechanisms are already in place to deal with challenges of food insecurity (Singh, 2018). Another scheme to help farmers protect their incomes is the Pradhan Mantri Fasal Bima Yojana which covers 30% of gross cropped area (Singh, 2018). The government has also put laws in place to subsidize grain production and farm inputs, providing minimum support price to farmers and reforming agricultural laws and regulations to open the Indian agricultural sector to global markets (Schneider, 2016).

The quinquennium of 2005–10 heralded the introduction of numerous legislations and policy measures targeted at protecting and promoting people's entitlements to land, employment, education, and allied aspects. 100 days of work on demand to every rural household was guaranteed

Table 7.3 SDG-related program measures in India

Goals	Policy measures
Goal 2: Achieve food security and improved nutrition and promote sustainable agriculture	• Ration cards being issued to senior female members of the household • *Mid-Day Meal Program*, for providing meals to 100 million primary school children
Goal 3: Ensure healthy lives and promote well-being for all at all ages	• Efforts in India to increase access to health care as well as improve the quality of care • Village-level Anganwadi Centres for providing primary health care, family planning, nutrition and health education, the reduction of maternal and infant and under-five mortality, immunizations, and referral services • Health insurance to families living below the poverty level
Goal 5: Achieve gender equality and empower all women and girls	• *Educate the Girl Child* and *Maternity Benefit Program* for childbearing and breastfeeding women. These programs are aimed at protecting wage loss during the first 6 months postpartum through a conditional cash transfer initiative • Establishment of Women Empowerment Centres on village level affiliated with the Anganwadi Centres to more fully meet this goal

by the National Rural Employment Guarantee Act (NREGA). Access to elementary schooling to every child was promised by the Right to Education Act (RTE). This is also the period where elementary education and primary health care were brought to the fore by the government through programs such as Sarva Siksha Abhiyan, ensued by the Right to Education and the National Rural Health Mission (NRHM). Universalization of cooked mid-day meals in schools, expansion in the Public Distribution System, and universalization of early childcare services through the Integrated Child Development Services (ICDS) were put in place (Joshi et al., 2017; Hertel, 2015). Passed in 2013, The National Food Security Act (NFSA) paved the way for an expanded public distribution system, which tried to capture poverty line beyond the quintessential consumption expenditure-based estimates. However, it cannot be denied that there are myriad gaps in the implementation of these programs, there is plenty of evidence to support the fact that these schemes serve as a lifeline for the poor people of India by providing employment during lean seasons and enabling access to at least one nutritious meal per day (Drèze & Khera, 2017). It is, thus, apt to conclude that some social welfare schemes have enabled a social safety net for the Indian poor.

7.6 Role of Public Distribution System

The National Food Security Act provides for the allocation of 5 kilos of food grains (consisting of wheat, rice, and millets) per person to 75% and 50% of the population in rural and urban areas, respectively, at very low rates (wheat at Rs. 2 per kilo, rice at Rs. 3 per kilo, and millets at Rs. 1 per kilo), disbursed through the Public Distribution System. Based on the above statistics, the central government disburses food grains to the states through the Food Corporation of India. The responsibility of identification of beneficiaries as well as the overall implementation of the scheme lies with the respective state governments (Sinha, 2020). Before the enactment of the NFSA, state governments were allotted food grains based on the population below poverty line (BPL) in the respective states, based on which BPL household was also identified. Owing to large exclusion and inclusion errors under the previous scheme, a large proportion of households remained deprived. The National Food Security Act ensures better selection and coverage, especially in economically backward states and rural areas, leading to increased inclusion and larger number of beneficiaries.

Under the Act, states were required to reform the functioning of the Public Distribution System (PDS). This ensured improved functioning and better implementation of PDS in states that were laggards, such as Bihar (Drèze & Khera, 2015). There is a dearth of more concurrent nationally representative data that can highlight trends on the leakages and coverage under PDS. This is also because the latest NSSO Consumer Expenditure Survey, used popularly to arrive at these estimates, was last conducted in 2011–12.

Households having ration cards under NFSA are being provided with additional 5 kilos of food grains (inclusive of 1 kilo of pulses per household) free of cost. Nearly 81 crore NFSA beneficiaries, constituting 60% of India's estimated population, fall under the ambit of this scheme. However, state ration card-holders and those not having ration cards have been excluded from the same (Sinha, 2020a). Reports suggest that an added 100 million population needs to be covered in order to be able to cover even the stipulated 67% population as per the latest population estimates (Scroll, 2020). In addition to the above, this requirement may be amplified due to the present crisis where they have lost their livelihoods.

The issue of access to food for those people who do not own ration cards is now becoming a policy focus for state governments. However, it is the concept of universal PDS that hasn't still been recognized sufficiently as a means to ensure maximum inclusion. Exclusion criteria can be put in place to identify that chunk of the population that does not need such coverage, such as those who are income tax payers (Himanshu & Sen, 2011). The PDS, in spite of all its limitations, has been a big relief for people, especially during the crisis situation induced by the pandemic and the ensuing national lockdown. Notwithstanding the already existing schemes, it is still crucial to have additional support mechanisms in place in the form of subsidized food grains to those people who are already NFSA beneficiaries, especially in the wake of the havoc wreaked by the pandemic and economy being in a downward spiral. A survey on COVID-19 conducted by the Azim Premji University found that while 20% of vulnerable households did not receive any rations during the lockdown, nearly half of them did not receive benefits from cash transfers (Lahoti et al., 2020). This evidently establishes the efficacy of PDS over other schemes and measures enacted during the lockdown. Another survey of over 3900 households in Chhattisgarh found that nearly 95% of the households received rations and, thus, recommend that it is imperative that PDS shops continue operating, especially in times following the pandemic (Pandey et al., 2020). Another study from rural Maharashtra showed that a mere 8% of seasonal migrant households were food secure, wherein 59% and 33% reported having food security without hunger and mild or moderate levels of hunger, respectively, with access to PDS being almost non-existent for them (Jaleel & Chattopadhyay, 2019). Evidence implies that despite facing efficacy issues, particularly pertaining to targeting food insecurity and poor population groups (George & McKay, 2019), India's Targeted Public Distribution System, providing nearly 800 million households with food grains and rations at lower prices through about 5 lakh fair price shops, is the world's biggest safety net program (Bhattacharya et al., 2018). Although evidence of the ramifications of the program on dietary diversity and nutrition is not completely clear, it is evident that PDS did show some positive impact on the intake of macronutrients (Rahman, 2016; Bhattacharya et al., 2018; George & McKay, 2019). The above evidence underpins the importance of PDS and states that it is the efficient way to reach people, especially in the present context.

7.7 The Mid-Day Meal (MDM) Scheme and Its Aftermath

The National Program of Nutritional Support to Primary Education (Mid-Day Meal Scheme) was catapulted as a centrally sponsored scheme on 15 August 1995. The scheme aimed at making primary education universal by pushing up enrolment rates, retaining more children in schools and increasing attendance rates concomitantly in a bid to bolster the nutrition levels of children. The program, in its initial days of launch, dealt solely with primary school children (classes 1st to 5th) enrolled in government, government-aided, and local body schools. The scheme was further expanded to bring children studying in the Education Guarantee Scheme (EGS) and Alternative and Innovative Education (AIE) Centres under its ambit as well in October 2002. The Ministry of Human Resource Development issued revised guidelines for scheme implementation in December 2004. These guidelines stressed on providing fully cooked meals consisting of a minimum of 300 cal and about 8–12 g of protein content. It also envisaged that there was a need to accord special attention on the enrolment, attendance, and retention of children belonging to the disadvantaged sections. In addition to the above, nutritional support to students at the primary stage in drought-affected areas was also to be provided during summer vacations. The importance of providing assistance for better management of the program, including its monitoring, and evaluation was also amply stressed upon. To bolster the inclusivity of the scheme, it was further extended to include children studying in upper primary classes and children studying in those Madarsas/Maktabs that were supported under the Sarva Shiksha Abhiyan.

As India attempts to make progressive strides towards nutrition security from food security, the MDMS can prove to be an ideal conduit through which the delivery of nutritious food can be bolstered. Some states have set an example by instilling policies particularly to revise the

MDMS to ameliorate nutritional outcomes. States have tweaked the scheme in myriad ways to make it more comprehensive and inclusive. A brief outline of such manoeuvres is elaborated as follows:

- In Uttar Pradesh (UP) and Tamil Nadu (TN), governments are piloting fortification of food grains, which are then served as a part of the MDM in some districts. The UP government has been fortifying food grains in Varanasi together with the Planet Food Program while the Tamil Nadu government is doing it independently. Such an intervention is advantageous because the WHO recommends food fortification as an effective way to scale back undernutrition. By buttressing the nutritional content of the food grains before serving them to the students, the governments of Tamil Nadu and Uttar Pradesh have certainly taken a massive step towards enhancing the nutritional outcomes of their students.
- In Uttarakhand, "apna kitchen, apna bhojan" is organized, under which kitchen helpers teach children to organize the MDM once every week. This intervention enables the students to be liable for their own food requirements and nutrition while imparting a crucial life skill for their future.
- The Gujarat government has bifurcated the MDM into two portions. According to the rules of the MDMS in Gujarat, schools need to provide 180 g of food grains to students in primary classes and 265 g of food grains to students in upper primary classes. When the required food grains are cooked, it expands to a weight that's an excessive amount for the first and upper primary classes to consume at one sitting. Thus, the meal is split into two meals and served as breakfast and lunch. The advantage of the above-mentioned intervention is that dividing the meal into two portions ensures that children eat the entire amount of food grains available. They eat both breakfast and lunch, which makes sure that they are not going hungry through the day.
- The governments of Andhra Pradesh, Karnataka, Tamil Nadu, and Telangana have further aggrandized the MDMS to cover students who study in classes 9 and 10. The funding for this expansion is done solely by the respective state governments. Findings of research studies have suggested that the scheme has led to increase in the rates of student retention and has played a monumental role in reducing dropout rates, especially among girls. The state governments hope to reap the same benefits by bringing the students of classes 9th and 10th under the ambit of MDMS.
- The Kerala government has undertaken an additional initiative wherein it provides a separate breakfast in the addition to the conventional MDM in approximately 3,000 schools within the state, all of which are funded by the state. The draft of the new education policy of the MHRD states that the morning time after a nutritious breakfast is often particularly productive. By ensuring that children receive not only the stipulated mid-day meal but also a nutritious breakfast, the Kerala government is making sure that students are well fed throughout the day, which enables them to focus better on their studies.
- The Chandigarh government has installed CCTV cameras in the kitchens. The advantage of this intervention is that it enables the concerned authorities to watch the kitchens in real time. It also serves as a medium to make sure that the kitchens adhere to the MDM guidelines and allow extenuation of any untoward incidents, like instances where children report falling sick after consuming a meal prepared in school.

Data from the MDM scheme from the past few years points out towards the fact that although a reasonable rise in the enrolment rate of children was observed under the scheme till 2017–18, it has registered a decline in the past few years. There is also evidence to suggest under-utilization of funds allocated for the scheme in states in the financial year 2018–19 (Report of the Comptroller and Auditor General of India, 2015). With number of children enrolled in schools going down from 150 to 140 million between 2009–10 and 2013–14, there has been a steady decline in the enrolment of students within the schools covered under the MDM scheme. On the other hand, enrolment rates in private schools have increased by 38% from 40 to 55 million during the same period. This goes on to suggest that the Mid-Day Meal scheme, although necessary, was not sufficient to ensure increased retention of children in schools, and that there was an ardent need to bolster the quality of education imparted in these schools (Report of the Comptroller and Auditor General of India, 2015). There have also been concerns about the quality and consistency of data recorded by the state governments. Significant differentials in coverage data of children have been observed in states, as per a Comptroller and Auditor General (CAG) report (Report of the Comptroller and Auditor General of India, 2015). This discrepancy severely limits the mechanism that has been put in place for data assimilation. This further limits any attempt to undertake any monitoring and evaluation activities to gauge the efficacy of the program.

7.8 Addressing the Issue of Food Security: The Role of Agriculture

The global population surpassed the 7.6 billion mark in 2018 (FAO United Nations Statistical Database) and is forecasted to touch 9.2 billion by 2050 (Silva, 2018), with a projected 59–102% increase in demand for food (Elferink & Schierhorn, 2016; Fukase & Martin, 2017). There is ample evidence to suggest the superiority of agricultural sector as compared to other sectors of economy in curtailing poverty rates and improving food security among the population (Irz et al., 2001; Majid, 2004). Owing to the above, it becomes pertinent to bolster agricultural production by about 60%–70% to provide for the dietary needs of the colossal global population in 2050 (Silva, 2018). There is increasing consensus among researchers that the food production will have to be nearly doubled by 2050 to meet the escalating demand (Foley et al., 2011; Tilman et al., 2011). The agricultural sector is the cornerstone for improving the availability of food and achieving food security (Smutka et al., 2009; Otsuka et al., 2013; Smutka et al., 2015; Wegren & Elvestad, 2018).

While there is general unanimity on the fact that a surreptitious increase is expected in the global demand for food in the coming decades, there is ambivalence when it comes to the capacity of global agriculture to cater to this increased demand through amplification in the food supply (Cook et al., 2011). Improved food provision made sure by strengthening agricultural productivity and extending the range of agricultural land use seems to be the plausible method to eradicate hunger (Stocking, 2003; Smyth et al., 2015). However, existing technological and ideological handicaps in low-income developing countries could prove to be a hurdle in their attempt to enhance their production capacities to meet the increased demand (Pinstrup-Andersen & Pandya-Lorch, 1998). The above discussion stresses on the fact that it is crucial that investments in research and development in agricultural and related systems are increased, especially in developing countries. This will ensure improved productivity both from agricultural lands and workers.

When classifying needs by severity and pertinence, Maslow accorded maximum importance to thirst and hunger, stating that it is the basic human need and absolutely essential for survival (Maslow, 1954). Malthus, in his seminal work, In An Essay on the Principle of Population, As It Affects the Future Improvement of Society, published in 1798, asserted that while agricultural production increased only arithmetically, the increase in population size is geometrical and beyond control (Malthus, 1798). As per Malthus, a decline in the productivity of agriculture could be expected if the population continued to grow while the supply of natural resources (especially land) remained constant. This could give rise to a situation wherein agricultural production would fall behind the rapidly rising population, while the contraction in supply was followed by famine. Despite being relevant in the contemporary context of the industrial revolution, Malthus' theory attracted a lot of criticism from researchers from disciplines. The important reason behind the failure of the Malthusian approach was his ignorance of technological advancements enabling rapid growth in rates of food production without having to acquire new land resources.

This issue was brought to the fore by Ester Boserup, who stated that owing to modernization and technological advancements, the rate of growth of food production would surpass that of the population growth (this became famous as the Boserupian model), hence breaking the Malthusian trap (Boserup, 1985). The 6th global nutrition report by the United Nations System Standing Committee on Nutrition (UNSCN), published in 2010, highlights the crucial role of agriculture in ensuring nutrition and food security (Progress in Nutrition, 2010).

Having dealt with the limitation of global food production capacity, another critical issue facing the global scientific community, now, is the problem of exhausting resources and sustainable food production methods. Some scientists have made an observation that accelerated and industrialized food production practices, which have been put in place to meet the increased global food demand (Hazel & Wood, 2008), have been accelerating environmental damage (Nellemann et al., 2019) and may chaperone ecological not just locally but also globally. There are extant studies that have acknowledged the presence of certain biophysical limits in the ecosystem, which may have cataclysmic repercussions for human beings (Rockström et al., 2009). A large proportion of population living in extreme destitution will be further deprived of any opportunity to assuage its decisive requirements and hunger issues due to environmental pollution and declining ecological stability of the biosphere. Another set of studies points out that, with manifested negative impacts on air and water quality, biodiversity, carbon sequestration, and transmission of infectious diseases, agriculture is not only the largest contributor to tropical deforestation but is also responsible for nearly 35% of global greenhouse gas emissions (Geist & Lambin, 2002; Foley et al., 2005; Foley et al., 2011).

It is ironic that despite historically high levels of food production in India, undernutrition and micronutrient deficiencies persist. Presently, nearly 3.4% and 36% of children under-five are overweight and stunted, respectively, with the former registering an increase in the last 5 years (IIPS, 2019–21). While undernutrition persists, latest estimates from the National Family Health Survey-5 reveal that about 24% and 23% of females and males, respectively, are overweight or obese (IIPS, 2019–21). While the issue of undernutrition and deprivation is not new in India, the increasing prevalence of overweight/obesity in recent years has further made matters worse for India. Registering rapid growth in both rural and urban areas, overweight and obesity rates have increased by more than double in the past decade in India. Women, in general, and especially urban residents are at increased risk of being overweight or obese than their male counterparts. It is crucial to observe people's dietary intake and how this pattern has evolved over time to be able to solve this problem. There is a plethora of evidence to suggest that Indian diets are traditionally cereal based and usually lacking in diversity. The reason behind historically high levels of nutritional anomalies and widespread micronutrient deficiencies is these kind of dietary practices coupled with food insecurity.

With a yield rate of 2.4 tons rice per hectare, India stands at the 27th position out of 47 rice-producing countries. From the 44 ha of land under rice cultivation, India produces 106 million tons of rice per annum. The yield rates of China and Brazil, at 4.7 t/ha and 3.6 t/ha, respectively, are much greater than India's. If India's production increased to China's and Brazil's levels, the production could be ramped up to 205.52 million tons and 160.01 million tons of rice, respectively. As far as the production of wheat is concerned, India has a higher yield rate for wheat as compared to rice, but it still lags behind countries. With nearly 30 million hectares under wheat cultivation, India produces 94 million tons of wheat with a yield rate of 3.15 t/ha. This places India at the 19th position out of 41 wheat-producing countries. It is also noteworthy that there has been an impressive increase in the agricultural productivity of wheat and rice in India over the years. Yield rates of wheat and rice have grown at exponential rates of 1.8% and 1.7% between 1983 and 2013. These growth rates are particularly encouraging considering that they make India rank 13th and 14th in rice and wheat production, respectively (Raghavan, 2014) (Fig. 7.5).

With increase in food production and improvement in access to better quality nutrition, the issue reckoning attention transitioned from food security to nutrition security. The current imbroglio demands an amelioration in the dietary diversity of the Indian population because compete reliance on cereals as a source of energy may lead to the co-existence of a micronutrient deficiency and macronutrient over-nutrition, the lack of dietary diversity being the prime reason behind the same and leading to increased nutritional anomalies.

The Second Sustainable Development Goal (*End Hunger and Achieve Food Security and Improved Nutrition*) stipulates that it is crucial to ensure continuous production of nutritious food, enhance its availability and accessibility, and buttress its affordability for the Indian population. The latest consumer expenditure survey (CES) of the NSSO (68th round) makes the following observations about the shift in dietary patterns of the Indian population:

- Increased intake of meat products, fat-intensive diets, and salty foods.
- Reduced intake of coarse grains.
- Increased rates of dining out.
- Massive increase in fast food consumption (Fig. 7.6).

The solution to the above-mentioned imbroglio lies in bolstering food availability and contributing sustainably to global food security by increasing agricultural productivity and resource efficiency, in addition to preserving natural resources and biodiversity (Basiago, 1995; Lee, 2005; Pretty et al., 2011; Zhang et al., 2011; Noleppa et al., 2013; Wang et al., 2015; Adnele et al., 2019). The above findings were reiterated by other studies that stated that it was a universal observation, with the findings being more relevant for developing and the least developed economies, suggesting that one of the prime

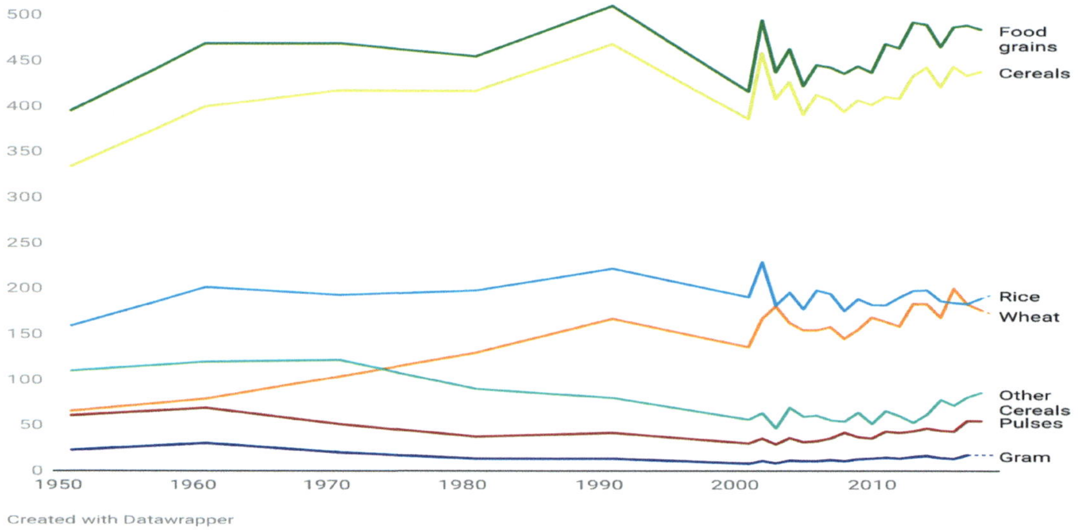

Fig. 7.5 Per capita net availabilities of food grains (per day), India (1951–2018). *Source* 1. Based on Pocket Book of Agricultural Statistics 2018, Directorate of Economics & Statistics, Ministry of Agriculture & Farmers Welfare, Govt. of India. (Website. http://eands.dacnet.nic.in), 2. Based on Agricultural Statistics at a Glance 2017, Directorate of Economics & Statistics, Ministry of Agriculture & Farmers Welfare, Govt. of India. (Website: http://eands.dacnet.nic.in)

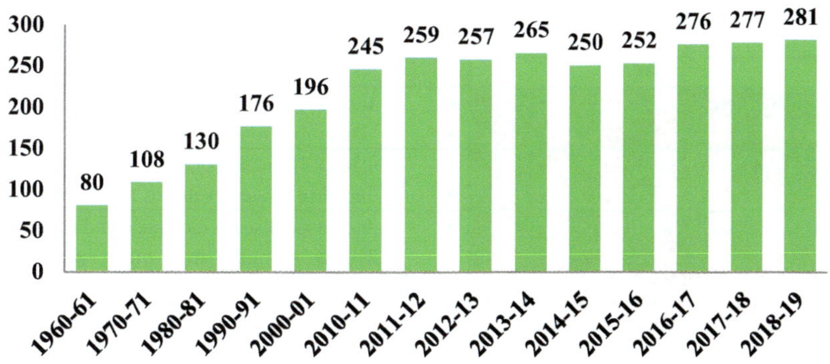

Fig. 7.6 Production of food grains (million tons), India (1960–2019). *Source* Based on Department of Agricultural, Cooperation, and Farmers Welfare, Annual Report, 2018–19

reasons for hunger being widespread is that food production systems around the world are unsustainable (McDonald, 2010). There is a plethora of evidence that suggests that a new orientation for agricultural development must be sought after (Goodland & Ledger, 1987; Pretty, 1995; Daly, 2007; Zegar, 2012; Vitunskiene & Dabkiene, 2016). This novel developmental trajectory in agriculture should accord importance to the sustainable development goals in all countries, with special focus on developing countries.

Pritchard et al. (2017), in a mixed-method study conducted on two communities in India, suggested that it is difficult to arrive at a one-stop solution to the agriculture-nutrition nexus because of the complex relationship between the two. There is a need to look at the bigger picture of the food system when formulating policies for nutrition and food security. This includes looking at the complete set of factors involved in the process, ranging from food production, transportation, and delivery to the end-product consumer. It is important to have concordance between different food system elements, ranging from food production, to processing, to distribution, to final consumption. Any ignorance of this synergy and a lack of vigilance on the part of food system actors can lead to exacerbation of nutritional adversities.

Invigorating the agriculture-nutrition linkages when considering food system development inIndia will play a decisive role in addressing the above-mentioned hurdles. The importantelements include the following:

- Ensuring that agriculture is adequately represented in national nutrition policy.
- Incentivizing the production of nutritional products for producers to create a healthychoice base for consumers.
- Using price and non-price mechanism for creating incentives for consumers.
- Handling safety and related concerns along the value chains for healthy, fresh foods.

7.9 COVID-19 and SDGs: The Bigger Picture

See Table 7.4.

The COVID-19 pandemic has only exacerbated the perils of countries falling short on their

Table 7.4 Short-term impact of COVID-19 on SDGs

SDGs	Impacts
SDG1: No poverty	• Increased poverty due to loss of jobs and lockdowns • Disproportionate impact on vulnerable groups
SDG2: Zero hunger	• Lack of food security due to disruption in global food supplies • Increase in hunger due to fall in incomes
SDG3: Good health and well-being	• Increased disease incidence and mortality due to COVID-19 • Higher mortality from other causes due to overburdening of health systems • Issues related to mental health
SDG4: Quality education	• Closure of schools and day-care centres • Setback in human capital development
SDG5: Gender equality	• Social impacts on women from the lockdown (domestic violence) • Increased mortality rates among men
SDG6: Clean water and sanitation	• Reduced access to clean water among disadvantaged groups
SDG7: Affordable and clean energy	• Setback in economic growth leading to a reduction in energy prices
SDG8: Decent work and economic growth	• Global economic crisis • Trade disruption • Mass unemployment
SDG9: Industry, innovation and infrastructure	• Decline in industrial outputs • Improved usage of digital technologies, for e-health, e-education, e-governance, and e-payments
SDG10: Reduced inequalities	• Skewed negative health and economic impacts on vulnerable groups • Loss of jobs of lower skilled, lower wage labour
SDGs	**Impacts**
SDG11: Sustainable cities and communities	• Rise in urban poverty and vulnerability • Shut down of public transports • Sharp short-term reduction in pollution levels
SDG12: Responsible consumption and production	• Short-term reduction in natural resource use • Increased plastic pollution
SDG13: Climate action	• Short-term reduction in global GHG emissions • Pressure to reduce environmental safeguards
SDG14: Life below water	• Short-term reduction in threats to marine
SDG15: Life on land	• Short-term reduction in threats to terrestrial biodiversity
SDG16: Peace, justice and strong institutions	• Increased public deficits and debt • Suspension of freedom-of-information laws and transparency policies
SDG17: Partnership for the goals	• Closing of borders • Slowdown in international trade

Source The Sustainable Development Report, 2020

(red) —Negative Impact	(orange) —Mixed or moderately negative impact
(grey) —Impact still unclear	(green) —Mainly positive impact

commitments towards SDGs. As per the *Sustainable Development Goals Report 2020*, pandemic-induced damages had already led to the derailing of all the progress made over the years towards the achievement of SDGs by the end of 2019 (Sachs et al., 2020).

7.10 The Way Forward: Policy Recommendations

India's current social protection programs cater to the traditional "safety net" definition of social protection, wherein restricted and suggestive measures are taken by institutions to only compensate for market failure (MacKinnon, 2002). With a massive reliance of India's social security system on cash transfers, it is imperative that the governments identify the down and out without precision. However, it is arduous to garner reliable data in a country where as low as 7% of its adult population files taxes (Ghosh, 2020). There is increasing evidence that brings to the fore adversities faced by susceptible groups due to omission errors, exclusions, delays in payment or payment failure, and misdirection of payments (Dhingra, 2020). To make these plans sustainably viable, it is imperative to adopt a transformational that addresses the underlying causes of poverty. The focal point of such programs should be on equity, empowerment, and well-defined rights for disparaged groups. There is also an ardent need to surmount targeting challenges to assure that no one is excluded. India's National Rural Employment Guarantee Act is another pertinent step towards achieving this objective. The lack of sufficient budgetary allocation, resulting in workers receiving less than minimum wage, has, however, posed major challenges to the objective of inclusion.

With more than 90% of the workforce engaged in informal sector and 80% of the above earning less than Rs. 15,000 per month, the capability of people to make ends meet with a continual source of income is negligible in India (Periodic Labour Force Survey, 2018). Additionally, the risk of India facing a severe crisis of hunger and undernutrition was high even during the pre-COVID-19 times, owing to high levels of undernutrition and lack of dietary diversity among a considerable proportion of the population. In such situations, government support in the form of direct benefit transfers could play an instrumental role in averting such a situation. Further, it will also be useful to increase expenditure made on welfare and transfer schemes and putting money directly into hands of those who have a high propensity to consume by pursuing an expansionary fiscal policy.

There are also lacunae in these schemes that need to be addressed. The important among them is non-universality of these schemes and the absence of a potential system to identify and limit exclusion errors. This became especially apparent during the pandemic when lakhs of migrant workers and households were left stranded with no respite because they either were excluded from beneficiary lists, or were not eligible because of document or quota issues. The systems of e-coupons created further confusion and chaos and only further proved that putting the burden of proof on the poor and marginalized will only exclude them further rather than including them. Additionally, it is imperative to accord necessary attention to interventions, such as the mid-day meals and ICDS that are universal and serve to improve nutrition status especially of women and children. The dilemma of universal coverage and higher entitlements are, therefore, particularly relevant, more important so in the current context. There is room for further improvement on the role played by these schemes in improving food and economic security for susceptible households. Transparency is the key to assuring this, wherein public portal and websites should share data related to these schemes so that independent assessments can be done.

There is an imminent need for a redesign in policy to move from a conventional attention on attaining self-sufficiency in food grains to tackling a more comprehensive group of nutrition-related goals. It is crucial to have a policy plan that ensures food and nutrition security and enhances affordability and access to a balanced diet not just in terms of proteins, micronutrients, and vitamins but also acts as a balanced source of energy. A nutrition security policy must place its focus not just on the incessant issue of micronutrient undernutrition and child undernutrition but also on the looming challenges of overweight and obesity. The solution to the above lies in shifting the policy focus from staple food items to a more comprehensive idea of food and nutrition. The following major changes could be introduced into the planning trajectory in order to spearhead India's journey in attaining SDG2.

Need to look beyond calories: The rapid dietary transition and changes in caloric consumption pattern are evidence which are enough to criticize the undue focus on calories. It is important to diversify food intake by including different sources, for example, millets for micronutrients, minerals and B-complex vitamins (Gavaravarapu & Nair, 2014), and pulses for proteins (Roy et al., 2016). There is a need to promote the consumption of these nutrient-rich items, given an increasing proportion of micronutrient-deficient population in the country. In a trailblazing manoeuvre, a customized version of the food security act was introduced by the Chhattisgarh State government, prior to the introduction of the National Food Security Act. It provided for the distribution of iodized salts and pulses, along with the general wheat and rice distribution that takes place under the Public Distribution System. There is, thus, a need to discard the old "one-size-fits-all" approach and tailor-made policies that are best suited as per local needs and grievances.

Life-cycle approach to nutrition: Problems of undernutrition such as stunting, wasting, and underweight set in early in life, some even during pregnancy, and could prevail throughout the life of an individual. Hence, it is pertinent for policies pertaining to nutrition to adopt a life-cycle approach (Rai et al., 2014). Important interventions in early stages of the life cycle such as nutritional supplements for women during their adolescence, pregnancy, and lactation together with early childhood nutrition interventions for children could play a massive role in curbing overall undernutrition rates. While the ICDS was designed with a life-cycle approach, it operationally unfolded into a food safety net program. Similarly, the NFSA professes to promote a life-cycle approach but programmatic aspects for making it one seems to be missing (Rai et al., 2014). Improved access to family planning, increased role of women in household decision-making, bolstered child care and nutrition practices, access to clean water and better sanitation practices, and a more alimental food system that is affordable to the poor are all fundamental elements of a life-cycle approach to enhanced nutritional status. While the NFSA covers these aspects, this nuance still needs to be put in the centre stage of policy focus and the ensuing debate.

Renewed focus on agriculture with an emphasis on diversification towards more nutritious crops and livestock products: Advocating a "crop-neutral" policy with sufficient market infrastructure, credit services, and input availability would go a long way in enabling smallholder farmers to respond proactively to the increased demand for non-staple food items. Promotion of nutritious crops through kitchen gardens and through the diversification of production system towards fruits and vegetables, livestock, and aquaculture could lead to better nutrition outcomes (Pandey et al., 2016). Pingali (2015) calls for a "crop-neutral" agricultural policy, one that creates a level playing field which enables farmers to respond to market signals, rather than an entire framework of policymaking that is prejudiced towards a particular set of crops. Diversifying of production is useful not only for the overall food production but is also instrumental in reducing poverty rates (Birthal et al., 2015).

Introduction of pulses, millets, and diverse crops in the PDS: It is a fact that the nutritious value of food provided through the PDS system could be greatly augmented by expanding its scope to include coarse grains and pulses. There are precedents where states like Karnataka and Tamil Nadu are already providing millets through PDS. The central government can also take cue from such initiatives by different state governments. For example, Chhattisgarh also provides iodized salt, black gram, and pulses to the poorer households in addition to stipulated grains. Similarly, Uttarakhand has also proposed to introduce pulses as part of the PDS (Pingali et al., 2017). Subsidized pulses can help diversify diets and bolster protein consumption. Rapid release and promulgation of all the bio-fortified crops should be encouraged as an added mechanism for promoting a more nutrition-sensitive food system. Procurement of bio-fortified pearl millet, rice, and wheat for the PDS systems would give these crops a rapid boost in terms of their scaling up, while taking care of the iron and zinc requirements at the population level.

Inter-sectoral and inter-departmental convergence on nutritional goals: There is an absence of a point of convergence on nutrition in the various programs spearheaded by the ministries of agriculture, and the food and public distribution programs. The supply-side focus of nutrition policy leads to conflicting priorities across various food, economic, and agricultural departments leading to a policy "inertia" which results in the perpetuation of the status quo of a calorie-centred stance of policymaking (Thow et al., 2016). The concurrence of myriad schemes such as ICDS with the National Rural Health Mission (NRHM) and the Total Sanitation Campaign (TSC) exists only as ideas on paper without any practical application (Mohmand, 2012; Thow et al., 2016). This very lack of coordination between the departments has often been stated as the reason for slow headway on nutritional status of the population. Hence, better nutrition as the common policy agenda provides these divergent programs a better operating framework for buttressed developmental consequences in the country. Contemporary achievements of the state-level nutrition missions and the ineptitude of governmental attempts at bringing about improvements in nutritional status underscore the need for decentralization of these programs with flexibility at the lower levels of administrative units to tailor it to their specific requirements.

7.11 Conclusion

While categorical in only one SDG, nutrition is a crucial factor that cuts across all the SDGs, in ways. The need of the hour is evidence-based data that can serve as a guideline for global change; however, added evidence from the scientific community is required to continue the examination of the linkages between diet, environment and human health, and to provide latest information. Other facets, such as education, work conditions, gender inequality, clean water, and sanitation, are also equally important. These factors are, as mentioned above, closely intertwined with different aspects of nutrition. Thus, improved nutrition would be a significant contributor to the achievement of various SDGs. Our key finding points towards a general lack of consistency in food security status as measured by the different indicators along the thoroughfare. This heterogeneity implies that it is not sufficient to have a food security policy with a singular focus, given that there are more detachments abounding along the agriculture-to-nutrition pathways than linkages. In a way, this explains the inadequacy of food security policies in India in curtailing the high rates of undernutrition for decades. In addition to the above, serious data gaps hinder efforts to tackle the problem of undernutrition. An integrated framework for measuring food and nutrition security, and implementing and monitoring relevant policies, is missing. Modernizations in survey methodology are needed to take into account the different aspects of food and nutrition security. More integrated and comparable surveys are required to arrive at improved policy conclusions and make informed decisions. Policy interventions need to be more broad based, evidence driven, and should take into account both short-term and long-term indicators of food security, going beyond mere calorie security. Without such all-inclusive and multi-pronged approaches, attaining the SDGs could be seriously compromised.

Key findings
India is ranked 101 of 116 countries on food security, with hunger levels categorized as "serious"
Nearly 8 percent adults aged 45 and above reported facing severe shortage in household availability of food in the last 1 year
States like Bihar, Jharkhand, Uttar Pradesh, Gujarat, and Madhya Pradesh are the *Aspirants,* which are lagging behind heavily in their progress to achieve *Zero Hunger*
States like Rajasthan and Punjab are *Performers* while Kerala and Tamil Nadu are *Front Runners* and are performing rather satisfactorily in achieving the goal of *Zero Hunger*

8 Policy Perspectives: A Level Framework

Abstract

Nutrition is key to National and Global Sustainable Development Goals. It is critical to prevent undernutrition and prevent growth and development issues that are irreversible and that act as impediments to maternal and child health, and sabotage numerous breakthroughs that have been achieved in learning outcomes, adult productivity, and gender equality. This chapter focuses on the levels of knowledge of parents on nutrition, availing of ICDS services, and consumption of IFA tablets by expectant mothers. Besides, the chapter throws light on different policies adopted by countries across the world in addressing undernutrition. Further, it discusses the state-specific interventions in India to tackle nutrition and suggestive measures. In addition to the above, the chapter deals with the gaps that are present in India's nutrition policies and suggests measures to address these issues.

Keywords

Policy analysis · SDGs · Anaemia · MCH · Ageing · India

8.1 MDGs to SDGs: Is India Still Lagging Behind?

The findings of the Global Nutrition Report, 2020 released by the World Health Assembly reveal that India is likely to miss the 2025 nutrition targets (Global Nutrition Report, 2020). The report suggests that with the highest rates of domestic inequalities, India is off-track in achieving the following four targets:

1. Stunting among children aged 5 years and below.
2. Anaemia among women of reproductive age.
3. Childhood overweight and obesity.
4. Exclusive breastfeeding.

The findings of the report state that despite a meagre reduction in the proportion of underweight children in India, the value is still considerably high as compared to the average values of Asia as a whole. In addition to the above, the report noted that there is a considerable proportion of population which is suffering from both undernutrition and over-nutrition, with one in two women of reproductive age anaemic and a surreptitious increase in the rate of overweight and obesity, leading to a host of severe and chronic health issues. It has also been observed that the rate of obesity in females is double than their male counterparts. The report further goes on to state that India, lying narrowly below

A. Chattopadhyay et al., *Undernutrition in India*, Sustainable Development Goals Series,
https://doi.org/10.1007/978-981-19-8182-1_8

Nigeria and Indonesia, is the third worst affected country, hit by the dual burden of overweight and stunting. Furthermore, one in three children under the age of 5 years in India is estimated to be stunted and one in five is estimated to be wasted, with the highest proportion of children in Uttar Pradesh. The vulnerability of the situation is further exacerbated by the stark inequalities between rural and urban areas and among different socio-economic strata in India (Global Nutrition Report, 2020).

8.2 Policies and Programs Addressing Nutrition in India

Despite the Government's unquestionable commitment towards countering the challenge of nutrition, it is astonishing that India is still experiencing inhibited expedition in enhancing its nutrition situation despite having a surfeit of food security and nutrition interventions. The subject of nutrition in India comes under the ambit of Ministry of Health and the Ministry of Women and Child Development. The focus of the interventions and schemes that have been launched so far is on targeting the immediate causes and symptoms of undernutrition through efforts addressed towards buttressing food allocation and distribution and revamping nutrition among children. In the above process, vital intermediate and underlying determinants of nutrition such as inequality, lack of empowerment, and insufficient access to integral sectorial resources remain unscathed. Despite having a well-founded nutrition policy, replete with amendments and modifications, India is still grappling with the issue of a sound implementation policy. In order to address the abovementioned lacunae, the National Nutrition Mission (NNM), the cutting-edge program of the National Institution for Transforming India (NITI) Aayog, was launched in 2017 envisioning a "Kuposhan Mukt Bharat, 2022" (Malnutrition Free India, 2022).

An important development in the spectrum of nutrition-based interventions is the National Nutrition Mission program (NNM). Although officially under the ambit of Ministry of Women and Child Development, this program has been designed to encourage confluence between other programs and missions focusing on nutrition and food security such as National Health Mission (NHM), Public Distribution System (PDS), Anganwadi Services, Scheme for Adolescent Girls (SAG) of MWCD, Swachh-Bharat Mission, Pradhan Mantri Matru Vandana Yojana (PMMVY), Janani Suraksha Yojana (JSY), and MGNREGA; all these programs are running under different ministries and departments such as food and public distribution and drinking water and sanitation. The above-mentioned programs are targeted at sub-groups of the population such as infants, young children, pregnant and breastfeeding women, adolescents, and tribal population. The following section deals with initiatives and interventions for different segments of the population.

8.2.1 Infant and Young Child Care, Nutrition, and Health

These interventions are primarily targeted on children under the age of 3 years by encouraging.

- Colostrum feeding (first milk formed immediately after delivery) and exclusive breastfeeding for the first 6 months.
- Up-to-the-minute and appropriate complementary feeding after 6 months, followed by continued breastfeeding until the age of 2 years or beyond.
- Using the Mother Child Protection card to counsel mothers and families about universal growth monitoring and promotion of young children using World Health Organization Child Growth Standards.

- Providing nutritional support to infants and young children through ICDS.
- Providing nutritional support to acutely or severely undernourished children through caregiving, better feeding practices, and timely management and interventions.
- Providing newborn care (especially to low birth weight babies) under health and family welfare scheme.
- Supplementing Vitamin A to children under 5 years of age twice a year.
- Complete, timely, and universal immunization (including booster dosages) of infants against preventable diseases.
- Micronutrient (iron folic acid) supplementation and deworming of children under 5 years of age and children under 2 years of age, respectively, twice a year as per regulatory guidelines.
- Tackling common neo-natal and childhood illnesses such as acute respiratory infections, diarrhoea, and nutritional inadequacies both at the community and institution levels through oral rehydration solution and zinc supplementation.

8.2.2 Maternal Care, Nutrition, and Health

The following initiatives have been taken to address the challenge of maternal nutrition:

- ICDS supported supplementary nutritional support, especially during pregnancy and breastfeeding.
- Screening and management of anaemia, antenatal care, and health counselling care for mothers, including IFA supplementation and consumption of iodized salt.
- Implementing PMVVY efficiently to offer ameliorated protection to mothers.
- Channelizing ASHA and ICDS workers for institutional deliveries, breastfeeding management, and giving newborn care.
- Health promotion practices such as increasing age at marriage, getting pregnant at the right age, inter-pregnancy gapping, and father's involvement in childcare and parenting.
- Focus on educating and empowering women.

8.2.3 Adolescent Care, Nutrition, and Health

- Proving equal care to girl children, focusing on the life-cycle approach, by linking it to the "Beti Bachao Beti Padhao" program.
- Providing health care, counselling support, educating about adolescent reproductive, and sexual health through schools and community intervention programs.
- Revamped access to nutritional interventions to current attendees through Mid-Day Meals in schools and to dropouts through SABLA scheme.
- Universal access to iron folic acid supplementation for both girls who are current attendees and dropouts.
- Increased focus on educating girls and developing skills.
- Modifying gender-based ideas—fostering gender-based harmony and life skills among adolescent boys and girls.
- Curbing child marriage—devising policies to increase the age at marriage among girls.

8.2.4 Tribal Nutrition and Health

Indian government has been implementing a number of programs that impact food and nutrition security (FNS) outcomes among the tribal population directly or indirectly. The direct programs encompass the Mid-Day Meal Scheme (MDMS) in primary schools (now under extension to secondary schools), targeted Public Distribution System (PDS), Integrated Child Development Services (ICDS), and the recent National Food Security Act. Addressing the issue of tribal undernutrition and over-nutrition indirectly, schemes such as MGNREGA and NRLM have been aimed at increasing household income and purchasing power for food security, particularly for those households that are living below the poverty line (BPL). Programs such as the National Rural Health Mission (NRHM) and Nirmal Bharat Abhiyan aim to provide health and community environmental hygiene services that are imperative for nutrition and well-being.

8.2.5 Community-Based Interventions

- Encouraging WASH practices with a special focus on making India free of open defecation through the Clean India Mission.
- Facilitating malaria prevention and treatment for malaria by encouraging the usage of mosquito nets and preventive therapies, especially in areas where malaria is endemic and by opting for state/district-specific control measures, with special focus on needs of a particular community.
- Improving household food security through social security schemes and safety net programs like the Annapurna scheme, the Antyoday Anna Yojna, and similar schemes.
- Information and education activities (including such information as a part of school and college curriculum) to foster knowledge about breastfeeding and child caring practices, diversifying consumption, WASH practices, and promotion of healthy practices.
- Targeted programs for those social and economic groups that are susceptible to undernutrition, especially nutritional inadequacies pertaining to massive seasonal fluctuations, outbreak of diseases, natural calamities, and other related scenarios.
- Creating a framework that is community specific as per the needs of a particular state or district to strengthen nutritional outcomes.

8.3 India's Association with Scaling Up Nutrition (SUN)

Since its inception in 2010, the Scaling up Nutrition (SUN) initiative has been instrumental in bringing together governments, international organizations such as the UN and WHO, civil societies, business organizations, and donors to put up a fight against hunger, food security, and undernutrition. It is a movement that is primarily run by countries and has 61 countries and 3 Indian states (Jharkhand, Maharashtra, and Uttar Pradesh) as participants. The movement works on the premise that there are very few issues faced by the world that match the intensity of undernutrition, a problem that affects one-third of the global population. Despite making significant strides towards reducing undernutrition rates, there is still a lot that needs to be done. One of the main focus areas of the initiative is to work in tandem with the United Nations towards the fulfilment of the Sustainable Development Goals and ensuring improved nutrition, especially during the first 3 years of life.

8.4 India and Hunger: Trends and Possible Solutions

The Global Hunger Index (GHI) is an instrument devised to exhaustively keep track of and quantify hunger at national and global levels. These scores are computed on an annual basis to gauge the developments and impediments in restraining hunger. The GHI is designed as a tool to increase the grasp and recognition of the skirmish against hunger, provide a way to compare the inter-country and inter-regional differentials in hunger, and reckon attention to those parts of the world where hunger levels are highest and where there is the greatest need for combined incremental efforts to combat hunger.

8.4.1 How are GHI Scores Calculated?

The index is calculated using a three-step process that is based on available data from myriad sources to consider the multifaceted idea of hunger. The indicators considered for the calculations of the first step are as follows:

1. **Undernourishment**: The proportion of the population whose calorie intake is inadequate.
2. **Child wasting**: Proportion of children aged 5 years and below who are wasted—an indicator for acute undernutrition.
3. **Child stunting**: Proportion of children aged 5 years and below who are stunted—an indicator for chronic undernutrition.
4. **Child mortality**: Mortality rate of children aged 5 years and below—accounting for the cataclysmic combination of deficient nutrition and unhealthy environments.

The second step involves standardizing each of the four components on a 100-point scale. This is based on the global maximum observed level for the given component in recent decades. The third step comprises the aggregation of these standardized scores to arrive at the final GHI score for each country, with each of the three dimensions (child stunting and wasting combined to form child undernutrition) given equal weight.

8.4.2 Where Does India Stand?

Figure 8.1 shows India's GHI score and performance on the four dimensions across different points in time. In essence, India's lackadaisical performance is being attributed to elevated levels of child stunting and wasting. While there has been a remarkable decline in the prevalence of child stunting in India from 54.2 to 34.7% in 2000 and 2020, respectively, it is still among the worst globally. The prevalence of wasting is reported to be at a global maximum of 17.7%. It is crucial to understand the reasons behind the continually high prevalence of child wasting in India despite a host of policies and measures in place. Although small improvements were registered during 2010–14, the prevalence escalated again in 2015–19. While comparing India's performance over the years, a caveat has to be noted. The GHI scores across different years cannot be compared given the difference in methodology and data sources in different years. Additionally, since different countries are included in the ranking, it would be incorrect to compare the rankings of a previous report from the current one. It must also be noted that change in India's ranking could also be a ramification of her being compared to a different set of countries in the current report.

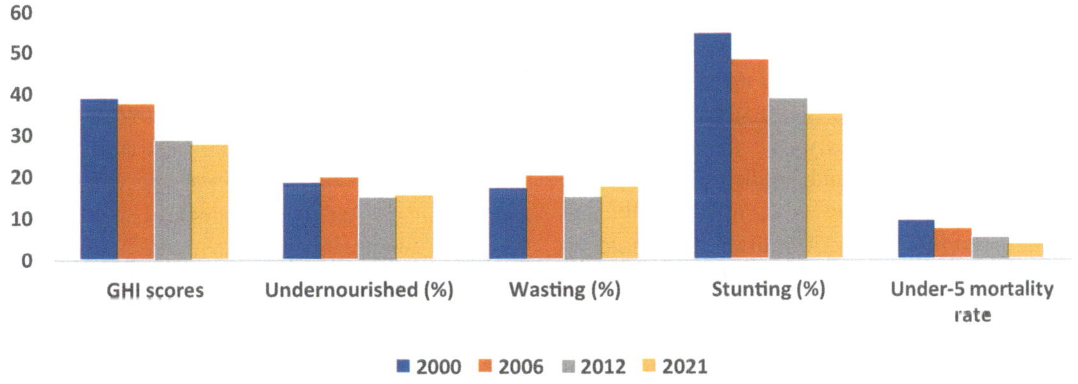

Fig. 8.1 Hunger and nutrition: India

8.4.3 What are the Data Sources?

- Data for undernourishment is obtained from Food and Agricultural Organization (FAO). The prevalence of undernourishment is estimated using the Food Balance Sheet (assessed based on the proportion of population with insufficient calorie intake).
- Data for child stunting and wasting have been taken from various data sources, including current estimates from UNICEF, WHO, World Bank, and Comprehensive National Nutrition Survey (CNNS).
- Estimates for U-5 mortality rates are taken from the United Nations Inter-Agency Group for Child Mortality Estimation (UN IGME).

8.4.4 India's Face-Off with Hunger Continues: Why?

Amartya Sen, in his work *Poverty and famines,* pioneered the idea of "exchange entitlement decline" as one of the causes for starvation and famines. Portrayed by a detrimental alteration in the exchange value of endowments for food, it fundamentally means that the employment of a certain proportion of people is not compensatory enough to be able to buy sufficient food. Although originally used in the context of famines, this theory could be extended to explain the high rates of hunger in India. Despite having surplus food, farmers with small or marginal land holding do not have access to adequate food. There are myriad reasons for the above. First, agricultural output from small and marginal land holdings has either been sluggish or deteriorating over the years, primarily due to declining soil fertility, fragmented land holdings, and varying prices of farm produces. This is especially pertinent given that nearly 50 million households in India are dependent on these holdings. Secondly, relative income of certain sections of the population has been on the downturn. This has detrimental impacts on their capability to purchase enough food, particularly when food prices have been on the upswing. Thirdly, there is a dearth of opportunities for engaging in remunerative works. Lastly, the benefits accruing from the public distribution system (PDS) are not accessible to some of the vulnerable sections of the population. It is also noteworthy that all the data used in GHI 2021 calculations pertain to the pre-pandemic period. Estimates from other sources of nationally representative data, like the Centre for Monitoring Indian Economy and various field surveys conducted by research organizations, academics, and civil society groups, suggest that the situation of food security in India was already worrisome by the end of 2020. One of the reasons behind the above could be the exclusion of poorer households from the Below Poverty Line (BPL) category mainly due to faulty exclusion criteria, political influence, and widespread corruption. In addition to the above, COVID-19 also caused disruptions in schemes like the Integrated Child Development Scheme (ICDS) and Midday Meals in areas, depriving a huge proportion of children of the one assured nutritious meal per day.

8.5 Gaps in Policies in India and Action Plans

India has a wide spectrum of programs and policies that are targeted at addressing maternal child, adolescent and tribal health and nutrition, which can play a major role in improving maternal and child health outcomes. Although massive strides have been made in curtailing the rates of infant and maternal mortality in the past years, the present rates of decline are hardly enough to reach the aspired targets (Chatterjee & Paily, 2011). One could argue why India has been able to reduce infant and child mortality by half in two decades, while at the same time, managed to lower the incidence of child undernutrition indicators only marginally. The impressive decline in infant and child mortality could be attributed to rising investments in health, improved access to medical services, and improvements in education and awareness (especially among mothers). When it comes to child nutrition, though, dietary diversity poses serious concerns. Despite having tons of excess stocks of grains and cereals, India still needs to diversify food production to produce more diversified and nutrient-rich food that covers the requirements of micro- and macronutrients of the general population. There are myriad hurdles that should be taken into account to buttress the quality of services in existing programs and knowledge gaps that need to be filled to help improve program design and implementation. The gaps that are extremely crucial to address and actions required are as follows:

1. **Quality of health services**

   - The supply of health services is quite deplorable, especially in rural and tribal areas.
   - Availability of doctors at PHCs is minimal in spite of the physical existence of a large number of Primary Health Centres (PHCs) across the states.
   - Limited availability of nurses/midwifes/staff nurses at PHCs and Community Health Centres (CHCs), more so in geographically inaccessible rural tribal areas.
   - Low utilization is another concern, primarily because of poor quality of services and lack of awareness.

2. **Loopholes in execution**

   - Health and nutrition policies in India face supply side, service delivery, and utilization challenges, more often at the community level.
   - India ranks 86 among 180 countries in terms of corruption (Economic Times, 2021).
   - Questions that need to be asked are: *Are the policies not reaching those who are in maximum need of support? Are the benefits/financial transfers being drained in the process of allocation or distribution? Is it that poverty is so deep-rooted that households are actually consuming such foods and supplements? Are there loopholes at the grass-root level that are not being resolved by the administration? Is there a limited understanding of the issue among the common people?*
   - These envisage bolstering monitoring and evaluation frameworks, advocating assimilation of services at levels, assuring efficient procurement mechanisms for micronutrient and food supplements, and establishing regional training facilities for ameliorated program implementation and guidance.

3. **Setting unrealistic targets**

   - Another puzzle that needs attention is the women's status and nutrition.
   - All programs will benefit by advancing the preference given to maternal nutrition in the National Rural Health Mission and the Integrated Child Development Services.
   - Discernible targets should be established for achieving reductions in maternal underweight, infant low birth weight, and teenage pregnancies. This will expedite results based on monitoring and evaluation strategies that climax in uninterrupted, solutions-oriented feedback.

4. **Lack of focus on women's status**

   - Women's status has bearings on the demand for quality services to improve their health and nutrition and the progeny that follows them.
   - Women are often not empowered enough to take required steps to bolster their nutritional status.
   - Family and peer influence is a strong hindrance to postponing marriage and first birth, birth spacing, and utilization of healthy nutrition practices.
   - Absence of literacy, awareness, decision-making power, and caveats to their freedom of movement acts as a huge impediment to their care and caregiving practices.

- Women from Scheduled Castes and Scheduled Tribes experience these problems even more acutely due to the all-pervasive caste discrimination. There are a number of programs focused on adolescent girls and women of reproductive age that could act as conduits for augmenting women's status.

5. **Food wastage**

- The estimates for India in this regard are non-existing, except few local studies.
- The latest estimate of UNEP (2021) indicates that though per capita wastage is low as compared to other Asian countries, Indian households wastes 68, 760 163 tons of food per year (United Nations Environment Program, 2021).
- Therefore, the food wastage in low- and middle-income countries, and in low-income populations within those countries, merits for more research.
- With widespread food insecurity for hundreds of millions, addressing food wastage is imperative for creating healthy and resilient food systems.
- India needs to pay ardent attention to minimizing food wastage at both household and community levels to minimize undernutrition.

6. **Neglecting nutritional needs of the urban population**

- There is an immense focus on maternal and child nutrition in rural areas. As a consequence, nutritional issues among the urban population are not adequately addressed.
- With increasing urbanization in India, urban poor, school-going children, and adolescents of all wealth classes have emerged as vulnerable sections warranting attention.
- Especially amid the continuously growing trends of consumerism, early morning school schedule that leads skipping of breakfast, growing slum population and the filthy environment that it inhabits, lack of open spaces for physical activities, and deteriorating urban quality of life.
- Healthy childhoods are crucial for a country like India, that is, looking to reap benefits accruing from its huge demographic dividend. This requires strong and cohesive partnership between the parents and children, along with schools, policymakers, and various stakeholders. India must, therefore, pay attention to the nutritional abnormalities of urban India before it is too late.

7. **Lack of sustained focus on maternal health**

- Detailed recommendations and guidelines must be used to address the core concerns surrounding anaemia, low birth weight, and low maternal BMI.
- Of these areas and recommendations are overlapping and call for increased assimilation across different sectors (health, nutrition, governance, etc.) and support for a culture of supportive supervision that would establish a system for supervising community health workers that is characterized by positive problem-solving and bidirectional flow of information.
- Curricula used by training institutes should be built on supportive managerial skills and training that can provide the health workers with an assistance in fostering a paradigm shift from various programs to integrated platforms.
- Community-based organizations, such as village health-nutrition-sanitation committees (VHSNCs), can be actively involved in planning and monitoring the delivery of essential health, nutrition, and sanitation initiatives in the community under the National Rural Health Mission.

8. **Neglecting the role of contraception**

- Contraception has never been discussed or thought of as a tool for abating anaemia.

- It is, however, important to start contemplating family planning programs in India.
- South Asian countries such as Bangladesh, having a predominantly Muslim population, have a far lower prevalence of anaemia as compared to India despite being economically much behind India.
- Findings from the book suggest that provision of a basket of contraceptive choices is essential at every corner of this country along with encouraging couples to choose modern contraception out of their free will.
- Although there are a few studies that link anaemia with sterilization, yet there is clear evidence of a strong unidirectional association of the two (Gautam et al., 2019; Ali et al., 2021; Rahman et al., 2021).
- It is noteworthy that Indian males are far less anaemic than their female counterparts, their anaemia level being identical to the average of certain European nations.
- It will be insightful to understand whether gender inequality explains the male–female differential in anaemia prevalence? Because if that was the case, similar trends would have been exhibited by India's neighbouring countries, but that is not the case. It is, therefore, crucial to identify the risk factors for anaemia among Indian women from a different angle.
- This might probably require a deviation from the target-oriented sterilization policy in India

9. **No focus on elderly nutrition**

- With all major policies targeted towards the abatement of maternal and child undernutrition, the nutritional needs of the elderly population are often not paid sufficient attention to.
- Through the book, we have tried to establish that there is a considerable proportion of elderly in India who suffer from undernutrition and should, therefore, be a focus of policymaking initiatives.
- The process of ageing results in changes in the physical, pathological, social, and psychological situations of a person.
- Nutrition is important to ensure good health among the elderly, and it has a huge bearing for the process of healthy ageing.
- The prevalence of both undernutrition and over-nutrition is increasing rapidly among the elderly, both globally and in India, and is associated with concomitant reductions in the functional status, anaemia, hindered muscle function, reduced bone mass, decreased cognitive function, immune dysfunction, dismal wound healing capacity, delayed recovery from surgery, higher hospitalization rates, and mortality.
- Due to the rapidly changing socio-economic environment, elderly people are often left alone to fend for themselves to maintain their health, which may prove to be an obstacle in the maintenance of a good nutritional status. Regular diagnosis of the nutritional status among older patients demands that there be increased awareness regarding nutritional status in older patients.

10. **Lack of basic entitlements**

- Last but not the least, every Indian should have the basic entitlements that guarantee healthy living.
- NFHS 5 reveals that in 2018, while 67% of the population did not have access to piped drinking water, 21% did not have access to toilets, and 40% did not have access to LPG connection. In urban areas, the heads of only about 21% of slum-dwelling households held a ration card.
- Workers in the unorganized sector, constituting 75% of the total workforce, are unable to use their ration card after having migrated to other states and, thus, get deprived of basic PDS access.

Table 8.1 Policy actions

Policy actions	Policy actions
All-round approach for tackling child and adolescent nutrition, in addition to focusing on economic development	Access to water and sanitation and diverse food production, adaptation of nutrition norms at schools
Enact policies specifically designed for adolescent and elderly health and nutrition, with special attention on screening tools and preventive methods	Large-scale surveys designed to capture the nutritional aspect of less focused population—elderly, school children, urban population
Discard target-oriented contraception policies and focus on the *cafeteria* approach to tackle anaemia among women	Regular update of anaemia prevalence and its determinants
Collaborative efforts including medical practitioners, academicians, and policymakers to tackle the issue of nutrition	Database management and comprehensive research to identify the markers of undernutrition
Ensure that policies and regulations are in place for micronutrient supplementation and food diversity	Regular update of micronutrient (supplementation) guidelines within the country and formal legislation related to food fortification for iodization of salt, and other relevant micronutrients
Stop food wastage and monitor distribution at varying levels	Enhance education, nutrition knowledge, work participation of women, asset holding direct CCT, promotion of child care/elderly care centres, provision of healthy food in community, and work places/schools

- It should be understood that it is difficult for any country to make sustainable progress if all citizens fail to get two square meals, access to health care, and education.
- There is a need to develop a self-sustaining system that caters to all the above-mentioned aspects and once such a system is developed, people would automatically be strong enough to take care of themselves. We believe in the saying "*If you give a man a fish, you feed him for a day. If you teach a man to fish, you feed him for a lifetime*" (Table 8.1).

8.6 Addressing Undernutrition and Micronutrient Deficiencies: Level Framework for Informed Policy Decisions

The right to food and nutrition is one of the elementary human entitlements and the important obligation of all states (De Schutter, 2014; UN CESCR, 1999). The governance of nutrition, which is crucial for the design and implementation of such policies to realize this right (Villarreal & Stloukal, 2005; Narula, 2005), is, therefore, among the crucial and deciding commitments of society. Pro-active governance, broadly defined, has the ability to improve facets of nutrition, for instance, by promoting collaborative actions between sectors and agencies, encouraging accountability of corporate actors, enhancing the food supply, promoting community ownership in intervention programs, revamping the responsiveness of government to the demand of citizens, thus being instrumental in upholding the right to food.

We propose a Level Framework for addressing undernutrition and micronutrient deficiencies among different age groups. This framework is in line with the *Systems approach to nutrition* promulgated by UNICEF (UNICEF, 2020). This avenue aspires to stimulate the five systems, food, health, water and sanitation, education, and social protection, with the maximum potential to deliver nutritious diets, indispensable nutrition services, and affirmative nutrition practices for children, adolescents, women, and elderly. Through the framework, our idea is to advocate mechanisms that help in buttressing the preparedness and accountability of these five systems towards nutritional requirements of individuals belonging to different age groups, sexes, and social strata. We identify intervention areas and targets for these systems at five levels, namely, individual, household, community, state, and world.

Conceptual frameworks deal with interventions both at the micro- and macro-levels to address the nutritional issues among children and women (UNICEF, 1990; UNICEF, 1998; Engle et al., 1999; Levitt et al., 2009; UNICEF, 2013; Black et al., 2013; Nguyen et al., 2017; UNICEF, 2020). However, none of the previous works has dealt with the underlying factors causing nutritional inadequacies among another vulnerable sub-section of the population—the elderly. Similarly, a lot of work has been done on the varied mechanisms that work in different ways towards aggravating undernutrition. However, not much work has been done to develop a conceptual framework that addresses contributing factors at each level of economy—the individual, the household, the community, the state, and the world. Our Level Framework, to the best of our knowledge, is the first such framework. The framework that we propose combines all the factors that have been dealt with previously, factoring in new variables that have remained unaddressed so far, and segregates them into action plans at different levels of policymaking. Thus, the framework moves from the smallest unit of consumption in the economy, the household, and moves upwards, incorporating the greater players and culminating into the largest unit—the world. This framework, hence, presents a micro- to macro- approach to nutrition among children, women, and elderly at differing levels.

Food consumption

- At the individual level, the timely consumption of food and the quality of food consumed is dependent on whether the food is prepared in a hygienic manner and is abundant in nutrients and minerals (household level), which in turn is dependent on the state of food security, accessibility, and affordability (community level).
- These factors are affected by myriad factors such as food distribution networks, storage and marketing, agricultural incentives at the state or country level and trade regulations, financial stability, climatic shocks and risk assessment, and international cooperation at the global level.
- Though not unanimous, there is evidence to suggest that access to healthy food is a pertinent contributor to a healthy diet. Policy documents in countries suggest that absence of such access in certain areas is one of the explanations for persistent inequities in diet and in health conditions (Moodie et al., 2009; Marmot et al., 2010).
- Findings from studies suggest that individuals who have proximity or improved access to large non-chain grocery stores (Zenk et al., 2009) and smaller food stores (Rose & Richards, 2004; Bodor et al., 2008) are able to avail higher intakes of fruits and vegetables.
- Additionally, shorter distances between grocery, fruit, and vegetable stores are also found to be linked to a healthier body mass index (BMI) (Rundle et al., 2009).
- In addition to the above, practices such as home gardening can play a crucial part in bolstering food and nutritional security during and after the COVD-19 pandemic, while also buttressing the quality of ecosystem services (i.e. plant biodiversity, microclimate, water runoff, water quality, and human health) (Lal, 2020).
- Research suggests that foods with high nutritional quality should contain optimal levels of essential nutrients including essential fatty acids, essential amino acids, vitamins, minerals, fibres, and bio-actives which are critical for maintaining health, reducing risk of chronic diseases, and promoting longevity in people (Pan, 2019).
- Estimates place the number of Indians who go hungry every day at nearly 194 million (FAO

et al., 2021). This issue is attributed to massive food wastage. Estimates place the monetary value of the food wasted in India annually at about US$14 billion (12.42 billion euro) (FAO et al., 2021).

- The global population is expected to range between 8 and 10.4 billion by 2050, with a median value of 9.1 billion (UNDESA, 2009). It is, thus, evident that the continual growth in population and consumption will pose a major threat to global food security, with the situation only worsening over the next 40 years (Godfray et al., 2010).
- Only 3 billion hectares of land, out of a total of 14 billion hectares globally, are arable and even this number has been dwindling in recent years. There has been an increase in demand for fodder, wood, and bio-energy in recent times, further reducing the land available for food production (Kampman et al., 2008).
- Climate change is a consequence of increasing average temperatures, changes in rainfall patterns, melting of glaciers, and other related changes. Increase in temperatures leads to heat stress in plants, thus heightening sterility and reducing overall productivity, besides increasing evaporation from plants and soils and lowering water availability (Parris, 2008).

Estimates state that India's fast food industry is growing at the rate of 40% annually.

Additionally, India is at the 10th position when it comes to per capita spending on fast food, with this expenditure constituting 2.1% of the annual total spending (Ashakiran & Deepthi, 2012).

The harmful effects of fast food are compounded by the fact that the energy density of fast foods is more than twice the recommended daily allowance for children (Printice & Jebb, 2003).

- The current childhood obesity pandemic is, hence, attributed to the increased consumption of fast foods (Ashakiran & Deepthi, 2012). This has led to rapid increase in life- threatening conditions, especially non-communicable diseases in developing countries (Ashakiran & Deepthi, 2012; Jaisheeba et al., 2012).
- The dense sugar content in fast foods is also causing dental cavities in school children (Nisar et al., 2009).
- In addition to the above, additives and preservatives used in preparation of these food stuffs are found to be carcinogenic and can cause allergic reactions such as asthma and rashes, also being increasingly observed among children (Ashakiran & Deepthi, 2012).
- In addition to the above, issues like poor hygiene practices during preparation, storage, and handling of fast foods in developing countries like India can lead to micro-organisms contamination (Kaushik et al., 2011).

Health condition and health behaviour

- Bandura's social cognitive theory (SCT) states that behaviour change is influenced by the co-action among personal and environmental factors, and attributes of an individual's behaviour (Bagherniya et al., 2018).
- The social cognitive determinants of dietary behaviours encompass knowledge, attitude, self-efficacy, social support, intention, and related factors (Sleddens et al., 2015).
- At the individual level, health condition and health behaviour are important determinants of one's nutritional status, which is impacted by the family's health history and support at the household level.
- Another issue is the rapidly growing consumption of fast foods globally. Edentulism is another factor that has huge impact on the nutrition status of the elderly. Edentulous elderly has a problem in chewing foods that are hard or rough in texture. To avoid difficulties, individuals often modify their diets to include softer and easily chewable foods.
- It is worth enquiring the modified diet of edentulous individuals' nutritious enough. Studies suggest that edentulous individuals lack certain specific nutrients and, as a consequence, may be exposed to nutritional deficiencies and health disorders (Hutton

et al., 2002; Nowjack-Raymer & Sheiham, 2003).

- This is further impacted by the prevalent health conditions and regional prevalence of diseases at the community level. At both national and global levels, strengthening public distribution systems, innovative approaches, and cooperation can help facilitate nutritional betterment in the population.
- A plethora of research identifies the role of Public Distribution System and National Food Security Act in improving food security and nutritional outcomes in India, especially among the deprived sections of the society through the provision of requisite number of calories (Bhattacharya et al., 2017; Pingali et al., 2017).

Mental health

- There is a lack of awareness on the nexus between mental health issues and nutritional status. Taking depression as an example, nutrition can play a crucial part in the onslaught as well as severity and duration of depression.
- Many of the readily ostensible food patterns that foreshadow depression are identical to those that happen during depression. These may encompass lack of appetite, increased frequency of skipping meals, and an increased craving for sugary foods (Rao et al., 2008).
- The common mental disorders that are currently prevalent in numerous countries are depression, bipolar disorder, schizophrenia, and obsessive- compulsive disorder (OCD) (Murray & Lopez, 1996).
- The pattern of dietary intake in Asian, African, and American countries is such that their diets are generally deficient in essential nutrients, particularly essential vitamins, minerals, and omega-3 fatty acids (Rao et al., 2008). Additionally, there are probable biological pathways through which diet quality could have ramifications for mental health, especially among children and adolescents.
- Firstly, a diet that is of poor quality and lacks nutrients can lead to nutrient deficiencies that have been significantly linked to mental health problems. For instance, evidence suggests that the dietary intake of nutrients such as magnesium, zinc, and folate is inversely proportional to the risk of having depressive disorders (Jacka et al., 2012), whereas dietary long-chain omega-3 fatty acids are inversely linked with anxiety disorders (Jacka et al., 2013).
- A noteworthy feature of the diets of patients suffering from mental disorders is the severity of deficiency in the above-mentioned nutrients.
- Studies have indicated that daily supplements of vital nutrients are often effective in reducing patients' symptoms (Shaheen & Vieira, 2008). Recent evidence suggests a link between low levels of serotonin and suicide (Rao et al., 2008).
- Depending on the local context, certain individuals and groups in society may be placed at a considerably high susceptibility to mental health issues. This may depend on the family history and the environment at home.
- The community-level factors to address this can include organization of counselling sessions, organizing drives for reduction of substance abuse, and alcohol addiction.
- Taking evidence-based decisions and expanding the reach of services, especially to low resource settings, at national level and strategies promoting universal access and equity in mental health and promotion of human rights at the international level can go a long way in addressing mental health concerns and buttressing nutritional outcomes for patients of mental health.

Occupation

- In the health impairment process, job demands (e.g. excessive work pressure, role uncertainty, emotional challenges) and various features of a job play a major role in depleting the physical and mental health of employees and result in health issues (Bakker and Demerouti, 2007, 2017; Lesener et al., 2019).

- This implies that workload, in itself, has a direct impact on health behaviours of individuals by draining physical and mental energy or by downsizing the time that an individual dedicates to engaging in healthy behavioural choices (Bowling and Kirkendall, 2012).
- Evidence from previous studies has pointed towards the fact that workload has a positive association with both mental health concerns such as depression and anxiety and physiological issues such as headache and stomach ache (Nixon et al., 2011; Spector and Jex, 1998).
- The impact of high workload is manifested in higher uptake of calories from fat sources, uncontrolled eating, and emotional eating. At the individual level, excessive workload can result in stress and, in turn, impair eating behaviours, calorie consumption, and can affect nutritional status of individuals.
- Strategies should incorporate ways to assess workload and exhaustion and address high workload or exhaustion through behavioural therapy.
- A solid evidence base is required to formulate strategies that minimize the effects of workload and exhaustion on eating behaviours and physical activity.
- This can be countered by worksite weight loss programs and weight management programs at the community level, supported by increased physical and social environment support at the national and international levels.

WASH practices

- Epidemiological studies have revealed that household access and quality of water, sanitation, and hygiene have a huge impact on child stunting, wasting, maternal health, and micronutrient deficiencies (Bartram et al., 2005; Fewtrell et al., 2005; Montgomery & Elimelech, 2007; Danaei et al., 2016; Zavala et al., 2021).
- A review of WASH interventions on the nutritional status of children states that WASH practices affect nutritional status of children via three disease pathways, namely, diarrhoea, helminth infections, and environmental enteric dysfunction (Dangour et al., 2013; Zavala et al., 2021).
- Estimates suggest that up to 45% of global undernutrition-related child deaths could be prevented by improving WASH conditions and practices (Curtis & Cairncross, 2003; Black et al., 2013; Mshida et al., 2018).
- One of the elementary solutions is to ensure supply of piped water, providing chlorinated water and well-covered drainage systems. This alone would lead to significant reductions in diarrhoea prevalence (Duflo, 2015; Bhalotra et al., 2017; Alsan & Goldin, 2019).
- Construction of septic tanks, availability of handwashing facilities near public toilets, and ensuring that sewage systems transfer excreta away from human interface to a more secure and remote location will also go a long way in ensuring improved nutrition outcomes (Zavala et al., 2021).

Genetics

- The genetics of height and excessive weight gain or obesity have been fundamental targets of genome-wide association studies in nutritionally sound populations (Duggal & Petri Jr., 2018).
- Primitive definitions of heritability, or the proportion of total variation that can be attributed to genetic disparity in a population, focused on height because studies have established that a child's height is linearly related to the heights of the parents (Galton, 1886; Fisher, 1918).
- Understanding of human nutrition remains incomplete without taking underlying genetic variations into account, which may be reflected as variations in nutritional processes such as absorption, metabolism, receptor action, and excretion (Velazquez & Bourges, 1984).
- Genetic factors affecting nutrition at individual and family level are need to be complemented by strengthening national and international policies, increasing inter-sectoral coherence in policies to allow a synergistic

approach to addressing nutritional challenges, as listed in the framework.

Contraception

- The agenda of the 65th World Health Assembly (WHA, 2012) was to find novel ways to tackle maternal and child undernutrition and one of those ways was identified as giving women the potential to plan their families and use of family planning by women or their husbands as an instrument to enhance the maternal and child nutrition (Allison et al., 2010; MIYCN-FP Integration Technical Working Group, 2011; Bongaarts, et al., 2012; Carr et al., 2012; Horton & Peterson, 2012; USAID, 2014; Ogutu, 2015; UNFPA, 2015).
- Previous studies have shown that contraceptive methods can have a considerable impact on women's haemoglobin status in myriad ways (UN, 1998; Skegg, 1999).
- Commonly, limiting or spacing births through any fertility management methods is probable to avert maternal depletion syndrome and anaemia (Skegg, 1999; Uche-Nwachi et al., 2010; Gebremedhin & Enqulassie, 2011).
- However, individual contraceptives may have differential impacts on iron status and, hence, have different impacts on the risk of anaemia (Skegg, 1999).
- Innately, the use of oral contraceptive pills (OCP), inclusive of iron supplements, helps in the prevention of iron deficiency anaemia (Haile et al., 2016; Bellizzi & Ali, 2018).
- Similarly, alterations in the regular menstrual flow—amenorrhea, irregular, lighter, or heavy bleeding—generally linked with hormonal and intrauterine device (IUD) methods may also have an impact on the risk of anaemia (UN, 1998; Skegg, 1999).
- Involvement of both the husband and the wife in making decisions related to contraceptives is an important correlation of self-determination among women.
- It not just gives them the right to regulate their fertility but the use of contraceptives has also been proven to reduce the risk of anaemia among women.
- Governments at community, national, and international levels can complement this by providing a basket of choices and forming global advocacy groups.

Menstruation and reproductive health

- Menstrual cleanliness is another important "hygiene" component. A large number of adolescent girls, especially in rural areas of India and in other Asian and African countries, resort to using cloth during menstruation (Esrey et al., 1991; Khanna et al., 2005; Adinma & Adinma, 2008; Dasgupta & Sarkar, 2008; Venkatraman & Patel, 2017).
- Latest estimates show that the condition is particularly worse in rural, poverty-stricken, and backward regions of the country compared to their urban counterparts (IIPS & ICF, 2017).
- Taboos regarding menstruation and sexual and reproductive health prove to be a big hurdle towards realizing the goal of improved nutrition among women, especially among adolescents.
- It is, therefore, crucial to discard taboos and stigma at the household, community, national, and international levels and provide services at the community level to address the issue of nutritional inadequacies among women, especially adolescents.
- Treating menorrhagia (heavy menstrual bleeding) among adolescents and women of childbearing ages is also an important step towards combatting iron deficiency anaemia (IDA) (Deli et al., 2013; Taylor & Rampton, 2015).

Common determinants

- In addition to all the above-mentioned determinants, there are certain determinants of nutrition that play a part in ensuring improved nutrition outcomes across all age groups and social classes.
- The role of economic stability in bolstering nutritional outcomes is well known. At both

micro- and macro-levels, economic factors play a key role in improving nutrition.

- Using child mortality as the dependent variable, one of the earliest attempts to link medical and socio-economic frameworks states that all social and economic determinants affecting children's health operate through a set of common determinants, also called the proximate determinants (Mosley & Chen, 1984).
- A plethora of research has been done on nutritional indicators and the common determinants identified for all age groups that have been identified have access to safe drinking water and sanitation facilities, access to health care, prevalence of parasitic and infectious diseases, health-seeking behaviour, race or ethnicity, rural residence, and social network and family support (Esrey et al., 1988; Gopalan, 1996; Frongillo et al., 1997; Jafar et al., 1998; Jacobs & Robert, 2004; Reyes et al., 2004).
- Demographic characteristics such as age and gender also play a very crucial role in determining the nutritional status of an individual (Vella et al., 2000).
- A number of studies have illustrated that individuals, especially children, from poorer households tend to be more undernourished than their counterparts in wealthier households (Zere & McIntyre, 2003; Thank & Popkin, 2003; Larrea & Freire, 2002; Wang et al., 2002; Doak et al., 2002). Social deprivation has also been linked with nutritional status of children (Armstrong et al., 2003). (Table 8.2).

8.7 Methodological Issues in the Measurement of Nutrition

1. **Issues with cut-offs for child nutrition indicators**

The estimates of nutrition indicators in India and countries globally are based on the WHO Multicenter Growth Reference Study (MGRS) (WHO, 2006). Stunting, a measure of chronic nutritional deficiency, is defined as a deficit in height relative to a child's age, that is, two standard deviations (SD) below the median height-for-age derived from the WHO (World Health Organization) child growth standards, whereas wasting, a measure of acute nutritional deficiency, is defined as a deficit in weight relative to a child's height, that is, two standard deviations (SD) below the median weight-for-height derived from the WHO (World Health Organization) child growth standards (WHO, 2006). These references are based on the anthropometric indices of children living in what is considered to be the "best case" for socio-economic conditions and nutritional benefits (WHO, 2006). In the MGRS, ample pretext for pooling data across countries to arrive at a global standard was provided by the very low ($\sim 3\%$) inter-country differentials of age-specific mean height, and a robust resemblance in the mean and standard deviation of linear growth of children from birth to 5 years of ages in samples from different countries (WHO, 2006).

The population estimate of nutrition indicators, especially child nutrition indicators such as wasting and stunting are sensitive to the dispersion of the height distribution in the population survey to which the standard is applied (Perumal et al., 2018). It can be both tricky and difficult to maintain the desired level of precision in length or height measurement in any large-scale survey. Low precision will result in over-dispersion and, hence, overestimate a dispersion-sensitive measure such as stunting or wasting (Grellety & Golden, 2016). Evidence from simulation exercises show that even miniscule random errors in height measurements can intensify the measure of dispersion and this increase in error can result in an exponential increase in the dispersion (Grellety & Golden, 2016). It has also been ostensibly demonstrated that this over-dispersion could, in turn, result in inflation of estimates of standard deviation cut-off-based undernutrition indicators. In addition to the over-dispersion caused by measurement error (Grellety & Golden, 2016; Corsi et al., 2017; Mejía-Guevara

Table 8.2 Addressing undernutrition and micronutrient deficiencies: level framework

Individual	Household	Community	State	World
Food on plate	• Hygienic method of cooking • Variety of food with adequate quantity • Timely consumption of healthy food • Home gardening • Children skipping food due to early morning schools, etc. • Consumption of fast foods	• Food security, • Proximity to food and ration shops • Affordability • Involvement of schools and education system to propagate healthy diets and practices • Provision of healthy food shops in locality	• Food distribution, pricing, incentives, variety, storage and marketing, population trends, incentivizing agriculture with a profitable market, proportion of arable land	• Food production, rules and regulations, trade protocols • Financial support • Healthy food promotion • International cooperation • Water resources, climatic risk assessment, and protection
Physical health condition and health behaviour	• Family health history and family support	• Community public health condition and health system support • Endemic disease condition • Nutrient dense foods low in trans-fat and saturated fats	• Strengthening public distribution and health system for all	• International cooperation in health and nutrition innovations
Mental and psychological health	• Family history • Family environment	• Reducing substance abuse and alcohol addiction • Counselling sessions	• Evidence-based practice • Expansion of mental health services	• Universal access and equity in mental health • Promotion of human rights
Occupation	• Amount of workload • Impact on food consumption	• Weight/calorie consumption management program	• Increase physical and social environmental support	• Global cooperation on quality of life
WASH practices	• WASH-related decision and practices	• Water and sanitation • Quality, availability, accessibility, and utilization	• Just water distribution, storage, recharge, irrigation, sustainable, and healthy practices • Ensuring basic facilities to all	• Just water distribution, storage, recharge, recycling of water
Genetics	• Family genetics	• Community health issues related to genetics	• Targeted approach	• International collaborative research and innovation
Contraception choice (adult women)	• Couple involvement in taking decision, • Encouraging spacing method,	• Providing basket of choice of FP at grass roots	• Providing basket of choice of FP	• Global advocacy groups, strategic plan formulation
Menstruation	• Knowledge provision and treatment of	• Involvement of community health	• Provision of hygienic materials, water and sanitation	• Global advocacy groups,
	problems since adolescent	workers and schools to address problems	facilities at every level, focus of adolescent health	strategic plan formulation
RH	• Treatment of problems since adolescent	• Provision of facilities • Breaking of taboos across age • Imparting knowledge to family on RH	• Provision of facilities • Breaking of taboos across age	• Global advocacy groups, strategic plan formulation

Common determinants:

Wealth

Education and knowledge promotion

Non-discriminatory social environment

Improved physical environment/climate conditions

Source Conceptualized by Chattopadhyay and Singh

et al., 2018), heterogeneity in population due to biological variations, socio-economic inequities, and unfavourable environmental exposure would independently lead to higher dispersion as compared to that of the standard population.

2. **Seasonality and wasting**

Another issue lies with the stunting and wasting data and the period of its collection. The abnormal fluctuation in levels of stunting and wasting can be attributed to the differentials in time period of data collection—the seasonality effect. In parts of India, hunger is primarily a seasonal experience, with agriculture being the prime source of livelihood for a considerable proportion of the population residing in rural areas. If the data is collected during lean periods (the time gap between the sowing and harvesting cycles), it is bound to register elevated levels of undernutrition. Increased prevalence of wasting in the fourth round of National Family Health Survey (NFHS) can be attributed to the fact that the data was collected after the harvesting period. These methodological concerns cast aspersions on the reliability of the estimate and demand adjustments to take into account the above-mentioned factors to arrive at a more robust estimate of hunger.

3. **Issues with anaemia data**

NFHS measures haemoglobin in a drop of capillary blood that oozes out from making a prick in the finger. This method has raised concerns, mainly because previous research suggests that this could lead to dilution of blood. Consequently, this could lead to a falsely lower value of anaemia and a high prevalence of anaemia. Reasons have been put forth to explain the dilution of blood, the important ones being different concentrations of white blood cells (WBCs) in different blood drops, blood getting contaminated from disinfectants, and "milking" or squeezing the finger to force blood out. Research suggests that a better alternative is to collect venous blood to obtain more robust estimates.

4. **Issues with Global Hunger Index (GHI) calculation**

The calculation of one of the indicators used in GHI, the undernourishment indicator, is based on the Food Balance Sheet published by the FAO. Despite painting an encompassing picture of a country's food supply during a specified reference period, there are some inherent issues with its construction. The first issue is the coverage or representativeness of data. The production statistics used for making Food Balance Sheet are limited to include major commercial food crops and exclude the production of non-commercial or subsistence crops. Another issue is the inaccuracy and incompleteness of food crops production data, especially in developing countries like India. While the production statistics for certain commodities may not be available, they may not always be reliable even when statistics are available. Additionally, certain kinds of food grains are not included in the national production statistics and are, hence, not included in the Food Balance Sheet. Certain adjustments are required in the construction of the Food Balance Sheet and the final results are derived as a residual, its reliability is heavily dependent on the availability and accuracy of data, which in India's case is a formidable issue. In addition to the above, since the final estimate of food available for consumption is derived as a residual, the error is unquantifiable and its direction is also unknown. Furthermore, using calories consumed to calculate undernourishment can be misleading because of reasons. Firstly, simply knowing the calorific intake does not give an account of the quality of diet consumed. Secondly, the national values of per capita calorie intake mask the widespread differentials in intra-country calorie consumption and distribution as a function of household characteristics. Thirdly, it could be misleading to assume that consuming calories beyond a minimum threshold signifies food security. But there have been issues like obesity becoming increasingly common among the poor with excessive consumption of calories coupled with levels of food security that are mild to moderate.

In addition to the above, there has been a lot of clamour about the FAO methodology used in the preparation of the Global Hunger Index report, 2021. The Indian government refused to recognize the report, dismissing the representativeness of the opinion poll used to collect data for the purpose of the report. Claiming that the report accorded no regard to numerous attempts by the government to ensure food security to the country's population during the coronavirus pandemic, the government also stated that the methodology used to measure undernourishment was "scientifically inaccurate". Concerns have been raised about the FAO methodology even earlier. The limitations of the methodology include the following:

(i) The quality of diet consumed is not considered.
(ii) The national average *per capita* caloric intake conceals intra-country caloric distribution as a function of household characteristics.
(iii) The method assumes consumption of calories beyond minimum caloric limit is an indicator of food security. But there have been issues like obesity becoming increasingly common among the poor with excessive caloric consumption coupled with mild-to-moderate levels of food insecurity (Townsend et al., 2001).
(iv) There is a high degree of measurement error in the numerator (the data used for the calculation is based on the amount of calories available but not necessarily consumed) and the denominator (indicating the population residing in the country in the year of origin). Summarily, the origin of data used by countries is often times arduous to comprehend and its validity is questionable. In addition to the above, almost no efforts are made to ensure data standardization and quality control across countries.
(v) There are myriad conceptual fallacies in establishing an average *per capita* caloric requirement cut-off point because, in reality, it is a function of factors including but not limited to physical activity levels, gender, and age.

8.8 Solutions to Data Quality Issues

The preceding discussion raises more questions than it provides answers to pertaining to approaches to measurement of food security and nutrition. It is clear that, among other considerations, the decision on what an appropriate approach must be is hugely dependent on two things:

(i) The conceptualization of the construct to be measured
(ii) The purpose of data collection.

Taking cues from issues surrounding data quality and its implications for nutrition-related indicators, tools, and methods have been put in place to assure improved quality assessment of anthropometric measures, especially curated for large-scale surveys at the time of data collection, reporting, and interpretation. Some of the common tools include standard methods such as the Standardized Monitoring and Assessment of Relief and Transitions (Erhardt et al., 2016). There is, however, no method currently that provides a quantitative assessment of the expected measurement errors. Such a measure could be instrumental in providing more robust estimates of nutrition indicators after considering the biases and uncertainty factors. Evidence pertaining to height distribution from 179 Demographic and Health Surveys (DHS) in 64 low- and middle-income countries reported the mean standard deviation of height-for-age (HAZ) scores to be 1.68 (range: 1.65–2.11), pointing towards the plausibility of increased uncertainty in these countries when using the WHO standard (Roth et al., 2017). Estimates from the same analysis showed that the mean height-for- age would register a reduction without a concomitant increase in the standard deviation if all children were exposed to the same growth hindering factors (Roth et al., 2017). The lower dispersion and higher stunting prevalence of stunting in Sub-Saharan Africa and Latin American countries could be attributed to the above (Ghosh et al., 2020). It is important to emphasize the crucial need for not compromising with precision in anthropometric measurements, particularly in large-scale surveys used to derive nutritional status indicators that are used to arrive at policy decisions.

In guiding the selection of suitable measures of food security and nutrition, it could be useful to ask the following questions:

1. What components pertaining to nutrition and food security (availability, access, utilization, stability) are to be measured?
2. Who will the data be of use to and what kind of data will be the appropriate for them?
3. What is the objective behind data collection? Is it for preparing a system for famine warning, addressing food assistance programs, identifying high-risk households for intervention purposes, monitoring changes in nutrition indicators/food security status over time, evaluating program usage, evaluating programs and policies, in general, or advocacy?
4. What is the periodicity to be evaluated?
5. What kind of indicators are being measured (chronic or acute)?
6. Will there be repeated data collection/ measurement?
7. At what point in the causal pathway does the measurement lie?
8. At what scale is the variable of concern being measured (individual, household, regional, national)?
9. What are the resources at disposal for planning, data collection, and analysis?
10. What is the intended application of the findings?

Analytical and methodical assessment of programs, coupled with a resolved usage of data, may prove to be beneficial for food security and nutrition-oriented programs. In certain circumstances, it will be appropriate to have an approach that ensures convergence of the evidence base. However, in the context of program evaluation, it is not advantageous to have a program that is positioned to concomitantly address all domains or loci of food security or nutrition in the conceptual pathway. It is, therefore, pertinent to identify mechanisms that are particularly well suited to the needs and resources of a program. This is not just crucial but also aids in the more competent and valid measurement of food security and nutrition. The diversification of categories and disciplines for nutrition-based indicators implies that the study and approaches used for policy formulation and program development and evaluation must remain equally diverse. Thus, there is a need to identify the need and adapt the diversity that is needed in not just policy formulation but also measurement approaches, the result of which will be a bolstered evidence base for all.

In conclusion, it can be said that India has made remarkable strides towards reducing all forms of nutritional inadequacies among different population groups. Despite certain lacunae in the implementation and operationalization of policies, India's achievements on public health front since seven decades after independence are to be applauded. Housing the world's second largest population and catering to the welfare of such diversified population can be an uphill task. The need of the hour is to channel our limited resources to areas as per their necessity and, thus, diversify the benefits of policymaking. Despite its continuing high levels of poverty and illiteracy, India has a huge demographic potential in the form of a budding young population. This leveraging position must be used as an upper hand by investing in nutrition education, household access to nutritious diets, sanitary environment, and a health-promoting lifestyle. This requires collaborative efforts by all the stakeholders, including governments, non-government organizations, academia, civil society organizations, and the common people as well.

References

Abriha, A., et al. (2014). Prevalence and associated factors of anaemia among pregnant women of Mekelle town: A cross sectional study. *BMC Research Notes, 2014*(7), 888.

Accorsi, S., Fabiani, M., Nattabi, B., et al. (2005). The disease profile of poverty: Morbidity and mortality in northern Uganda in the context of war, population displacement and HIV/AIDS. *Transactions of the Royal Society of Tropical Medicine and Hygiene, 99*, 226–233.

Adenle, A. A., Weding, K., & Azadi, H. (2019). Sustainable agriculture and food security in Africa: The role of innovative technologies and international organizations. *Technology in Society, 58,* 1–17.

Adinma, E. D., & Adinma, J. I. (2008). Perceptions and practices on menstruation amongst Nigerian secondary school girls. *African Journal of Reproductive Health, 12*(1), 74–83.

Adish, A. A., Esrey, S. A., Gyorkos, T. W., & Johns, T. (1999). Risk factors for iron deficiency anaemia in preschool children in northern Ethiopia. *Public Health Nutrition, 2*(3), 243–252.

Adjiwanou, V., & LeGrand, T. (2014). Gender inequality and the use of maternal healthcare services in rural sub-Saharan Africa. *Health & Place, 29*, 67–78.

Agarwal, B. (1997). "Bargaining" and gender relationships: Within and beyond the household. *Feminist Economics, 3*(1), 1–51.

Agrawal, S. (2013). Disadvantageous situation of tribal women and children of Orissa, India: A special reference to their health and nutritional status. *Journal of Community Nutrition & Health, 2*(1).

Agarwal, E., Miller, M., Yaxley, A., et al. (2013). Malnutrition in the elderly: A narrative review. *Maturitas, 2013*(76), 296–302.

Agrawal, S., Kim, R., Gausman, J., et al. (2019). Socio-economic patterning of food consumption and dietary diversity among Indian children: Evidence from NFHS-4. *European Journal of Clinical Nutrition, 73*, 1361–1372. https://doi.org/10.1038/s41430-019-0406-0

Ahmad, N. (2011). Impact of institutional credit on agricultural output: A case study of Pakistan. *Theoretical and Applied Economics, 2011*(18), 99–120.

Ahmed, T., & Haboubi, N. (2010). Assessment and management of nutrition in older people and its importance to health. *Clinical Interventions in Aging, 5*, 207–216.

Aijaz, R. (2017). Preventing hunger and malnutrition in India. *ORF Issue Brief, 182.*

Alderman, H., & Headey, D. D. (2017). How important is parental education for child nutrition? *World Development, 94,* 448–464. https://doi.org/10.1016/j.worlddev.2017.02.007

Alderman, H., Haddad, L., Headey, D. D., & Smith, L. (2014). Economic growth and early childhood nutrition. *The Lancet Global Health, 2*, e500.

Ali, A. (1992). Nutrition. In Voluntary Health Association of India (Ed.), *State of India's Health* (pp 1–50). VHAI.

Ali, S. S., & Goudar, S. (2014). The impact of nutrition on child development at 3 years in a rural community of India. *International Journal of Preventive Medicine, 5*, 494–499.

Allendorf, K. (2007). Do women's land rights promote empowerment and child health in Nepal? *World Development, 35*(11), 1975–1988.

Allison, B. (2011). *Certain foods linked to long-term weight gain.* National Institutes of Health, 11 July 2011.

Allison, A., Anthony-Kouyate, R., Blanchard, H., Deller, B., Foreman, M., Galloway, R. et al. (2010). *Maximizing synergy between maternal, infant and young nutrition and pregnancy prevention* (A discussion paper prepared for maternal, infant and young child nutrition (MIYCN) and family planning (FP). Integration Technical Meeting).

Alsop, R., Bertelsen, M. F., & Holland, J. (2006). *Empowerment in practice: From analysis to implementation*. World Bank.

Anderson, A. L., Harris, T. B., Tylavsky, F. A., et al. (2011). Dietary patterns and survival of older adults. *Journal of the American Dietetic Association, 111*, 84–91.

Anele. (2017). *Nigeria has the third highest infant mortality rate in the world—WHO* [Internet]. Listwand. http://listwand.com/2017/10/nigeria-has-the-third-highest-infant-mortality-rate-inthe-world-who/

A. Chattopadhyay et al., *Undernutrition in India*, Sustainable Development Goals Series,
https://doi.org/10.1007/978-981-19-8182-1

Armstrong, J., Dorosty, A. R., Reilly, J. J., & Emmett, P. M. (2003). Coexistence of social inequalities in undernutrition and obesity in preschool children: Population based cross sectional study. *Achieves Diseases of Childhood, 88*, 671–675.

Ashakiran, D. R. (2012). Fast foods and their impact on health. *Journal of Krishna Institute of Medical Sciences University., 1*, 7–15.

Aturupane, H., Deolalikar, A. B., & Gunewardena, D. (2011). Determinants of child weight and height in Sri Lanka: A quantile regression approach. In *Health inequality and development* (pp. 64–88). Springer.

Avenell, A., & Handoll, H. H. (2003). A systematic review of protein and energy supplementation for hip fracture aftercare in older people. *European Journal of Clinical Nutrition, 57,* 895e903.

Ayensu, J., Annan, R., Lutterodt, H., Edusei, A., & Peng, L. (2020). Prevalence of anaemia and low intake of dietary nutrients in pregnant women living in rural and urban areas in the Ashanti region of Ghana. *PLoS ONE, 15*(1), e0226026. https://doi.org/10.1371/journal.pone.0226026

Aziz Ali, S., Feroz, A., Abbasi, Z., Aziz Ali, S., Allana, A., Hambidge, K. M., et al. (2021). Perceptions of women, their husbands and healthcare providers about anaemia in rural Pakistan: Findings from a qualitative exploratory study. *PLoS ONE, 16*(4), e0249360. https://doi.org/10.1371/journal.pone.0249360

Babu, S., Gajanan, S. N., & Hallam, J. A. (2016). *Nutrition economics: Principles and policy applications*. Academic Press.

Bach, A., Serra Majem, L., Carrasco, J. L., Roman, B., Ngo, J., Bertomeu, I., et al. (2006). The use of indexes evaluation the adherence to the Mediterranean diet in epidemiological studies: A review. *Public Health Nutrition, 9,* 132e46.

Bagherniya, M., Taghipour, A., Sharma, M., Sahebkar, A., Contento, I. R., Keshavarz, S. A., et al. (2018). Obesity intervention programs among adolescents using social cognitive theory: A systematic literature review. *Health Education Research, 33*, 26–39.

Bahamondes, L., Valeria Bahamondes, M., & Shulman, L. P. (2015). Noncontraceptive benefits of hormonal and intrauterine reversible contraceptive methods. *Human Reproduction Update, 21*, 640–651.

Baker, P., Gill, T., Friel, S., et al. (2017). Generating political priority for regulatory interventions targeting obesity prevention: An Australian case study. *Social Science and Medicine, 177*, 141–149.

Bakker, A. B., & Demerouti, E. (2007). The job demands-resources model: State of the art. *Journal of Managerial Psychology, 22*(3), 309–328.

Bakker, A. B., & Demerouti, E. (2017). Job demandsresources theory: Taking stock and looking forward. *Journal of Occupational Health Psychology, 22*(3), 273–285.

Balarajan, Y. (2014). Creating political priority for micronutrient deficiencies: A qualitative case study from Senegal. *British Medical Journal Open, 4*, e004784.

Balarajan, Y., & Reich, M. R. (2016). Political economy of child nutrition policy: A qualitative study of India's Integrated Child Development Services (ICDS) scheme. *Food Policy, 62*, 88–98.

Balgir, R. S., Mishra, R. K., & Murmu, B. (2003). Clinical and hematological profile of hemoglobinopathies in two tribal communities of Sundargarh District in Orissa, India. *International Journal of Human Genetics, 3*, 209–216.

Banerjee, A. (2014). The Indian health paradox: Lessons from Bangladesh. *Medical Journal of Dr. D.Y. Patil University, 7*, 411. https://doi.org/10.4103/0975-2870.135250

Barker, D. J. (1995). Fetal origins of coronary heart disease. *BMJ, 311,* 171–174.

Barosso, C., & Jacobson, J. L. (2000). Population policy and women's empowerment: Challenges and opportunities. In H. B. Presser & G. Sen (Eds.), *Women's empowerment and demographic processes.* Oxford University Press.

Bartram, J., Lewis, K., Lenton, R., & Wright, A. (2005). Focusing on improved water and sanitation for health. *Lancet, 365*(9461), 810–812.

Basiago, A. D. (1995). Sustainable development in Indonesia: A case study of an indigenous regime of environmental law and policy. *International Journal of Sustainable Development & World Ecology, 2,* 199–211.

Basu, S. K. (1993). Health status of tribal women in India. *Social Change, 23*(4), 19–39.

Beker, V. A. (2016). Growth, inequality and poverty: What do we know? Available at SSRN: https://ssrn.com/abstract=2727231 or https://doi.org/10.2139/ssrn.2727231

Bellizzi, S., & Ali, M. M. (2018). Effect of oral contraception on anemia in 12 low- and middle-income countries. *Contraception, 2018*(97), 236–242.

Benson, T. (2007). Cross-sectoral coordination failure: How significant a constraint in national efforts to tackle Undernutritionin Africa? *Food and Nutrition Bulletin, 28*(Suppl), S323–S330.

Bentley, M. E., & Griffiths, P. L. (2003). The burden of anaemiaanaemia among women in India. *European Journal of Clinical Nutrition, 2003*(57), 52–60.

Bershteyn, A., Lyons, H. M., Sivam, D., et al. (2015). Association between economic growth and early childhood nutrition. *The Lancet Global Health, 3*, e79-80.

Bezanson, K., & Isenman, P. (2010). Scaling up nutrition: A framework for action. *Food Nutrition Bulletin, 31* (1), 178–186. https://doi.org/10.1177/156482651003100118

Bhagowalia, P., Menon, P., Quisumbing, A. R., & Soundararajan, V. (2012). *What dimensions of women's empowerment matter for child nutrition? Evidence using nationally representative data from Bangladesh.*

Bharati, P., Som, S., Chakrabarty, S., Bharati, S., & Pal, M. (2008). Prevalence of anaemia and its determinants among nonpregnant and pregnant women in India. *Asia-Pacific Journal of Public Health, 20*(4), 347–359. https://doi.org/10.1177/1010539508322762

Bhattacharya, S., Falcao, V. L. & Puri, R. (2018). The public distribution system in India: Policy evolution and program delivery trends. In H. Alderman, U. Gentillini, & R. Yemtsov (Eds.), *The 1.5 billion people question* (pp. 43–105). World Bank.

Bhutta, Z. A. (2006). Effect of infections and environmental factors on growth and nutritional status in developing countries. *Journal of Pediatric Gastroenterology and Nutrition, 43*, S13–S21.

Bhutta, Z. A. (2016). What does India need to do to address childhood malnutrition at scale? *Social Science & Medicine, 157,* 186±8. https://doi.org/10.1016/j.socscimed.2016.02.038. PMID: 27080066.

Bhutta, Z. A., Das, J. K., Rizvi, A., et al. (2013). Evidence-based interventions for improvement of maternal and child nutrition: What can be done and at what cost? *Lancet, 382*, 452–477.

Bhutta, Z. A., Gupta, I., De'Silva, H., Manandhar, D., Awasthi, S., Hossain, S. M., et al. (2004) Maternal and child health: Is South Asia ready for change? *BMJ (Clinical Research Ed.) 328,* 816–819.

Biadgilign, S., Shumetie, A., & Yesigat, H. (2016). Does economic growth reduce childhood undernutrition in Ethiopia? *PLoS ONE, 11*, e0160050.

Birthal, P. S., Roy, D., & Negi, D. S. (2015). Assessing the impact of crop diversification on farm poverty in India. *World Development, 72*(i), 70–92. https://doi.org/10.1016/j.worlddev.2015.02.015

Bishai, D. M., Cohen, R., Alfonso, Y. N., et al. (2016). Factors contributing to maternal and child mortality reductions in 146 low- and middle-income countries between 1990 and 2010. *PLoS ONE, 11*, e0144908.

Black, R. E., Victora, C. G., Walker, S. P., et al. (2013). Maternal and child undernutrition and overweight in low-income and middle-income countries. *Lancet, 382*, 427–451.

Blackburn, G., & Thornton, P. (1979). Nutritional assessment of the hospitalized patient. *Medical Clinics of North America, 63,* 1103e15.

Bloom, D. E., Hu, P., Arokiasamy, P., Risbud, A., Sekher, T. V., Mohanty, S. K., Kale, V., O'Brien, J., Chien, S., & Lee, J. (2014). *Longitudinal aging study in India: Biomarker data documentation*. Harvard University Program on the Global Demography of Aging.

Bodnar, L. M., Cogswell, M. E., & McDonald, T. (2005). Have we forgotten the significance of postpartum iron deficiency? *American Journal of Obstetrics and Gynecology, 193*(1), 36–44. https://doi.org/10.1016/j.ajog.2004.12.009

Bodnar, L. M., Scanlon, K. S., Freedman, D. S., Siega-Riz, A. M., & Mary, E. (2001). Cogswell, high prevalence of postpartum anaemia among low-income women in the United State. *American Journal of Obstetrics and Gynecology, 185*(2), 438–443. https://doi.org/10.1067/mob.2001.115996. ISSN 0002-9378

Bodor, J., Rose, D., Farley, T., Swalm, C., & Scott, S. (2008). Neighbourhood fruit and vegetable availability and consumption: The role of small food stores in an urban environment. *Public Health Nutrition, 11*, 413–420.

Bongaarts, J., Cleland, J. C., Townsend, J., Bertrand, J. T., & Gupta, M. D. (2012). *Family planning programs for the 21st century: Rationale and design*. Population Council Inc.

Boosalis, M. G., Ott, L., Levine, A. S., Slag, M. F., Morley, J. E., Young, B., & McClain, C. J. (1989). Relationship of visceral proteins to nutritional status in chronic and acute stress. *Critical Care Medicine, 17*, 741–747.

Bora, J. K., & Saikia, N. (2018). Neonatal and under-five mortality rate in Indian districts with reference to sustainable development goal 3: An analysis of the National Family Health Survey of India (NFHS), 2015–2016. *PLoS ONE, 13*(7), e0201125. https://doi.org/10.1371/journal.pone.0201125

Boserup, E. (1981). *Population and technology*. Basil Blackwell.

Bowling, N. A., & Kirkendall, C. (2012). Workload: A review of causes, consequences, and potential interventions. In J. Houdmont, S. Leka, & S. S. Sinclair (Eds.), *Contemporary occupational health psychology: Global perspectives on research and practice* (Vol. 2, pp. 221–238). Wiley-Blackwell.

Brennan, L., McDonald, J., & Shlomowitz, R. (2004). Infant feeding practices and chronic child malnutrition in the Indian states of Karnataka and Uttar Pradesh. *Economics and Human Biology, 2*, 139–158.

Buisman, L. R., Van de Poel, E., O'Donnell, O., et al. (2019). What explains the fall in child stunting in sub-Saharan Africa? *SSM Population Health, 8*, 100384.

Burke, R. M., Leon, J. S., & Suchdev, P. S. (2014). Identification, prevention and treatment of iron deficiency during the first 1000 days. *Nutrients, 6*, 4093–4114.

Buvinic, M., & Furst-Nichols, R. (2016). *Promoting women's economic empowerment: What works?* The World Bank Research Observer.

Carr, B., Gates, M. F., Mitchel, A., & Shah, R. (2012). Giving women the power to plan their families. *The Lancet, 380*(9837), 80–82.

Casey, B., et al. (2003). *Policies for an ageing society: Recent measures and areas for further reform*. OECD.

Cederholm, T., Barazzoni, R., Austin, P., et al. (2017). ESPEN guidelines on definitions and terminology of clinical nutrition. *Clinical Nutrition, 36*, 49–64.

Cederholm, T., Bosaeus, I., Barazzoni, R., Bauer, J., Van Gossum, A., Klek, S., Muscaritoli, M., Nyulasi, I., Ockenga, J., Schneider, S. M., et al. (2015). Diagnostic criteria for malnutrition—An ESPEN consensus statement. *Clinical Nutrition, 34*, 335–340.

Cha, S. (2017). The impact of the worldwide millennium development goals campaign on maternal and under-five child mortality reduction: 'Where did the worldwide campaign work effectively?' *GlobHealth Action, 10*, 1267961.

Chakrabarti, A. (2019). Understanding female autonomy in India through their family headship status. *Journal of Population and Social Studies, 27*(3), 266–285. https://doi.org/10.25133/JPSSv27n3.0017

Chandra, R. K. (2002). Nutrition and the immune system from birth to old age. *European Journal of Clinical Nutrition, 56,* 73e6.

Chandra, J., Jain, V., & Narayan, S. (2002). Folate and cobalamin deficiency in megaloblastic anaemia in children. *Indian Pediatrics, 39*(5), 453–457.

Charney, P. (1995). Nutritional assessment in the 1990s: Where are we now? *Nutrition in Clinical Practice, 10*, 131–139.

Chatterjee, A., & Paily, V. (2011). Achieving millennium development goals 4 and 5 in India. *BJOG: An International Journal of Obstetrics & Gynaecology.* https://doi.org/10.1111/j.1471-0528.2011.03112.x

Chattopadhyay, A., Sethi, V., Nagargoje, V. P., et al. (2019). WASH practices and its association with nutritional status of adolescent girls in poverty pockets of eastern India. *BMC Women's Health, 19*, 89. https://doi.org/10.1186/s12905-019-0787-1

Checkley, W., Buckley, G., Gilman, R. H., Assis, A. M., Guerrant, R. L., Morris, S. S., et al. (2008). Multi-country analysis of the effects of diarrhoea on childhood stunting. *International Journal of Epidemiology, 37*(4), 816–830.

Chen, Y., & Li, H. (2009). Mother's education and child health: Is there a nurturing effect? *Journal of Health Economics, 28*(2), 413–426.

Chhotray, G. P. (2003). Health status of primitive tribes of Orissa. *ICMR Bulletin, 33*.

Choudhary, M., & Dashora, R. (2015). Effect of nutritional status on prevalence of anaemia among females. *Food Science Research Journal, 6*(1), 1–7.

Chowa, G. A. N., Masa, R. D., Wretman, C. J., & Ansong, D. (2013). The impact of household possessions on youth's academic achievement in the Ghana Youthsave experiment: A propensity score analysis. *Economics of Education Review, 33*(C), 69–81.

Chung, A., Shill, J., Swinburn, B., et al. (2012). An analysis of potential barriers and enablers to regulating the television marketing of unhealthy foods to children at the state government level in Australia. *BMC Public Health, 12*, 1123.

Clayton, M. L., Frattaroli, S., Palmer, A., et al. (2015). The role of partnerships in U.S. food policy council policy activities. *PLoS One, 10,* e0122870.

Collins, C. E., Kershaw, J., & Brockington, S. (2005). Effect of nutritional supplements on wound healing in home-nursed elderly: A randomized trial. *Nutrition, 21,* 147e55.

Conley, D. (2001). Capital for college: Parental assets and postsecondary schooling. *Sociology of Education, 74* (1), 59–72.

Cook, D. C., Fraser, R. W., Paini, D. R., Warden, A. C., Lonsdale, W. M., & De Barro, P. J. (2011). Biosecurity and yield improvement technologies are strategic complements in the fight against food insecurity. *PLoS ONE, 6,* e26084.

Corish, C. A., & Bardon, L. A. (2018). Malnutrition in older adults: Screening and determinants. *The Proceedings of the Nutrition Society, 78*, 372–379.

Cornwall, A., & Anyidoho, N. A. (2010). Introduction: Women's empowerment: Contentions and contestations. *Development, 53*, 144–149.

Cornwall, A., & Edwards, J. (2010). Introduction: Negotiating empowerment. *IDS Bulletin, 41*, 1–9.

Corsi, D. J., Perkins, J. M., & Subramanian, S. V. (2017). Child anthropometry data quality from demographic and health surveys, multiple indicator cluster surveys, and national nutrition surveys in the west Central Africa region: Are we comparing apples and oranges? *Global Health Action, 10*(1), 1328185. https://doi.org/10.1080/16549716.2017.1328185

Coyte, P. C., Goodwin, N., & Laporte, A. (2008). *How can the settings used to provide care to older people be balanced?* WHO Regional Office for Europe.

Craig, R. L., Felix, H. C., Walker, J. F., et al. (2010). Public health professionals as policy entrepreneurs: Arkansas's childhood obesity policy experience. *American Journal of Public Health, 100*, 2047–2052.

Crichton, M., Craven, D., Mackay, H., Marx, W., de van der Schueren, M., & Marshall, S. (2018). A systematic review, meta-analysis and meta-regression of the prevalence of protein-energy malnutrition: Associations with geographical region and sex. *Age Ageing, 48*, 38–48.

Cunningham, K., Headey, D., Singh, A., Karmacharya, C., & Rana, P. P. (2017). Maternal and child nutrition in Nepal: Examining drivers of progress from the mid1990s to 2010s. *Global Food Security, 13*(2), 30–37.

Curtis, V., & Cairncross, S. (2003). Effect of washing hands with soap on diarrhoea risk in the community: A systematic review. *The Lancet Infectious Diseases, 3*, 275–281.

Cusick, S. E., & Georgieff, M. K. (2016). The role of nutrition in brain development: The golden opportunity of the "first 1000 days." *Jpediatr, 175*, 16–21.

Dalton, E. T. (1872). *Descriptive ethnography of Bengal Calcutta.*

Daly, H. E. (2007). *Ecological economics and sustainable development. Selected essays of Herman Daly.* Edward Elgar.

Dangour, A. D., Green, R., Häsler, B., Rushton, J., Shankar, B., Waage, J., et al. (2012). Linking agriculture and health in low- and middle-income countries: An interdisciplinary research agenda. *The Proceedings of the Nutrition Society, 71*(2), 222–228.

Dangour, A. D., Watson, L., Cumming, O., Boisson, S., Che, Y., Velleman, Y., Cavill, S., Allen, E., & Uauy, R. (2013). Interventions to improve water quality and supply, sanitation and hygiene practices, and their effects on the nutritional status of children. *Cochrane Database of System Review, 8,* Art. No.: CD009382. https://doi.org/10.1002/14651858.CD009382.pub2

Das, S. (2019). *The indigenous colour of India—The Indian Tribes*. https://www.tourmyindia.com/blog/the-indigenous-colour-of-india-the-indian-tribes/

Das, P. K., Bhavani, R. V., & Swaminathan, M. S. (2014). A farming system model to leverage agriculture for nutritional outcomes. *Agricultural Research, 3*, 193–203.

Dasgupta, A., & Sarkar, M. (2008). Menstrual hygiene: How hygienic is the adolescent girl? *Indian Journal of Community Medicine, 33*(2), 77–80.

Daviglus, M., et al. (2005). Cardiovascular risk profile earlier in life and medicare costs in the last year of life. *Archives of Internal Medicine, 165*, 1028–1034.

De Onis, M., & Habicht, J. P. (1996). Anthropometric reference data for international use: Recommendations from a World Health Organization expert committee. *American Journal of Clinical Nutrition, 64*, 650–658.

De Schutter, O. (2014). *UN special Rapporteur on the right to food. Report on agroecology and the right to food.*

De, M., Halder, A., Podder, S., Sen, R., Chakrabarty, S., Sengupta, B., Chakraborty, T., Das, U., & Talukder, G. (2006). Anaemia and hemoglobinopathies in tribal population of Eastern and North-eastern India. *Hematology (Amsterdam, Netherlands), 11*(5), 371–373. https://doi.org/10.1080/10245330600840180

Deaton, A. (2001). *Health, inequality, and economic development.* Working Group 1 of the WHO Commission on Macroeconomics and Health.

Deaton, A. (2006). *Global patterns of income and health: Facts, interpretations, and policies*. NBER Working Paper No. 12735.

Deaton, A., & Dreze, J. (2009). Food and nutrition in India: Facts and interpretation. *Economic & Political Weekly, XLVI*(7), 42–65.

Delil, R., Tamiru, D., & Zinab, B. (2018). Dietary diversity and its association with anaemia among pregnant women attending public health facilities in South Ethiopia. *Ethiopian Journal of Health Sciences, 28*(5), 625–634. https://doi.org/10.4314/ejhs.v28i5.14

Deng, S., Huang, J., Jin, M., & Sherraden, M. (2014). Household assets, school enrollment, and parental aspirations for children's education in rural China: Does gender matter? *International Journal of Social Welfare, 23*(2), 185–194.

Department of Agriculture, Cooperation and Farmers' Welfare. (2019). *Annual report*. Ministry of Agriculture & Farmers Welfare, Govt. of India. http://eands.dacnet.nic.in

Department of Health. (2004). *Better health in old age*. Department of Health.

Department of Women and Child Development, Ministry of Human Resource Development, Government of India. (1993). National Nutrition Policy. Government of India. http://childlineindia.org.in/CP-CR-Downloads/national%20nutrition%20policy.pdf

Development Initiatives. (2017). *Global nutrition report 2017: Nourishing the SDGs*. www.globalnutritionreport.org

Deyshapppriya, N. R. R. (2018). *Examining poverty trends*. London School of Economics. https://blogs.lse.ac.uk/southasia/2018/07/31/examining-poverty-trends-in-south-asian-countries-where-is-sri-lanka-among-its-south-asian-counterparts/

Dhingra, S. (2020). *Protecting informal workers in urban India: The need for a universal job guarantee*. https://voxeu.org/article/protecting-informal-workers-urban-india

Directorate of Economics & Statistics. (2017). *Agricultural statistics at a glance*. Ministry of Agriculture & Farmers Welfare, Govt. of India. http://eands.dacnet.nic.in

Directorate of Economics & Statistics. (2018). *Pocket book of agricultural statistics*. Ministry of Agriculture & Farmers Welfare, Govt. of India. http://eands.dacnet.nic.in

Doak, C., Adair, L., Bentley, M., Fengying, Z., & Popkin, B. (2002). The underweight/overweight household: An exploration of household sociodemographic and dietary factors in China. *Public Health Nutrition, 5*, 215–221.

Doku, D. T., Bhutta, Z. A., & Neupane, S. (2020). Associations of women's empowerment with neonatal, infant and under-5 mortality in low- and/middle-income countries: Meta-analysis of individual participant data from 59 countries. *BMJ Global Health, 5*(1), e001558. https://doi.org/10.1136/bmjgh-2019-001558

Donini, L. M., Poggiogalle, E., Molfino, A., Rosano, A., Lenzi, A., Rossi Fanelli, F., & Muscaritoli, M. (2016). Mini-nutritional assessment, malnutrition universal screening tool, and nutrition risk screening tool for the nutritional evaluation of older nursing home residents. *Journal of the American Medical Directors Association, 17*, 959.e11-959.e18.

Doss, C. (2006). The effects of intrahousehold property ownership on expenditure patterns in Ghana. *Journal of African Economies, 15*(1), 149–180.

Drèze, J. (2015). Man made starvation. *The Times of India*, 21 December 2015.

Drèze, J., & Khera, R. (2015). Thought for food. Outlook. https://www.outlookindia.com/magazine/story/thought-for-food/295144

Drèze, J., & Khera, R. (2017). Recent social security initiatives in India. *World Development, 98*, 555–572.

Duggal, P., & Petri, W. A., Jr. (2018). Does malnutrition have a genetic component? *Annual Review of Genomics and Human Genetics, 2018*(19), 247–262.

e Pioneer. *Thumbs down to packaged food under ICDS*, 22 February 2015.

Economics Times. (2021). *India falls to 86th rank in corruption perception index 2020.*

Elferink, M., & Schierhorn, F. (2016). Global demand for food is rising. Can we meet it? *Harvard Business Review*, 7 April 2016. Retrieved June 2, 2021, from https://hbr.org/2016/04/global-demand-for-food-is-rising-can-wemeet-it

Elia, M. (2003a). *Screening for malnutrition: A multidisciplinary responsibility. Development and use of the*

'Malnutrition Universal Screening Tool' ('MUST') for adults. Malnutrition Advisory Group (MAG), a Standing Committee of BAPEN. BAPEN.
Elia, M. (2003b). *The MUST report: Nutritional screening for adults: A multidisciplinary responsibility*. BAPEN (MAG).
Elliott, W., & Sherraden, M. (2013). Assets and educational achievement: Theory and evidence. *Economics of Education Review, 33*, 1–7.
England, P. (2000). Conceptualizing women's empowerment in countries of the north. In H. Presser & G. Sen (Eds.), *Women's empowerment and demographic processes*. Oxford University Press.
Engle, P. L., Menon, P., & Haddad, L. (1997). *Care and nutrition: Concepts and measurement* (pp. 1–60). International Food Policy Research Institute.
Erhardt, J., Golden, M. H., Seaman, J., & Bilukha, O. (2016). *ENA for SMART*. http://www.nutrisurvey.de/ena/ena.html
Esrey, J. P., Habicht, J. P., & Latham, M. C. (1988). Drinking water source, diarrheal morbidity, and child growth in villages with both traditional and improved water supplies in rural Lesotho, Southern Africa. *American Journal of Public Health, 78*, 1451–1455.
Esrey, S. A., Potash, J. B., Roberts, L., & Shiff, C. (1991). Effects of improved water supply and sanitation on ascariasis, diarrhoea, dracunculiasis, hookworm infection, schistosomiasis, and trachoma. *Bulletin of the World Health Organization, 69*(5), 609.
European Commission. (2006). *Commission communication: The demographic future of Europe—From challenge to opportunity*. EuropeanCommission.
Evandrou, M. (1996). Unpaid work, carers and health. In D. Blane, E. Brunner, & R. Wilkinson (Eds.), *Health and social organisation: Towards a health policy forthe 21st century* (pp. 204–231). Routledge.
Ezeh, O., Agho, K., Dibley, M., et al. (2014). The impact of water and sanitation on childhood mortality in Nigeria: Evidence from demographic and health surveys, 2003–2013. *International Journal of Environmental Research and Public Health, 11*, 9256–9272.
FAO. (1996a). *Report of the world food summit*. http://www.fao.org/3/w3548e/w3548e00.html
FAO. (1996b). *Rome Declaration on World Food Security*.
FAO. (2019). *The state of food security and nutrition in the world*. www.fao.org/state-of-food-security-nutrition/en
FAO United Nations Statistical Database. *Annual population*. http://www.fao.org/faostat/en/#data/OA
FAO, IFAD, UNICEF, WFP and WHO. (2021). The State of Food Security and Nutrition in the World 2021. Transforming food systems for food security, improved nutrition and affordable healthy diets for all. *FAO*. https://doi.org/10.4060/cb4474en
FAO, IFAD, & WFP. (2015). *e State of food insecurity in the world* (p. 2015). FAO.
Fávaro-Moreira, N., Krausch-Hofmann, S., Matthys, C., et al. (2016). Risk factors for malnutrition in older adults: A systematic review of the literature based on longitudinal data. *Advances in Nutrition, 7*, 507–522.
Fears, R., ter Meulen, V., & von Braun, J. (2018). Scientific opportunities for food and nutrition security. *Lancet Planet Health, 2*, 2–3.
Fewtrell, L., Kaufmann, R. B., Kay, D., Enanoria, W., Haller, L., & Colford, J. M., Jr. (2005). Water, sanitation, and hygiene interventions to reduce diarrhoea in less developed countries: A systematic review and meta-analysis. *The Lancet Infectious Diseases, 5* (1), 42–52.
Filmer, D., & Pritchett, L. H. (2001). Estimating wealth effects without expenditure data–or tears: An application to educational enrollments in states of India. *Demography, 38*(1), 115–132.
Fisher, R. A. (1918). The correlation between relatives on the supposition of Mendelian inheritance. *Transactions of the Royal Society of Edinburgh, 52*, 399–433.
Fleck, A. (1988). Acute phase response: Implications for nutrition and recovery. *Nutrition, 4*, 109–117.
Foley, J. A., DeFries, R., Asner, G. P., Barford, C., Bonan, G., Carpenter, S. R., Chapin, F. S., Coe, M. T., Daily, G. C., Gibbs, H. K., et al. (2005). Global consequences of land use. *Science, 309*, 570–574.
Foley, J. A., Ramankutty, N., Brauman, K. A., Cassidy, E. S., Gerber, J. S., Johnston, M., Mueller, N. D., O'Connell, C., Ray, D. K., West, P. C., et al. (2011). Solutions for a cultivated planet. *Nature, 478*, 337–342.
Food and Agriculture Organization of the United Nations IFfAD, the United Nations Children's Fund, World Food Programme, WHO. (2018). *The State of Food Security and Nutrition in the World*. World Health Organization.
Food Security Information Network. (2019). *Global report on food crisis*. https://reliefweb.int/report/world/global-report-food-crises-2019
Forbes, G. B., & Reina, J. C. (1970). Adult lean body mass declines with age: Some longitudinal observations. *Metabolism, 19*, 653e63.
Fratiglioni, L., et al. (2000). Influence of social networks on occurrence of dementia: A community-based longitudinal study. *Lancet, 355*, 1315–1319.
Freedman, V., et al. (2006). Trends in the use of assistive technology and personal care for late-life disability, 1992–2001. *The Gerontologist, 46*, 124–127.
Fries, J. (2005). Frailty, heart disease, and stroke: The Compression of Morbidity paradigm. *American Journal of Preventive Medicine, 29*(5 Suppl 1), 164–168.
Frongillo, E. A., Onis, M., & Hanson, K. M. P. (1997). Socioeconomic and demographic factors are associated with worldwide pattern of stunting and wasting of children. *Journal of Nutrition, 127*, 2302–2309.
Fukase, E., & Martin, W. J. (2017). *Economic growth, convergence, and world food demand and supply*. Policy Research Working Paper 8257; World Bank

Group, Development Research Group Agriculture and Rural Development Team.
Fulhan, J., Collier, S., & Duggan, C. (2003). Update on pediatric nutrition: Breastfeeding, infant nutrition, and growth. *Current Opinion in Pediatrics, 15*, 323–332.
Galton, R. (1886). Regression towards mediocrity in hereditary stature. *Journal of the Royal Anthropological Institute, 15*, 246–262.
Gandjour, A. (2009). Aging diseases—Do they prevent preventive health care from saving costs? *Health Economics, 18*(3), 355–362.
Gandjour, A., & Lauterbach, K. (2005). Does prevention save costs? Considering deferral of the expensive last year of life. *Journal of Health Economics, 24*, 715–724.
Gariballa, S. E. (2000). Nutritional support in elderly patients. *Journal of Nutrition, Health and Aging, 4*, 25e7.
Gautam, S., Min, H., Kim, H., & Jeong, H.-S. (2019). Determining factors for the prevalence of anaemia in women of reproductive age in Nepal: Evidence from recent national survey data. *PLoS ONE, 14*(6), e0218288. https://doi.org/10.1371/journal.pone.0218288
Gavaravarapu, S. R. M., & Nair, K. M. (2014). Millets in meeting Nutrition security: Issues and way forward for India millets in meeting nutrition security. *The Indian Journal of Nutrition and Dietetics,* (August), 306–321.
GBD. (2017). Risk factors collaborators. Global, regional, and national comparative risk assessment of 84 behavioural, environmental and occupational, and metabolic risks or clusters of risks for 195 countries and territories, 1990–2017: A systematic analysis for the Global Burden of Disease Study 2017. *Lancet, 92*, 1923–1994.
Gebremedhin, S., & Asefa, A. (2018). *BMJ Sex Reprod Health Published Online First*. https://doi.org/10.1136/bmjsrh-2018-200178
Gebremedhin, S., & Enquselassie, F. (2011). Correlates of anaemia among women of reproductive age in Ethiopia: Evidence from Ethiopian DHS 2005. *Ethiopian Journal of Health Development, 25*, 22–30.
Geist, H. J., & Lambin, E. F (2002). Proximate causes and underlying driving forces of tropical deforestation: Tropical forests are disappearing as the result of pressures, both local and regional, acting in various combinations in different geographical locations. *BioScience, 52*, 143–150.
George, N. A., & McKay, F. H. (2019). The public distribution system and food security in India. *International Journal of Environmental Research and Public Health, 16*(17), 3221.
Ghosh, P. (2020). *We need a Marshall plan to fight Covid-19*. Ideas for India. https://www.ideasforindia.in/topics/macroeconomics/we-need-a-marshall-plan-to-fight-covid-19.html
Ghosh, S. (2021). Socio-economic review, 2020–21: Health programme, nutrition schemes take a hit in Gujarat amid pandemic. *The Indian Express*.
Ghosh, S., Shivakumar, N., Bandopadhyay, S., Sachdev, H. S., Kurpad, A. V., & Thomas, T. (2020). An uncertainty estimate of the prevalence of stunting in national surveys: The need for better precision. *BMC Public Health, 20*, 1634. https://doi.org/10.1186/s12889-020-09753-8
Ghosh-Jerath, S., Singh, A., Magsumbol, M. S., Lyngdoh, T., Kamboj, P., & Goldberg, G. (2016). Contribution of indigenous foods towards nutrient intakes and nutritional status of women in the Santhal tribal community of Jharkhand, India. *Public Health Nutrition, 19*(12), 2256–2267. https://doi.org/10.1017/S1368980016000318
Gillespie, S., & Haddad, L. (2003). *The double burden of malnutrition in Asia. Causes, consequences and solutions*. International Food Policy Research Institute and Sage Publications.
Gillespie, S., van den Bold, M., Hodge, J., et al. (2015). Leveraging agriculture for nutrition in South Asia and East Africa: Examining the enabling environment through stakeholder perceptions. *Food Security, 7*, 463–477.
Giridhar, G., Sathyanarayana, K. M., & James, K. S. (2014). Introduction. In G. Giridhar, K. M. Sathyanarayana, S. Kumar, K. S. James, & M. Alam (Eds.), *Population ageing in India*. Cambridge University Press.
Glewwe, P. (1999). Why does mother's schooling raise child health in developing countries? Evidence from Morocco. *The Journal of Human Resources, 34*, 124–159.
Global Nutrition Report. (2020a). *Country nutrition profiles*. https://globalnutritionreport.org/resources/nutrition-profiles/
Global Nutrition Report. (2020b). *Global nutrition report: Action on equity to end malnutrition*. Development Initiatives.
Godfray, H. C. J., Beddington, J. R., Crute, I. R., Haddad, L., Lawrence, D., Muir, J., et al. (2010). Food security: The challenge offeeding 9 billion people. *Science, 327*, 812–818.
Goldman, D., et al. (2005). Consequences of health trends and medical innovation for the future elderly. *Health Affairs, 24*(Suppl 2), W5R-17.
Goldman, D. P., et al. (2006). The value of elderly disease prevention. *Forum for Health Economics & Policy, 9* (2). Retrieved November 10, 2008, from http://www.bepress.com/fhep/biomedical_research/1
Goodland, R., & Ledec, G. (1987). Neoclassical economics and principles of sustainable development. *Ecological Modelling, 38*, 19–46.
Gopalan, C. (1996). Current food and nutrition situation in south Asian and south-east Asian countries. *Biomedical and Environmental Sciences, 9*, 102–116.
Goswmai, S., & Das, K. K. (2015). Socio-economic and demographic determinants of childhood anaemia. *Journal De Pediatria, 2015*(91), 471–477.
Government of Madhya Pradesh, Women and Child Development Department. Atal Bihari Bajpai Child

Health and Nutrition Mission. http://www.mpwcd.nic.in/web/wcd/sc-ic-abm

Green, S. H., Wang, C., Ballakrishnen, S. S., Brueckner, H., & Bearman, P. (2019). Patterned remittances enhance women's health-related autonomy. *SSM Population Health, 9*, 100370. https://doi.org/10.1016/j.ssmph.2019.100370

Grellety, E., & Golden, M. H. (2016). The effect of random error on diagnostic accuracy illustrated with the anthropometric diagnosis of malnutrition. *PloS ONE, 11*(12). https://doi.org/10.1371/journal.pone.0168585

Grosso, G., Mateo, J., Rangelov, N., Buzeti, T., & Birt, C. (2020). Nutrition in the context of the sustainable development goals. *European Journal of Public Health, 30*(Supplement 1), i19–i23.

GSS. Ghana demographic and health survey 2014. Ghana Health Service (GHS), and ICF Macro. 2015.

Guigoz, Y., Lauque, S., & Vellas, B. J. (2002). Identifying the elderly at risk for malnutrition. The mini nutritional assessment. *Clinics in Geriatric Medicine, 18*, 737e57.

Gulati, J. K. (2010). Child malnutrition: Trends and issues. *Anthropologist, 12*(2), 131–140.

Gulati, A., Kumar, A. G., Sreedhar, G., & Nandkumar, T. (2012). Agriculture and malnutrition in India. *Food and Nutrition Bulletin, 33*(1), 74–86.

Habyarimana, F., Zewotir, T., & Ramroop, S. (2018). Spatial distribution and analysis of risk factors associated with anaemia among women of reproductive age: Case of 2014 Rwanda demographic and health survey data. *The Open Public Health Journal, 11*(1).

Haddad, L. (1999). Women's status: Levels, determinants, consequences for malnutrition, interventions, and policy. *Asian Development Review, 17*(1/2), 96–131.

Haddad, L., Achadi, E., Bendech, M.A., Ahuja, A., Bhatia, K., Bhutta, Z., Blössner, M., Borghi, E., Colecraft, E.,de Onis, M., et al (2015). The global nutrition report 2014: Actions and accountability to accelerate the world's progress on nutrition. *Journal of Nutrition, 145*, 663–671.

Haddad, L., Nisbett, N., Barnett, I., et al. (2014). *Maharashtra's child stunting declines: What is driving them? Findings of a multidisciplinary analysis.* Institute of Development Studies.

Haile, Z. T., Kingori, C., Teweldeberhan, A. K., & Chavan, B. (2017). The relationship between history of hormonal contraceptive use and iron status among women in Tanzania: A population-based study. *Sexual & Reproductive Healthcare: Official Journal of the Swedish Association of Midwives, 13*, 97–102. https://doi.org/10.1016/j.srhc.2017.07.003

Haile, Z. T., Teweldeberhan, A. K., & Chertok, I. R. (2016). Association between oral contraceptive use and markers of iron deficiency in a cross-sectional study of Tanzanian women. *International Journal of Gynaecology and Obstetrics, 132*(1), 50–54.

Hajeebhoy, N., Rigsby, A., Mccoll, A., et al. (2013). Change strategies to protect, promote, and support infant and young child feeding. *Food and Nutrition Bulletin, 34*(Suppl), S181–S194.

Häkkinen, U., et al. (2008). Aging, health expenditure, proximity to death, and income in Finland. *Health Economics, Policy and Law, 3*(Pt 2), 165–195. *Policy Brief, 28.*

Hall, K., Whiting, S. J., & Comfort, B. (2000). Low nutrient intake contributes to adverse clinical outcomes in hospitalized elderly patients. *Nutrition Reviews, 58*, 214e7.

Harttgen, K., Klasen, S., & Vollmer, S. (2013). Economic growth and child undernutrition in sub-Saharan Africa. *Population and Development Review, 39*, 397–412.

Hawkes, C., Brazil, B. G., Castro, I. R., et al. (2016). How to engage across sectors: Lessons from agriculture and nutrition in the Brazilian school feeding program. *Revista De Saude Publica, 50*, 38.

Hazell, P., & Wood, S. (2008). Drivers of change in global agriculture. *Philosophical Transactions of the Royal Society B: Biological Sciences, 363*, 495–515.

Headey, D. (2013). Developmental drivers of nutritional change: A cross-country analysis. *World Development, 42*(2), 76–88.

Headey, D., & Palloni, G. (2019). Water, sanitation, and child health: Evidence from sub-national panel data in 59 countries. *Demography, 56*, 729–752.

Hertel, S. (2015). Hungry for justice: Social mobilization on the right to food in India. *Development and Change, 46*(1), 72–94.

Hertzman, C., Frank, J., & Evans, R. G. (1994). Heterogeneities in health status and the determinants of population health. In R. G. Evans, M. L. Barer, & T. R. Marmor (Eds.), *Why are some people healthy and others not. The determinants of health of the populations* (pp. 67–92). Aldine de Gruyter.

Hickson, M. (2006). Malnutrition and ageing. *Postgraduate Medical Journal, 82*, 2–8.

Himanshu, S. A. (2011). Why not a universal food security legislation. *Economic and Political Weekly, 46*(12), 16.

Hirve, S., & Ganatra, B. (1994). Determinants of low birth weight: A community based prospective cohort study. *Indian Pediatrics, 31*, 1221–1225.

Hoddinott, J., & Adam, C. (1998). *Testing Nash bargaining household models with time series data: Divorce law reform and female suicide in Canada.* Food Consumption and Nutrition Division Discussion Paper 52. International Food Policy Research Institute.

Hoey, L., & Pelletier, D. L. (2011). Bolivia's multisectoral zero Undernutritionprogram: Insights on commitment, collaboration, and capacities. *Food and Nutrition Bulletin, 32*(Suppl), S70-81.

Horton, R., & Peterson, H. B. (2012). The rebirth of family planning. *The Lancet, 380*(9837), 77.

Houghton, L. A., Trilok-Kumar, G., McIntosh, D., Haszard, J. J., Harper, M. J., Reid, M., Erhardt, J., Bailey, K., & Gibson, R. S. (2019). Multiple micronutrient status and predictors of anaemiaanaemia in young children aged 12–23 months living in New Delhi, India. *PLOS ONE, 14*, e0209564.

Huang, J. (2011). *Asset effects for children with disabilities: Analysis of educational and health outcomes*. Ph.D. Dissertation, Washington University of St. Louis.

Huang, J. (2013). Intergenerational transmission of educational attainment: The role of household assets. *Economics of Education Review, 33*, 112–123.

Huicho, L., Segura, E. R., Huayanay-Espinoza, C. A., et al. (2016). Child health and nutrition in Peru within an antipoverty political agenda: A countdown to 2015 country case study. *The Lancet Global Health, 4*, e414–e426.

Human Rights Council. (2017). *Third universal periodic review of India* (p. 17). 18 January 2017.

Hurley, K. M., Yousafzai, A. K., Lopez-Boo, F., et al. (2016). Early child development and nutrition: A review of the benefits and challenges of implementing integrated interventions. *Advances in Nutrition, 7*, 357–363.

Hutton, J. H. (1921). *The Sema Naga*. Macmillan.

Hutton, B., Feine, J., & Morais, J. (2002). Is there an association between edentulism and nutritional state? *Journal of the Canadian Dental Association, 68*(3), 182–187.

Ibrahim, S., & Alkire, S. (2007). Agency and empowerment: A proposal for internationally comparable indicators. *Oxford Development Studies, 35*, 379–403.

IDPAS. (Iron Deficiency project Advisory Service)—CD Rom. International Nutrition Foundation. (2001).

IFPRI. (2016). *Global nutrition report 2016: From promise to impact: Ending undernutrition by 2030*. International Food Policy Research Institute.

India State-Level Disease Burden Initiative Malnutrition Collaborators. (2019). *The burden of child and maternal malnutrition and trends in its indicators in the states of India: The Global Burden of Disease Study 1990–2017*. Lancet Child Adolescent Health. https://doi.org/10.1016/S2352-4642(19)30273-1.2

Indian Council of Medical Research, Public Health Foundation of India, and Institute fir Health metrics and Evaluation. (2017). *India: Health of the Nation's States—The India State-level Disease Burden Initiative*. ICMR, PHFI and IHME.

Institute for Health Metrics and Evaluation. (2018). *GBD Compare data visualization*. Institute for Health Metrics and Evaluation, University of Washington. http://vizhub.healthdata.org/gbd-compare

Integrated Support Service on Food and Nutrition Security and Sustainable Agriculture (ISS FANSSA), the Nutrition Advisory Service, and the European Commission's Directorate-General for International Cooperation and Development (DG DEVCO). (2018). *Gender equality matters for nutrition*. EuropeAid, Directorate Sustainable Growth and Development.

International Food Policy Research Institute. (2016). *Global nutrition report 2016: From promise to impact: Ending malnutrition by 2030*. International Food Policy Research Institute.

International Institute for Population Sciences (IIPS) and ICF. (2017). *National Family Health Survey (NFHS 4), 2015–16*. IIPS. http://rchiips.org/NFHS/NFHS-4Reports/India.pdf

International Institute for Population Sciences and Women and Child Development Department, Government of Gujarat. (2014). *Comprehensive Nutrition Survey in Gujarat (CNSG)*. http://iipsindia.org/pdf/FactsheetCNSG14.pdf .

Irz, X., Lin, L., Thirtle, C., & Wiggins, S (2001). Agricultural productivity growth and poverty alleviation. *Development Policy Review, 19*, 449–466.

Ismail, I. M., Kahkashan, A., Antony, A., & Sobhith, V. K. (2016). Role of socio-demographic and cultural factors on anaemiaanaemia in a tribal population of North Kerala, India. *International Journal of Community Medicine and Public Health, 2016*(3), 1183–1188.

Jacka, F. N., Maes, M., Pasco, J. A., Williams, L. J., & Berk, M. (2012). Nutrient intakes and the common mental disorders in women. *Journal of Affective Disorders, 141*(1), 79–85.

Jacka, F. N., Pasco, J. A., Williams, L. J., Meyer, B. J., Digger, R., & Berk, M. (2013). Dietary intake of fish and PUFA, and clinical depressive and anxiety disorders in women. *British Journal of Nutrition, 109*(11), 2059–2066.

Jacobs, B., & Robert. (2004). Baseline assessment for addressing acute malnutrition by public health staff in Cambodia. *Journal of Health, Population and Nutrition, 22*, 212–219.

Jacobs, D. R., Jr., & Kromhout, D. (2019). Education, diet, and incident cardiovascular disease: Ecological interactions and conclusions. *Lancet Global Health, 7*, e684–e685.e5.

Jaffar, S., Jepson, A., Leach, A., Greenwood, A., Whittle, H., & Greenwood, B. (1998). Causes of mortality in twins in a rural region of The Gambia, West Africa. *Annals of Tropical Paediatrics, 18*, 231–238.

Jaisheeba, A. A., Sornaraj, R., & Gayathri, K. (2012). Influence of westernized culture and changed dietary habits on the BMI status of the school children of Tirunelveli. *International Journal of Pharm Tech Research, 4*(1), 1065–1077.

Jaleel, A. C. P., & Chattopadhyay, A. (2019). Livelihood crisis and distress seasonal migration in beed district of Maharashtra. *Economic & Political Weekly, IV*(41).

James-Hawkins, L., Peters, C., VanderEnde, K., Bardin, L., & Yount, K. M. (2018). Women's agency and its relationship to current contraceptive use in lower- and middle-income countries: A systematic review of the literature. *Global Public Health, 13*(7), 843–858. https://doi.org/10.1080/17441692.2016.1239270

Jayachandran, S., & Pande, R. (2017). Why are Indian children so short? The role of birth order and son preference. *The American Economic Review, 107*, 2600–2629.

Jeejeebhoy, K. N., Detsky, A. S., & Barker, J. P. (1990). Assessment of nutritional status. *Journal of Parenteral and Enteral Nutrition, 14*, 193–196.

Jemal, H. N. H., & Urga, K. (1999). Iron deficiency anaemia in pregnant and lactating mothers in rural Ethiopia. *East African Medical Journal, 1999*(76), 618–622.

Jethmalani, M. (2018). *Public investment for health care in Gujarat*. Pathey Trust (Pathey Budget Center).

Jeyaseelan, V., Jeyaseelan, L., & Yadav, B. (2016). Incidence of, and risk factors for, malnutrition among children aged 5±7 years in South India. *Journal of Biosocial Science, 48,* 289±305.

Jijau, R. (NA). *Mother-child health and nutrition mission Government of Maharashtra*. http://www.mahnm.in/about

Johri, A. (2020). *As lockdown returns, migrant families in India are going without food*. Scroll. https://scroll.in/article/967731/as-lockdown-returns-migrant-families-in-india-are-going-without-food

Joosten, E., Vanderelst, B., & Pelemans, W. (1999). The effect of different diagnostic criteria on the prevalence of malnutrition in a hospitalized geriatric population. *Aging Clinical and Experimental Research, 11*, 390–394.

Joshi, A. (2011). Community based screening and management of adolescent anaemiaanaemia in tribal areas of India key to reduction in maternal mortality. *Journal of Adolescent Health, 48*(2), Supplement 1:S23.

Joshi, A., Patnaik, B., & Sinha, D. (2017). Demanding accountability for hunger in India. In *Food riots, food rights and the politics of provisions* (pp. 116–135). Routledge.

Kabagambe, E. K., Baylin, A., Allan, D. A., Siles, X., Spiegelman, D., & Hannia, C. (2001). Application of the method of triads to evaluate the performance of food frequency questionnaires and biomarkers as indicators of long-term dietary intake. *American Journal of Epidemiology,154,* 1126e35.

Kabeer, N. (1999). Resources, agency, achievements: Reflections on the measurement of Women's empowerment. *Development and Change, 30*(3), 435–464. https://doi.org/10.1111/1467-7660.00125

Kamath, R., Majeed, J. A., Chandrasekaran, V., & Pattanshetty, S. M. (2013). Prevalence of anaemia among tribal women of reproductive age in Udupi Taluk, Karnataka. *Journal of Family Medicine and Primary Care, 2*(4), 345–348. https://doi.org/10.4103/2249-4863.123881

Kampman, B., Brouwer, F., & Schepers, B. (2008). *Agricultural land availability and demand in 2020. A global analysis of drivers and demand for feedstock and agricultural land availability*. CE Delft.

Kane, R. L., Ouslander, J. G., & Abrass, I. B. (1995). *Essentials of clinical geriatrics* (3rd ed.). McGraw-Hill.

Kar, B. R., Rao, S. L., & Chandramouli, B. A. (2008). Cognitive development in children with chronic protein energy malnutrition. *Behavioral and Brain Functions, 4*, 31.

Katz, E. (1997). The intrahousehold economics of exit and voice. *Feminist Economics, 3*(3), 25–46.

Kaushik, J. S., Narang, M., & Parakh, A. (2011). Fast food consumption in Children. *Indian Pediatrics, 48*, 97–101.

Keese, M., Hirsch, D., & Bednarzik, R. (2006). *Live longer, work longer*. OECD.

Kendrick, S., & Conway, M. (2006). Demographic and social change: Implication for use of acute care services by older people in Scotland. *European Journal of Population, 22*, 281–307.

Kennedy, E., Tessema, M., Hailu, T., et al. (2015). Multisector nutrition program governance and implementation in Ethiopia: Opportunities and challenges. *Food and Nutrition Bulletin, 36*, 534–548.

Kevane, M. (2000). Extrahousehold norms and intrahousehold bargaining: Gender in Sudan and Burkina Faso. In A. Spring (Ed.), *Women farmers and commercial ventures: Increasing food security in developing countries*. Lynne Rienner Publishers.

Khan, J., & Mohanty, S. K. (2018). Spatial heterogeneity and correlates of child undernutrition in districts of India. *BMC Public Health, 18,* 1027.

Khanna, A., Goyal, R. S., & Bhawsar, R. (2005). Menstrual practices and reproductive problems: A study of adolescent girls in Rajasthan. *Journal of Health Management, 7*(1), 91–107.

Khera, R. (2017). *Impact of Aadhaar in welfare programmes*. Available at SSRN 3045235.

Kim, Y., & Sherraden, M. (2011). Do parental assets matter for children's educational attainment?: Evidence from mediation tests. *Children and Youth Services Review, 33*(6), 969–979.

Kishor, S. (1999). *Women's empowerment and contraceptive use in Egypt*. Paper presented at the Annual Meetings of the Population Association of America, March, New York.

Klebanoff, M., Shiono, P., Selby, J., Trachtenberg, A., & Graubard, B. (1991). Anaemia and spontaneous preterm birth. *American Journal of Obstetrics and Gynecology, 164*, 59–63.

Koblinsky, M., Anwar, I., Mridha, M. K., et al. (2008). Reducing maternal mortality and improving maternal health: Bangladesh and MDG 5. *Journal of Health, Population and Nutrition, 26*, 280–294.

Kondrup, J., Allison, S. P., Elia, M., Vellas, B., & Plauth, M. (2003). ESPEN guidelines for nutrition screening. *Clinical Nutrition, 22*, 415–421.

Kotecha, P. V. (2011). Nutritional anaemia in young children with focus on Asia and India. *Indian Journal of Community Medicine: Official Publication of Indian Association of Preventive & Social Medicine, 36*(1), 8–16. https://doi.org/10.4103/0970-0218.80786

Krishna, V (2016). e Maharashtra nutrition mission. *Seminar, 681*.

Kugelberg, S., Jönsson, K., & Yngve, A. (2012). Understanding the process of establishing a food and nutrition policy: The case of Slovenia. *Health Policy, 107*, 91–97.

Kumar, N., & Quisumbing, A. (2012). Beyond "Death do us part": The long-term implications of divorce perceptions on women's well-being and child schooling in rural Ethiopia. *World Development, 40* (12), 2478–2489.

Kumud, K., & Priyanka, K. (2020). Demographical determinants associated with undernutrition and anaemia among tribal women of Malkangiri District of Odisha: A cross sectional survey. *European Journal of Molecular & Clinical Medicine, 7*(8), 2738–2749.

Lahoti, R., Basole, A., Abraham, R., Kesar, S., & Nath, P. (2020). Hunger grows as India's lockdown kills jobs: Results of a survey from 12 states. *The India Forum*. https://www.theindiaforum.in/article/hunger-grows-india-s-lockdown-kills-jobs

Lal, R. (2020). *Home gardening and urban agriculture for advancing food and nutritional security in response to the COVID-19 pandemic*. https://doi.org/10.1007/s12571-020-01058-3

Lancet. (2013). Executive summary of the Lancet maternal and child nutrition series. *The Lancet*.

Lanker, C., Yonzan, N., Mahler, D. G., Aguilar, A. C., & Wu, H. (2021). *Updated estimates of the impact of COVID-19 on global poverty: Looking back at 2020 and the outlook for 2021*. World Bank Blogs.

Lansey, S., Waslien, C., Mulvihill, M., & Fillit, H. (1993). The role of anthropometry in the assessment of malnutrition in the hospitalized frail elderly. *Gerontology, 39*, 346–353.

Lapping, K., Frongillo, E. A., Studdert, L. J., et al. (2012). Prospective analysis of the development of the national nutrition agenda in Vietnam from 2006 to 2008. *Health Policy and Planning, 27*, 32–41.

Larrea, C., & Freire, W. (2002). Social inequality and child malnutrition in four Aden countries. *Revista Panamericana De Salud Publica, 11*, 356–364.

Laxmaiah, K. M., Rao, R. H., Kumar, N., Arlappa, K. V., & Brahmam, G. N. V. (2007). Diet and nutritional status of tribal population in ITDA project areas of Khammam District, Andhra Pradesh. *Journal of Human Ecology, 21*(2), 79–86. https://doi.org/10.1080/09709274.2007.11905954

Lee, D. R. (2005). Agricultural sustainability and technology adoption: Issues and policies for developing countries. *American Journal of Agricultural Economics, 87*, 1325–1334.

Lee, G. (1985). Kinship and social support of the elderly: The case of the United States. *Ageing and Society, 5*, 19–38.

Lee, J. S., & Frongillo, E. A. (2001). Factors associated with food insecurity among U.S. elderly persons: Importance of functional impairments. *Journal of Gerontology, 56*, S94–S99.

Lesener, T., Gusy, B., & Wolter, C. (2019). The job demands-resources model: A meta-analytic review of longitudinal studies. *Work and Stress, 33*, 76–103.

Levinson, F. J., Balarajan, Y., & Marini, A. (2013). *Addressing undernutrition multisectorally: What have we learned from recent international experience*. UNICEF and MDG Achievement Fund.

Levitt, E. J., Pelletier, D. L., Dufour, C., et al. (2011). Harmonizing agriculture and health sector actions to improve household nutrition: Policy experiences from Afghanistan (2002–2007). *Food Security, 3*, 363–381.

Levitt, E. J., Pelletier, D. L., & Pell, A. N. (2009). Revisiting the UNICEF malnutrition framework to foster agriculture and health sector collaboration to reduce malnutrition: A comparison of stakeholder priorities for action in Afghanistan. *Food Policy, 34*, 156–165. https://doi.org/10.1016/j.foodpol.2008.07.004

Lievre, A., et al. (2007). Healthy working life expectancies at age 50 in Europe: A new indicator. *Journal of Nutrition, Health and Ageing, 11*(6), 508–514.

Loke, V. (2013). Parental asset accumulation trajectories and children's college outcomes. *Economics of Education Review, 33*, 124–133.

MacKinnon, R. (2002). Social risk management: A conceptual fallacy of composition. *Risk Management, 4*(2–3), 21–31.

Mahadevia, D. (2000). Health for all in Gujarat: Is it achievable? *Economic and Political Weekly, 35* (35/36), 3193–3197+3199–3204

Maiti, S., Unisa, S., & Agrawal, P. K. (2005). Health care and health among tribal women in Jharkhand: A situational analysis. *Studies of Tribes and Tribals, 3* (1), 37–46. https://doi.org/10.1080/0972639X.2005.11886518

Majid, N. (2004). *Reaching millennium goals: How well does agricultural productivity growth reduce poverty?* Employment Strategy Paper No. 12; International Labour Organization.

Majumdar, D. N. (1973). *A glimpse of Garo politics in North Eastern affairs*. Longman.

Malhotra, A., & Schuler, S. R. (2005). Women's empowerment as a variable in international development. *Measuring Empowerment: Cross-Disciplinary Perspectives, 1*, 71–88.

Malthus, T. R. (1798). *An essay on the principle of population, as it affects the future improvement of society*. Printed for J. Johnson.

Mangin, D., Sweeney, K., & Heath, I. (2007). Preventive care in elderly people needs rethinking. *British Medical Journal, 335*, 285–287.

Marmot, M., Allen, J., Goldblatt, P., Boyce, T., McNeish, D., Grady, M., & Geddes, I. (2010). *Fair society, healthy lives*. The Marmot Review. University College London.

Martins, V. J. B., Toledo Florêncio, T. M. M., Grillo, L. P., et al. (2011). Long-lasting effects of undernutrition. *International Journal of Environmental Research and Public Health, 8*, 1817–1846.

Martorell, R. (1996). The role of nutrition in economic development. *Nutrition Reviews, 54*, S66-71.

Mary, S. (2018). How much does economic growth contribute to child stunting reductions? *Economies, 6*, 55.

Maslow, A. (1954). *Motivation and personality* (3rd ed.). Addison-Wesley.

Mason, K. (1986). The status of women: Conceptual and methodological issues in demographic studies. *The Eastern Sociological Society, 1*(2), 284–300.

Mason, K. (1993). The impact of women's position on demographic change during the course of development. In N. Federici, K. Mason, & S. Sogner (Eds.), *Women's position and demographic change*. Clarendon Press.

Mathur, O. P. (2014). *Urban poverty in Asia*. Asian Development Bank. https://www.adb.org/sites/default/files/publication/59778/urban-poverty-asia.pdf

McDonald, B. L. (2010). *Food security*. Polity Press.

McElroy, M. (1990). The empirical content of Nash-bargained household behavior. *Journal of Human Resources, 25*(4), 559–583.

McElroy, M., & Horney, M. (1981). Nash-bargained household decisions: Toward a new generalization of the theory of demand. *International Economic Review, 22*(2), 333–349.

McGovern, M. E., Krishna, A., Aguayo, V. M., et al. (2017). A review of the evidence linking child stunting to economic outcomes. *International Journal of Epidemiology, 46*, 1171–1191.

Mejia-Costa, A. (2011). *Examining the political, institutional and governance aspects of delivering a national multi-sectoral response to reduce maternal and child undernutrition*. Institute of Development Studies.

Meija-Costa, A., & Fanzo, J. (2012). *Fighting maternal and child undernutrition: Analysing the political and institutional determinants of delivering a national multisectoral response in six countries*. Institute of Development Studies.

Mejía Acosta, A., & Haddad, L. (2014). The politics of success in the fight against undernutrition in Peru. *Food Policy, 44*, 26–35.

Mejía-Guevara, I., Corsi, D. J., Perkins, J. M., et al. (2018). Variation in anthropometric status and growth failure in low-and middle-income countries. *Pediatrics, 141*(3), e20172183. https://doi.org/10.1542/peds.2017-2183

Menon, N., Van Der Meulen Rodgers, Y., & Nguyen, H. (2014). Women's land rights and children's human capital in Vietnam. *World Development, 2014*(54), 18–31.

Ministry of Consumer Affairs, Food & Public Distribution, Government of India. (2015). National Food Security Act (NFSA), 2013. Food & Public Distribution. http://dfpd.nic.in/nfsa-act.htm

Ministry of Health and Family Welfare (MoHFW). (2016). *Annual report 2015–16, Chapter 3 Maternal and adolescent healthcare* (p. 26). Department of Health and Family Welfare.

Ministry of Health and Family Welfare and Ministry of Tribal Affair. (2018). *Tribal health in India: Bridging the gap and roadmap for the future*. http://nhm.gov.in/nhm_components/tribal_report/Executive_Summary.pdf

Ministry of Home Affairs, Govt. of India. (2010). *Sample registration system statistical report* (pp. 11–28).

Ministry of Human Resource Development (MHRD). (1993). *National nutrition policy* (pp. 3–6). Department of Women and Child Development.

Ministry of Human Resource and Development. (2015). *Performance audit of mid day meal scheme (2009–10 to 2013–14)*. Report No. 36 of the Comptroller and Auditor General of India.

Ministry of Statistics and Program Implementation, GOI. (2018). *Periodic Labor Force Survey*.

Ministry of Women and Child Development, Government of India. (2019). *POSHAN Abhiyaan (National Nutrition Mission)*. Ministry of Women and Child Development, Government of India. https://icds-wcd.nic.in/nnm/home.htm

Ministry of Women and Child Development. 'Universal Food Fortication', Press Information Bureau, 5 August 2016.

Mishell, D. R. (1993). Noncontraceptive benefits of oral contraceptives. *Journal of Reproductive Medicine, 38* (Suppl. 12), 1021–1029.

Mistry, R., Galal, O., & Lu, M. (2009). Women's autonomy and pregnancy care in rural India: A contextual analysis. *Social Science and Medicine, 69* (6), 926–933. https://doi.org/10.1016/j.socscimed.2009.07.008

Mittal, P. C., & Srivastava, S. (2006). Diet, nutritional status and food related traditions of Oraon tribes of New Mal (West Bengal), India. *Rural and Remote Health, 6*(1), 385.

MIYCN-FP Integration Technical Working Group. (2011). *Systematic review of integration of maternal, neonatal, and child health and nutrition and family planning*. USAID.

Mohanty, S. K., & Pathak, P. K. (2008). Rich-poor gap in utilization of reproductive and child health services in India. *Journal of Bio Social Science, 41*(03), 381–398.

Mohmand, S. K. (2012). *Policies without politics: Analysing nutrition governance in India*. Analysing Nutrition Governance: India Country Report.

Montgomery, M. A., & Elimelech, M. (2007). Water and sanitation in developing countries: Including health in the equation. *Environmental Science and Technology, 41*(1), 17–24.

Moodie, R., Daube, M., Carnell, K., Connors, C., Larkin, S., Roberts, L., Segal, L., Selvey, L., & Zimmet, P. (2009). *Australia: The healthiest country by 2020 National Preventative Health Strategy—The roadmap for action*. Australian Government Preventative Health Taskforce.

Morley, J. E. (1986). Nutritional status of the elderly. *American Journal of Medicine, 81*, 679e95.

Mosley, H., & Chen, L. C. (1984). An analytical framework for the study of child survival in developing countries. *Population and Development Review, 10* (Suppl.), 25–45.

MoSPI. (2016). *Statistical year book India 2016, Chapter 45 Millennium development goals*.

Mshida, H. A., Kassim, N., Mpolya, E., & Kia, M. (2018). Water, sanitation, and hygiene practices associated with nutritional status of under-five children in semi-pastoral communities Tanzania. *American Journal of Tropical Medicine and Hygiene, 98*, 1242–1249.

Murray, C. J. L., & Lopez, A. D. (1996). *The global burden of disease* (p. 270). World Health Organization.

Murthi, M., Guio, A.-C., & Dreze, J. (1995). *Mortality, fertility and gender bias in India: A district level analysis*. The Development Economics Research Programme, No. 61, London School of Economics.

Murty, J. S., & Ramesh, A. (1978). Selection intensities among the tribal population of Adilabad district, Andhra Pradesh. *Society of Biology, 25*, 302–305.

Naher, F., Barkat-e-Khuda, A. S. S., & Hossain, M. (2014). How nutrition-friendly are agriculture and health policies in Bangladesh? *Food and Nutrition Bulletin, 35*(1), 133–146.

Naik, R. R. K., & Venkatesha, K. R. (2019). Prevalence of nutritional anaemia in pediatric age group a cross sectional study. *International Journal of Pediatric Research, 6*(01), 17–21. https://doi.org/10.17511/ijpr.2019.i01.03

Nankinga, O., & Aguta, D. (2019). Determinants of Anaemia among women in Uganda: Further analysis of the Uganda demographic and health surveys. *BMC Public Health, 19*(1), 1–9.

Narula, S. (2005). The right to food: Holding global actors accountable under international law. *Columbia Journal of Transnational Law, 44*, 691.

Natalicchio, M., Garrett, J., Mulder-Sibanda, M., et al. (2009). *Carrots and sticks: The political economy of nutrition policy reforms*. World Bank.

Natarajan, V. S., Meclenan, W. J., & Hall, M. R. P. (1995). High prevalence of nutritional disorders and nutrient deficits in the elderly in a rural community in Tamil Nadu, India. *Antiseptic, 92,* 105e8.

Nathan, S. A., Develin, E., Grove, N., et al. (2005). An Australian childhood obesity summit: The role of data and evidence in 'public' policy making. *Australia and New Zealand Health Policy, 2*, 17.

NCD Risk Factor Collaboration (NCS-RisC). (2017). Worldwide trends in body-mass index, underweight, overweight, and obesity from 1975 to 2016: A pooled analysis of 2416 population-based measurement studies in 1289 million children, adolescents, and adults. *Lancet, 390*, 2627–2642.

NCD Risk Factor Collaboration (NCS-RisC). (2019). Rising rural body-mass index is the main driver of the global obesity epidemic in adults. *Nature, 569*, 260–264.

Nellemann, C., Macdevetta, M., Manders, T., Eickhout, B., Svihus, B., Prins, A. G., & Kaltenborn, B. P. (2019). *The environmental food crisis: The environment's role in averting future food crises*. A UNEP Rapid Response Assessment; United Nations Environment Programme, GRID-Arendal. Retrieved June 2, 2021, from http://www.grida.no/publications/154

Ng, M., Fleming, T., Robinson, M., et al. (2014). Global, regional, and national prevalence of overweight and obesity in children and adults during 1980–2013: A systematic analysis for the Global Burden of Disease Study 2013. *The Lancet,* 384(9945). www.thelancet.com/journals/lancet/article/PIIS0140-6736(14)60460-8/fulltext

Nguyen, P. H., Sanghvi, T., Kim, S. S., Tran, L. M., Afsana, K., Mahmud, Z., et al. (2017). Factors influencing maternal nutrition practices in a large scale maternal, newborn and child health program in Bangladesh. *PLoS ONE, 12*(7), e0179873. https://doi.org/10.1371/journal.pone.0179873

Nikolaus, T., Specht-Leible, N., & Bach, M. (1999). A randomized trial of comprehensive geriatric assessment and home intervention in the care of hospitalized patients. *Age and Ageing, 28*, 543–550.

NIMS, ICMR and UNICEF. (2016). *Infant and child mortality in India levels, trends and determinants, fact sheet*. Ministry of Health and Family Welfare. Annual Report 2015–16.

Nisar, N., Qadri, M. H., Fatima, K., & Perveen, S. J. (2009). Dietary habits and life style among the students of a Private Medical University, Karachi. *Journal of Pakistan Medical Association, 59*, 98–101.

Nisbett, N., Wach, E., Haddad, L., et al. (2015). What drives and constrains effective leadership in tackling child undernutrition? Findings from Bangladesh, Ethiopia, India and Kenya. *Food Policy, 53*, 33–45.

NITI Aayog. (2017). *A concept note on The National Consultation on SDG 2—Zero Hunger "End hunger, achieve food security and improved nutrition and promote sustainable agriculture"*. NITI Aayog, Government of India.

NITI Aayog. (2021). *SDG India index 7 dashboard: Partnerships in the decade of action*. NITI Aayog, Government of India.

Nixon, A. E., Mazzola, J. J., Bauer, J., et al. (2011). Can work make you sick? A meta-analysis of the relationships between job stressors and physical symptoms. *Work and Stress, 25*(1), 1–22.

Noleppa, S., von Witzke, H., & Cartsburg, M. (2013). *The social, economic and environmental value of agricultural productivity in the European Union*. Impacts on Markets and Food Security, Rural Income and Employment, Resource Use, Climate Protection, and Biodiversity HFFA Working Paper No. 3; Humboldt Forum for Food and Agriculture e.V. (HFFA).

Nolte, E., & McKee, M. (Eds.). (2008). *Caring for people with chronic conditions. A health system perspective*. Open University Press.

Nowjack-Raymer, R. E., & Sheiham, A. (2003). Association of edentulism and diet and nutrition in US adults. *Journal of Dental Research, 82*(2), 123–126. https://doi.org/10.1177/154405910308200209

NSO. (2021). *Elderly in India*. National Statistical Office, Ministry of Statistics & Programme Implementation, Government of India.

Nutritional Institute for Health and Clinical Excellence (NICE). (2006). *Nutritional support in adults*. NICE.

O'Connell, S. A., & Smith, C. (2016). Economic growth and child undernutrition. *The Lancet Global Health, 4*, e901–e902.

O'Neil, D., Hastie, I., & Williams, B. (2004). Developing specialist healthcare for older people: A challenge for the European Union. *Journal of Nutrition, Health andAging, 8*, 109–112.

Ocke, M., & Kaaks, R. (1997). Biochemical markers as additional measurements in dietary validity studies: Application of the method of triads with examples from the European prospective investigation into cancer and nutrition. *American Journal of Clinical Nutrition, 65*, 1240Se5S.

Ogutu, A. (2015). *Integrating maternal, infant, and young child nutrition and family planning services in Bondo sub-county, Kenya*. Jhpiego.

Oliveira Martins, J., et al. (2005). *The impact of ageing on demand, factor markets and growth economies*. OECD.

Onishi, N. (2004). *Love of U.S. food shortening Okinawans' lives/life expectancy among islands' young men takes a big dive* (p. 4). New York Times.

Ortiz-Ospina, E., & Roser, M. (2019). *Global extreme poverty*. Our World Data, 2019. https://ourworldindata.org/extreme-poverty

Osamor, P. E., & Grady, C. (2016). Women's autonomy in health care decision-making in developing countries: A synthesis of the literature. *International Journal of Women's Health, 8*, 191. https://doi.org/10.2147/IJWH.S105483

Osler, M., & Schroll, M. (1997). Diet and mortality in a cohort of elderly people in a north European community. *International Journal of Epidemiology, 26*, 155e9.

Otsuka, K. (2013). Food insecurity, income inequality, and the changing comparative advantage in world agriculture. *Agricultural Economics, 44*, 7–18.

Oxley, H. (2009). *Policies for healthy ageing: An overview*. OECD.

Pan, Y. (2019). Food quality and health. 3rd World Congress on Food Tech 2019 May 13–14, 2019. Advances in Food Science, Processing and Technology. *Journal of Food Processing & Technology, 10*. https://doi.org/10.4172/2157-7110-C2-112

Pandey, S. (2020). *Lockdown sees record spike in NREGA jobs, but 1.7 crore applicants fail to get one. The Print*. https://theprint.in/india/governance/lockdown-sees-record-spike-in-nrega-jobs-but-1-7-crore-applicants-fail-to-get-one/460818/

Pandey, V., Mahendra Dev, S., & Jayachandran, U. (2016). Impact of agricultural interventions on the nutritional status in South Asia: A review. *Food Policy, 62*, 28–40. https://doi.org/10.1016/j.foodpol.2016.05.002

Parris, B. (2008). Climate change threat to food security. *Global Future, 3*, 000–000.

Pasricha, S. R., Black, J., Muthayya, S., Shet, A., Bhat, V., Nagaraj, S., Prashanth, N. S., Sudarshan, H., Biggs, B. A., & Shet, A. S. (2010). Determinants of anaemiaanaemia among young children in rural India. *Pediatrics, 126*(1), e140–e149. https://doi.org/10.1542/peds.2009-3108

Patel, N. (2018). Figure of the week: Understanding poverty in Africa, *Brookings*, November 21, 2018.

Pawlak, R., & Bell, K. (2017). Iron status of vegetarian children: A review of literature. *Annals of Nutrition & Metabolism, 70*(2), 88–99. https://doi.org/10.1159/000466706

Pelletier, D., & Pelto, G. (2013). From efficacy research to large-scale impact on undernutrition: The role of organizational cultures. *Advances in Nutrition, 4*, 687–696.

Pelletier, D. L., Frongillo, E. A., Gervais, S., et al. (2012). Nutrition agenda setting, policy formulation and implementation: Lessons from the mainstreaming nutrition initiative. *Health Policy and Planning, 27*, 19–31.

Pelletier, D. L., Menon, P., Ngo, T., et al. (2011). The nutrition policy process: The role of strategic capacity in advancing national nutrition agendas. *Food and Nutrition Bulletin, 32*(Suppl), S59–69.

Perier, C., Triouleyre, P., Terrat, C., Chomette, M. C., Beauchet, O., & Gonthier, R. (2004). Energy and nutrient intake of elderly hospitalized patients in a steady metabolic status versus catabolic status. *Journal of Nutrition, Health and Aging, 8*, 518e20.

Perumal, N., Bassani, D. G., & Roth, D. E. (2018). Use and misuse of stunting as a measure of child health. *Journal of Nutrition, 148*, 311–315. https://doi.org/10.1093/jn/nxx064

Peters, D. H., Yazbeck, A. S., Sharma, R. R., Ramana, G. N. V., Pritchett, L. H., & Wagstaff, A. (2002). *Better health systems for India's Poor: Findings, analysis, and options*. The World Bank.

Pew Research Center. (2013). *Changing patterns of global migration and remittances*. Pew Research Center, December 2013.

Pickett, K. E., & Wilkinson, R. G. (2015). Income inequality and health: A causal review. *Social Science & Medicine, 128*, 316–326.

Pingali, P. (2015). Agricultural policy and nutrition outcomes—Getting beyond the preoccupation with staple grains. *Food Security, 7*, 583–591. https://doi.org/10.1007/s12571-015-0461-x

Pingali, P., Mittra, B., & Rahman, A. (2017). The bumpy road from food to nutrition security—Low evolution of India's food policy. *Global Food Security, 15*, 77–84. https://doi.org/10.1016/j.gfs.2017.05.002

Pinstrup-Andersen, P., & Pandya-Lorch, R. (1998). Food security and sustainable use of natural resources: A 2020 vision. *Ecological Economics, 26*, 1–10.

Pinstrup-Andersen, P., & Watson, D. D., II. (2011). *Food policy for developing countries: The role of government in global, national, and local food systems*. Cornell University Press.

Poel, V. D., & Speybroeck, N. (2009). Decomposing undernutrition inequalities between scheduled castes and tribes and the remaining Indian population. *Ethnicity and Health, 14*(3), 271–287. https://doi.org/10.1080/13557850802609931

Pratley, P. (2016). Associations between quantitative measures of women's empowerment and access to care and health status for mothers and their children: A systematic review of evidence from the developing world. *Social Science and Medicine, 169*, 119–131. https://doi.org/10.1016/j.socscimed.2016.08.001

Press Information Bureau. 'Bad quality food supply for Aanganwadis', 7 August 2013.

Preston, S. H. (1975). The changing relation between mortality and level of development. *Population Studies, 29*(2), 239–248.

Pretty, J., Toulmin, C., & Williams, S. (2011). Sustainable intensification in African agriculture. *International Journal of Agricultural Sustainability, 9*, 5–24.

Pretty, J. N. (1995). Participatory learning for sustainable agriculture. *World Development, 23*, 1247–1263.

Printice, A. M., & Jebb, S. A. (2003). Fast foods, energy density and obesity: A possible mechanistic link. *Obesity Reviews, 4*, 187–194.

Progress in Nutrition. (2010). In *6th Report on the world nutrition situation*. The United Nations System Standing Committee on Nutrition.

Qamra, S., Roy, J., & Mishra, D. (2009). *Food consumption pattern and associated habits of the Bhil Tribe of Dhar District of Madhya Pradesh*.

Quisumbing, A., & Maluccio, J. (2003). Resources at marriage and intra household allocation: Evidence from Bangladesh, Ethiopia, Indonesia, and South Africa. *Oxford Bulletin of Economics and Statistics, 3*(0305–9049), 283–327.

Raghavan, T. C. A. S. (2014). *India's agriculture yield suffers from low productivity*. The Mint.

Rahman, A. (2016). Universal food security program and nutritional intake: Evidence from the hunger prone KBK districts in Odisha. *Food Policy, 63*, 73–86.

Rahman, M. A., Rahman, M. S., Aziz Rahman, M., Szymlek-Gay, E. A., Uddin, R., & Islam, S. M. S. (2021). Prevalence of and factors associated with anaemia in women of reproductive age in Bangladesh, Maldives and Nepal: Evidence from nationally-representative survey data. PLoS ONE, *16*(1), e0245335. https://doi.org/10.1371/journal.pone.0245335. PMID: 33411804; PMCID: PMC7790421.

Rai, R. K., Kumar, S., Sekher, M., Pritchard, B., & Rammohan, A. (2014). A life-cycle approach to food and nutrition security in India. *Public Health Nutrition, 18*(5), 1–6. https://doi.org/10.1017/S1368980014001037

Raj, A., Saggurti, N., Winter, M., Labonte, A., Decker, M. R., Balaiah, D., & Silverman, J. G. (2010). The effect of maternal child marriage on morbidity and mortality of children under 5 in India: Cross sectional study of a nationally representative sample. *BMJ, 340*.

Rakesh, P. S. (2017). Prevalence of anaemia in Kerala State, Southern India—A systematic review. *Journal of Clinical and Diagnostic Research, JCDR, 11*(5), LE01–LE04. https://doi.org/10.7860/JCDR/2017/24681.9951

Ramachandran, V. K. (1997) On Kerala's development achievements. In J. Dreze & A. Sen (Eds.), *Indian development: Selected regional perspectives* (pp. 205–356). Oxford University Press.

Ramakrishnan, U., Lowe, A., Vir, S., Kumar, S., et al. (2012). Public health interventions, barriers, and opportunities for improving maternal nutrition in India. *Food and Nutrition Bulletin, 33*(supplement 2). The United Nations University.

Ramalingaswami, V., Jonsson, U., & Rohde, J. (1996a). *Commentary: The Asian enigma*.

Ramalingaswami, V., Jonsson, U., & Rohde, J. (1996b). *"The Asian Enigma," the progress of nations* (pp. 11–17). United Nations International Children's Emergency Fund.

Rammohan, A., Awofeso, N., & Robitaille, M.-C. (2012). Addressing female iron-deficiency anaemia in India: Is vegetarianism the major obstacle? *International Scholarly Research Notices, 2012*, Article ID 765476, 8 pp. https://doi.org/10.5402/2012/765476

Ranhoff, A., Gjøen, A., & Mowé, M. (2005). Screening for malnutrition in elderly acute medical patients: The usefulness of MNA-SF. *Journal of Nutrition, Health and Aging, 9*, 221e5.

Rao, T. S. S., Asha, M. R., Ramesh, B. N., & Rao, K. S. J. (2008). Understanding nutrition, depression and mental illnesses. *Indian Journal of Psychiatry, 50*(2), 77–82. https://doi.org/10.4103/0019-5545.42391

Ray, S., Chandra, J., Bhattacharjee, J., Sharma, S., & Agarwala, A. (2016). Determinants of nutritional anaemia in children less than five years age. *International Journal of Contemporary Pediatrics, 3*, 403–408.

Razavi, S. (2003). Introduction: Agrarian change, gender and land rights. *Journal of Agrarian Change, 2003*(3), 2–32.

Reddy, K. N., & Selvaraju, V. (1994). *Health care expenditure by Government in India, 1974–75 to 1990–91*. Seven Hills Publication.

Rehman, A., Ping, Q., & Razzaq, A. (2019). Pathways and associations between women's land ownership and child food and nutrition security in Pakistan. *International Journal of Environmental Research and Public Health, 2019*(16), 3360.

Reich, M., & Balarajan, Y. (2012). *Political economy analysis for food and nutrition security*. World Bank.

Reyes, H., Perez-Cuevas, R., Sandoval, A., Castillo, R., Santos, J. I., Doubova, S., & Gutierrez, G. (2004). The family as a determinant of stunting in children living in conditions of extreme poverty: A case-control study. *BMC Public Health, 4*, 57.

Riley, N. (1997). Gender, power, and population change. *Population Bulletin, 52*(1), 2–46.

Ritsatakis, A. (Ed.). (2008). *Demystifying the myths of ageing*. WHO Regional Office for Europe.

Rivers, H. H. (1973). *The Todas*. Macmillan.

Roberts, J. T. (2001). Global inequality and climate change. *Society & Natural Resources, 14*, 501±9. https://doi.org/10.1080/089419201184905002193201 5000309. PMID: 26440753.

Rockström, J., Steffen, W., Noone, K., Persson, Å., Chapin, F. S., III, Lambin, E. F., Lenton, T. M.,

Scheffer, M., Folke, C., Schellnhuber, H. J., et al. (2009). A safe operating space for humanity. *Nature, 461,* 472–475.

Rogers, B. (1996). The implications of female household headship for food consumption and nutritional status in the Dominican Republic. *World Development, 24* (1), 113–128.

Rokade, S., Mog, M., & Mondal, N. (2020). Nutritional status among tribal women in Maharashtra, India: Spatial variations and determinants. *Clinical Epidemiology and Global Health, 8.* https://doi.org/10.1016/j.cegh.2020.05.012

Roos, N. T., Shapiro, E., & Tate, R. (1989). Does a small minority of elderly account for a majority of health care expenditures? A sixteen year perspective. *The MilbankQuarterly, 67,* 347–356.

Rose, D., & Richards, R. (2004). Food store access and household fruit and vegetable use among participants in the U.S. Food Stamp Program. *Public Health Nutrition, 7,* 1081–1088.

Rosenthal, A. J., Sanders, K. M., McMurtry, C. T., Jacobs, M. A., Thompson, D. D., Gheorghiu, D., Little, K. L., & Adler, R. A. (1998). Is malnutrition overdiagnosed in older hospitalized patients? Association between the soluble interleukin-2 receptor and serum markers of malnutrition. *Journal of Gerontology, 2,* 81–86.

Roth, D. E., Krishna, A., Leung, M., Shi, J., et al. (2017). Early childhood linear growth faltering in low-income and middle-income countries as a whole population condition: Analysis of 179 demographic and health surveys from 64 countries (1993–2015). *Lancet Global Health, 5,* e1249–57. https://doi.org/10.1016/S2214-109X(17)30418-7

Roy, D., Kishore, A., Joshi, P. K., & Mishra, B. (2016). Pulses for food and nutritional security: The technology perspective. *Indian Society of Genetics and Plant Breeding, 76*(4), 375. https://doi.org/10.5958/0975-6906.2016.00057.2

Rudman, D., & Feller, A. G. (1989). Protein-caloric malnutrition in the nursing home. *Journal of the American Geriatrics Society, 37,* 173e83.

Ruel, M. T., Alderman, H., Maternal and Child Nutrition Study Group. (2013). Nutrition-sensitive interventions and programmes: How can they help to accelerate progress in improving maternal and child nutrition? *Lancet, 382,* 536–551.

Rundle, A., Neckerman, K., Freeman, L., Lovasi, G., Purciel, M., Quinn, J., Richards, C., Sircar, N., & Weiss, C. (2009). Neighborhood food environment and walkability predict obesity in New York City. *Environmental Health Perspectives, 117,* 442–447.

Sachdev, H. P. S. (2018). Undersized Indian children: Nutrients-starved or hungry for development? *Proceedings of the Indian National Science Academy.* Published online Nov 13. https://doi.org/10.16943/ptinsa/2018/49438

Sachs, J., Schmidt-Traub, G., Kroll, C., Lafortune, G., Fuller, G., & Woelm, F. (2020). *The sustainable development goals and COVID-19. Sustainable development report 2020.* Cambridge University Press.

Safilios-Rothschild, C. (1982). Female power, autonomy and demographic change in the Third World. In R. Ankar, M. Buvinic, & N. Youssef (Eds.), *Women's roles and population trends in the Third World.* Croom Helm.

Sample registration System. (2018). *SRS report.* Registrar General of India.

Sánchez, A. (2017). The structural relationship between early nutrition, cognitive skills and non-cognitive skills in four developing countries. *Economics and Human Biology, 27,* 33–54.

Schelleman, H., et al. (2004). Prevalence and determinants of undertreatment of hypertension in the Netherlands. *Journal of Human Hypertension, 18*(5), 317–324.

Scherhaufer, S., Moates, G., Hartikainen, H., et al. (2018). Environmental impacts of food waste in Europe. *Waste Management, 77,* 98–113.

Schloz, B., Gross, R., Schultink, W., & Sastroamidjojo, S. (1997). Anaemia is associated with reduced productivity of women workers even in physically-strenuous tasks. *British Journal of Nutrition, 77,* 47–57.

Schneider, M. (2016). Dragon head enterprises and the State of Agribusiness in China. *Journal of Agrarian Change, 17*(1), 3–21. https://doi.org/10.1111/joac.12151

Scrimshaw, N. (1991). Iron deficiency. *Scientific American, 4,* 46–52.

Scroll. (2020). *100 million Indians fall through gaps in food safety net, economists urge rethink on Covid-19 relief.* https://scroll.in/article/959235/100-million-indians-fall-through-gaps-in-food-safety-neteconomists-urge-rethink-on-covid-19-relief

Sen, A. (1985). Well-being, agency and freedom: The Dewey Lectures 1984. *Journal of Philosophy, 82*(4), 169–221.

Sen, A. (1990). Gender and cooperative conflicts. In I. Tinker (Ed.), *Persistent inequalities: Women in world development.* Oxford University Press.

Sen, G., & Batliwala, S. (2000). Empowering women for reproductive rights. In H. Presser & G. Sen (Eds.), *Women's empowerment and demographic processes.* Oxford University Press.

Sendhilkumar, M., & Muthuperumal, P. (2017). Ethnography of Koya Tribe in Eastern Ghats—Holistic approach. *International Journal of Innovative Research in Computer and Communication Engineering, 6,* 8516. https://doi.org/10.15680/IJIRSET.2017.0605204

Sethuramanb Sivakumar, P., et al. (2015). *Food consumption patterns of North Eastern Communities.* https://agritech.tnau.ac.in/itk/indi_farm_food_consumption.html

Shadap, A. M. W. K., & Pala, V. (2017). Nutritional intake and consumption pattern in the states of Himachal Pradesh and Meghalaya. *The NEHU Journal, 15*(2), 15–28.

Shaheen, L. S. E., & Vieira, K. F. (2008). Nutritional therapies for mental disorders. *Nutrition Journal, 7*, 2.

Shankar, B., Agrawal, S., Beaudreault, A. R., et al. (2017). Dietary and nutritional change in India: Implications for strategies, policies, and interventions. *Annals of the New York Academy of Sciences, 1395*, 49–59.

Shanks, T. R. W. (2007). The impacts of household wealth on child development. *Journal of Poverty, 11* (2), 93–116.

Shariff, A., & Ahn, N. (1995). Mother's education effect on child health: An econometric analysis of child anthropometry in Uganda. *Indian Economic Review, 30*(2), 203–222.

Sharma, H. (2020). *Only 13% of allocated free food grain handed out to returning migrant workers, reveals govt data. Indian Express*. https://indianexpress.com/article/india/only-13-of-allocated-free-food-grain-handed-out-to-returning-migrant-workers-reveals-govt-data-6485982/

Silva, G. (2018). *Feeding the world in 2050 and beyond —Part 1: Productivity challenges*. Michigan State University Extension—3 December 2018. Retrieved June 2, 2021 from https://www.canr.msu.edu/news/feeding-the-world-in-2050-and-beyond-part-1

Simcox, J. A., & McClain, D. A. (2013). Iron and diabetes risk. *Cell Metabolism, 17*(3), 329–341.

Singh, A. (2014). Why are economic growth and reductions in child undernutrition so weakly correlated—And what can public policy do? *The Lancet Global Health, 2*, e185–e186.

Singh, S. (2018). Doubling farmers' incomes mechanisms and challenges. *Economic & Political Weekly, lIiI*(7).

Sinha, D. (2020a). Hunger and food security in the times of Covid-19. *Journal of Social and Economic Development*. https://doi.org/10.1007/s40847-020-00124-y

Sinha, D. (2020b). *That foodgrain stocks lie in public godowns while people are going hungry is a scandal*. Indian Express. https://indianexpress.com/article/opinion/columns/india-coronavirus-lockdown-foodstock-supply-pds-scheme-6476514/

Skegg, D. C. (1999). Safety and efficacy of fertility-regulating methods: A decade of research. *Bulletin of the World Health Organization, 77*, 713–721.

Sleddens, E. F., Kroeze, W., Kohl, L. F., Bolten, L. M., Velema, E., Kaspers, P. J., et al. (2015). Determinants of dietary behavior among youth: An umbrella review. *International Journal of Behavioral Nutrition and Physical Activity, 12*, 7.

Slotzfus, R. J., Dreyfuss, M. L., Nutrition Foundation; INCAG. (1998). *Guidelines for the Iron Supplements to prevent and treat iron-deficiency anaemiaanaemia: A draft document prepared for the International Nutritional AnaemiaAnaemia Consultative Group (INCAG)*, 17th July 1997.

Smetana, S. M., Bornkessel, S., & Heinz, V. (2019). A path from sustainable nutrition to nutritional sustainability of complex food systems. *Frontiers in Nutrition, 6*, 39.

Smith, L., Ramakrishnan, U., Ndiaye, A., Haddad, L., & Martorell, R. (2003). *The importance of women's status for child nutrition in developing countries*. International Food Policy Research Institute, Department of International Health, Emory University.

Smith, L. C., & Haddad, L. J. (2015). Reducing child undernutrition: Past drivers and priorities for the post-MDG era. *World Development, 68*, 180–204.

Smutka, L., Steininger, M., Maitah, M., & Škubna, O (2015). The Czech Agrarian Foreign Trade—Ten years after the EU accession. In L. Smutka, & H. Rezbová (Eds.), *Agrarian Perspectives XXIV: Proceedings of the 24th International Scientific Conference, Czech University of Life Sciences Prague*, Faculty of Economics and Management, Prague, Czech Republic, 16–18 September 2015 (pp. 385–392). CAB Direct.

Smutka, L., Steininger, M., & Miffek, O. (2009). World agricultural production and consumption. *Agris On-line Papers in Economics and Informatics, 1*, 3–12.

Smyth, S. J., Phillips, P. W. B., & Kerr, W. A. (2015). Food security and the evaluation of risk. *Global Food Security, 4*, 16–23.

Spears, D. (2013). *How much international variation in child height can sanitation explain?* Policy Research Working Paper, World Bank.

Spears, D., Ghosh, A., & Cumming O. (2013). *Correction: Open defecation and childhood stunting in India: An ecological analysis of new data from 112 districts.*

Spector, P. E., & Jex, S. M. (1998). Development of four self-report measures of job stressors and strain: Interpersonal conflict at work scale, organizational constraints scale, and quantitative workload inventory. *Journal of Occupational Health Psychology, 3*(4), 356–367.

Steinberg, B., et al. (2008). Nine-year trends in achievement of risk factor goals in the US and European outpatients with cardiovascular disease. *American HeartJournal, 156*(4), 719–727.

Stevens, G. A., Finucane, M. M., De-Regil, L. M., Paciorek, C. J., Flaxman, S. R., Branca, F., Nutrition Impact Model Study Group. (2013). Global, regional, and national trends in haemoglobin concen-tration and prevalence of total and severe anaemia in children andpregnant and non-pregnant women for 1995–2011: A systematicanalysis of population-representative data. *The Lancet Global Health, 1*(1), e16–e25.

Stevens, G. A., Finucane, M. M., Paciorek, C. J., Flaxman, S. R., White, R. A., Donner, A. J., et al. (2012). Trends in mild, moderate, and severe stunting and underweight, and progress towards MDG 1 in 141 developing countries: A systematic analysis of population representative data. *Lancet, 380*(9844), 824–834.

Stiller, C. K., Golembiewski, S. K. E., Golembiewski, M., Mondal, S., Biesalski, H.-K., & Scherbaum, V. (2020). Prevalence of undernutrition and anaemia among Santal Adivasi Children, Birbhum District, West Bengal, India. *International Journal of*

Environmental Research and Public Health, 17(1), 342. MDPI AG. https://doi.org/10.3390/ijerph17010342

Stocking, M. A. (2003). Tropical soils and food security: The next 50 years. *Science, 302,* 1356–1359.

Stratton, R. J., Hackston, A., & Longmore, D., et al. (2004). Malnutrition in hospital outpatients and inpatients: Prevalence, concurrent validity and ease of use of the "Malnutrition Universal Screening Tool" (MUST) for adults. *British Journal of Nutrition, 92,* 799–808.

Strauss, J., & Thomas, D. (1995). Human resources: Empirical modeling of household and family decisions. In *Handbook of development economics* (Vol. 3). Elsevier.

Streicher, M., Zwienen-Pot, J., Bardon, L., Nagel, G., Teh, R., Meisinger, C., Colombo, M., Torbahn, G., Kiesswetter, E., Flechtner-Mors, M., et al. (2018). Determinants of incident malnutrition in community dwelling older adults: A MaNuEL multicohort meta-analysis. *Journal of the American Geriatrics Society, 66,* 2335–2343.

Suhrcke, M., et al. (2006). Investment in health could be good for Europe's economies. *British Medical Journal, 333,* 1017–1019.

Suhrcke, M., et al. (Eds.). (2008). *The economic costs of ill health in the European Region*. Copenhagen.

Sundar, R. (1995). *Household survey of health care utilisation and expenditure*. Working Paper No. 53, National Council of Applied Economic Research.

Sunny, J., Bheemeshwar, R. A., & Mayank, A. (2018). Child undernutrition in India: Assessment of prevalence, decline and disparities. *Economic and Political Weekly, 53,* 63–69.

Suri, S. (2019). Breakout nation: The nutrition transformation of Bangladesh. *ORF Issue Brief, 323.*

Swaminathan, M. S. (2001). Food security and sustainable development. *Current Science, 81,* 948–954.

Symreng, T., Anderberg, B., Kagedal, B., Norr, A., Schildt, B., & Sjodahl, R. (1983). Nutritional assessment and clinical course in 112 elective surgical patients. *Acta Chirurgica Scandinavica, 149,* 657–662.

Tabloski, P. A. (2006). Nutrition and ageing. In P. A. Tabloski (Ed.), *Gerontological nursing* (p. 110e46). Prentice Hall.

Tangka, F. K., Jabbar, M. A., & Shapiro, B. I. (2000). *Gender roles and child nutrition in livestock production systems in developing countries: A critical review*. Socio-economics and Policy Research Working Paper 27. International Livestock Research Institute.

Taylor, P. (2004). Age and work: International perspectives. *Social Policy and Society, 3*(2), 163–170.

Taylor, S. A., Perez-Ferrer, C., Griffiths, A., et al. (2015). Scaling up nutrition in fragile and conflict-affected states: The pivotal role of governance. *Social Science and Medicine, 126,* 119–127.

Teshale, A. B., Tesema, G. A., Worku, M. G., Yeshaw, Y., & Tessema, Z. T. (2020). Anaemia and its associated factors among women of reproductive age in eastern Africa: A multilevel mixed-effects generalized linear model. *PLoS ONE, 15*(9), e0238957. https://doi.org/10.1371/journal.pone.0238957

Thang, N. M., & Popkin, B. M. (2003). In an era of economic growth, is inequity holding back reduction in child malnutrition in Vietnam? *Asian Journal of Clinical Nutrition, 12,* 405–410.

Thomas, D. (1997). Incomes, expenditures, and health outcomes: Evidence in intrahousehold resource allocation. In L. Haddad, J. Hoddinott, & H. Alderman (Eds.), *Intrahousehold resource allocation in developing countries: Models, methods and policy* (pp. 142–164). Johns Hopkins University Press.

Thow, A. M., Kadiyala, S., Kandelwal, S., Menon, P. D., & Reddy, K. S. (2016). Toward food policy for the dual burden of malnutrition: An exploratory policy space analysis in India. *Food and Nutrition Bulletin, 37*(3), 261–274.

Thow, A. M., Swinburn, B., Colagiuri, S., et al. (2010). Trade and food policy: Case studies from three Pacific Island countries. *Food Policy, 35,* 556–564.

Thuluvath, P. J., & Triger, D. R. (1995). How valid are or reference standards of nutrition? *Nutrition, 6,* 731–733.

Tilman, D., Balzer, C., Hill, J., & Befort, B. L. (2011). Global food demand and the sustainable intensification of agriculture. *Proceedings of the National Academy of Sciences of the United States of America, 108,* 20260–20264.

Times of India. *Grains rotting with FCI could have fed 8L for a year*, 2 May 2016.

Townsend, M. S., Peerson, J., Love, B., Achterberg, C., & Murphy, S. P. (2001). Food insecurity is positively related to overweight in women. *Journal of Nutrition, 131*(6), 1738–1745.

Tripathi, M., et al. (2014). Perceived responsibilities and operational diculties of anganwadi workers at a coastal south Indian city. *Medical Journal, D.Y. Patil University, 7*(4), 468–472.

Uche-Nwachi, E. O., Odekunle, A., Jacinto, S., et al. (2010). Anaemia in pregnancy: Associations with parity, abortions and child spacing in primary healthcare clinic attendees in Trinidad and Tobago. *African Health Sciences, 10,* 66–70.

UN. (1998). task force for epidemiological research on reproductive health, United Nations. Effects of contraceptives on hemoglobin and ferritin. *Contraception, 58,* 262–273.

UN. (2015a). *India and the MDGs: Towards a sustainable future for all.* UN ESCAP, 2015.

UN. (2015b). UN population prospects 2015. http://esa.un.org/unpd/wpp/

UN. (2016). *Gender inequality index (Human development reports).* http://hdr.undp.org/en/composite/GII

UN. (2017a). *Sustainable development knowledge platform: India.* https://sustainabledevelopment.un.org/memberstates/india

UN. (2017b). *Zero hunger.* www.un.org/sustainabledevelopment/hunger